Diagnosis and Management of Acute Respiratory Failure

Editors

PHILIP YANG
ANNETTE M. ESPER

CRITICAL CARE CLINICS

www.criticalcare.theclinics.com

Consulting Editor
GREGORY S. MARTIN

April 2024 • Volume 40 • Number 2

ELSEVIER

1600 John F. Kennedy Boulevard • Suite 1800 • Philadelphia, Pennsylvania, 19103-2899

http://www.theclinics.com

CRITICAL CARE CLINICS Volume 40, Number 2
April 2024 ISSN 0749-0704, ISBN-13: 978-0-443-12917-9

Editor: Joanna Gascoine
Developmental Editor: Saswoti Nath

Critical Care Clinics (ISSN: 0749-0704) is published quarterly by Elsevier Inc., 360 Park Avenue South, New York, NY 10010-1710. Months of issue are January, April, July, and October. Business and Editorial Offices: 1600 John F. Kennedy Blvd., Suite 1800, Philadelphia, PA 19103-2899. Customer Service Office: 6277 Sea Harbor Drive, Orlando, FL 32887-4800. Periodicals postage paid at New York, NY and additional mailing offices. Subscription prices are $279.00 per year for US individuals, $100.00 per year for US students and residents, $317.00 per year for Canadian individuals, $362.00 per year for international individuals, $100.00 per year for Canadian students/residents, and $150.00 per year for foreign students/residents. For institutional access pricing please contact Customer Service via the contact information below. To receive student/resident rate, orders must be accompanied by name of affiliated institution, date of term, and the signature of program/residency coordinator on institution letterhead. Orders will be billed at individual rate until proof of status is received. Foreign air speed delivery is included in all *Clinics* subscription prices. All prices are subject to change without notice. POSTMASTER: Send address changes to *Critical Care Clinics*, Elsevier Periodicals Customer Service, 11830 Westline Industrial Drive, St. Louis, MO 63146. **Customer Service: 1-800-654-2452 (US). From outside of the US, call 1-314-447-8871. Fax: 1-314-447-8029. E-mail: journalscustomerservice-usa@elsevier.com (for print support) or journalsonlinesupport-usa@elsevier.com (for online support).**

Reprints. For copies of 100 or more of articles in this publication, please contact the Commercial Reprints Department, Elsevier Inc., 360 Park Avenue South, New York, NY 10010-1710. Tel.: 212-633-3874; Fax: 212-633-3820; E-mail: reprints@elsevier.com.

Critical Care Clinics is also published in Spanish by Editorial Inter-Medica, Junin 917, 1er A, 1113, Buenos Aires, Argentina.

Critical Care Clinics is covered in *MEDLINE/PubMed (Index Medicus), EMBASE/Excerpta Medica, Current Concepts/ Clinical Medicine, ISI/BIOMED*, and *Chemical Abstracts*.

Contributors

CONSULTING EDITOR

GREGORY S. MARTIN, MD, Msc
Professor, Division of Pulmonary, Allergy, Critical Care and Sleep Medicine, Research Director, Emory Critical Care Center, Director, Emory/Georgia Tech Predictive Health Institute, Co-Director, Atlanta Center for Microsystems Engineered Point-of-Care Technologies (ACME POCT), President, Society of Critical Care Medicine, Atlanta, Georgia

EDITORS

PHILIP YANG, MD, MSc
Assistant Professor of Medicine, Division of Pulmonary, Allergy, Critical Care, and Sleep Medicine, Emory University, Atlanta, Georgia

ANNETTE M. ESPER, MD, MSc
Professor of Medicine, Division of Pulmonary, Allergy, Critical Care, and Sleep Medicine, Emory University, Atlanta, Georgia

AUTHORS

KAREN E.A. BURNS, MD, FRCPC, MSc
Professor of Medicine, Clinician Scientist, Interdepartmental Division of Critical Care Medicine, University of Toronto, Department of Medicine, Division of Critical Care, Li Ka Shing Knowledge Institute, Unity Health Toronto, St. Michael's Hospital, Department of Health Research Methods, Evidence and Impact, McMaster University, Hamilton, Ontario, Canada

LINGYE CHEN, MD
Division of Pulmonary, Allergy, and Critical Care Medicine, Assistant Professor, Department of Medicine, Duke University Medical Center, Durham, North Carolina

SHEWIT P. GIOVANNI, MD, MSc
Assistant Professor, Division of Pulmonary, Allergy and Critical Care Medicine, Oregon Health and Science University, Portland, Oregon, USA

CATHERINE L. HOUGH, MD, MSc
Professor, Division of Pulmonary, Allergy and Critical Care Medicine, Oregon Health & Science University, Portland, Oregon

MADELINE LAGINA, MD, MPH
Fellow, Division of Pulmonary and Critical Care, Department of Medicine, University of Michigan, Ann Arbor, Michigan

STEPHEN E. LAPINSKY, MBBCh, MSc, FRCPC
Mount Sinai Hospital, Professor of Medicine, Interdepartmental Division of Critical Care Medicine, University of Toronto, Toronto, Ontario, Canada

ELIZABETH LEVY, MD
Fellow, Division of Pulmonary, Allergy and Critical Care Medicine, Department of Medicine, Philadelphia, Pennsylvania

VICTOR LIN, MD
Assistant Professor, Department of Neurology, University of Washington, Seattle, Washington

BEN MESSER, MBChB
Consultant, North East Assisted Ventilation Service, Royal Victoria Infirmary, Newcastle-upon-Tyne NHS Hospitals NHS Foundation Trust, Newcastle upon Tyne, United Kingdom

BHAKTI K. PATEL, MD
Assistant Professor, Department of Medicine, Section of Pulmonary and Critical Care, University of Chicago, Chicago, Illinois

NIDA QADIR, MD
Associate Clinical Professor, Division of Pulmonary Critical Care and Sleep Medicine, Department of Medicine, David Geffen School of Medicine, University of California, Los Angeles, Los Angeles, California

CRAIG R. RACKLEY, MD
Associate Professor, Department of Medicine, Duke University Medical Center, Durham, North Carolina

JOHN P. REILLY, MD, MSCE
Assistant Professor, Department of Medicine, University of Pennsylvania, Perelman School of Medicine, Philadelphia, Pennsylvania

ZACHARY ROBATEAU, MD
Resident, Department of Neurology, University of Washington, Seattle, Washington

BRAM ROCHWERG
Department of Health Research Methods, Evidence and Impact, McMaster University, Assistant Professor, Departments of Medicine and Critical Care, Hamilton Health Sciences, Juravinski Hospital, Hamilton, Ontario, Canada

LOUISE ROSE, BN, MN, PhD
Professor, Florence Nightingale Faculty of Nursing, Midwifery and Palliative Care, King's College London, Department of Critical Care and Lane Fox Unit, Guy's & St Thomas' NHS Foundation Trust, King's College London, London, United Kingdom

ANDREW J.E. SEELY
Department of Critical Care, Ottawa Hospital, Professor, Division of Thoracic Surgery, Department of Surgery, University of Ottawa, Clinical Epidemiology Program, Ottawa Hospital Research Institute, University of Ottawa, Ottawa, Ontario, Canada

KEVIN P. SEITZ, MD, MSc
Research Fellow, Department of Allergy, Pulmonary, and Critical Care Medicine, Vanderbilt University Medical Center, Nashville, Tennessee

MICHAEL W. SJODING, MD, MSc
Associate Professor of Medicine, Division of Pulmonary and Critical Care Medicine, University of Michigan, Ann Arbor, Michigan

JENNIFER C. SZAFRAN, MD
Assistant Professor, Department of Medicine, Section of Pulmonary and Critical Care, The University of Chicago, Chicago, Illinois

JONATHAN TAYLOR, MD
Division of Pulmonary, Critical Care, and Sleep Medicine, Mount Sinai Hospital, Icahn School of Medicine at Mount Sinai, New York, New York

MEGAN TRIEU, MD
Fellow Division of Pulmonary Critical Care Sleep Medicine and Physiology, Department of Medicine, University of California, San Diego, San Diego, California

THOMAS S. VALLEY, MD, MSc
Associate Professor, Division of Pulmonary and Critical Care, Department of Medicine, Center for Bioethics and Social Sciences in Medicine, University of Michigan Medical School, Institute for Healthcare Policy and Innovation, University of Michigan, Department of Veterans Affairs, VA Ann Arbor Healthcare System, Ann Arbor, Michigan

DANIELA N. VASQUEZ, MD
ICU Head of Department, Sanatorio Anchorena, City of Buenos Aires, Argentina

SARAH WAHLSTER, MD, FNCS
Assistant Professor, Departments of Neurology, Neurological Surgery, and Anesthesiology and Pain Medicine, University of Washington, Seattle, Washington

MARY ELIZABETH WILCOX, MD, PhD
Associate Professor, Department of Critical Care Medicine, Faculty of Medicine and Dentistry, University of Alberta, Edmonton, Canada

PHILIP YANG, MD, MSc
Assistant Professor of Medicine, Division of Pulmonary, Allergy, Critical Care, and Sleep Medicine, Emory University, Atlanta, Georgia

Contents

exists within the ARDS population. Treatment requires prompt recognition of ARDS and an understanding of which patients may benefit most from specific pharmacologic interventions. The key to finding effective pharmacotherapies for ARDS may rely on deeper understanding of pathophysiology and bedside identification of ARDS subphenotypes.

Fluid management in acute respiratory failure is an area of uncertainty requiring a delicate balance of resuscitation and fluid removal to manage hypoperfusion and avoidance of hypoxemia. Overall, a restrictive fluid strategy (minimizing fluid administration) and careful attention to overall fluid balance may be beneficial after initial resuscitation and does not have major side effects. Further studies are needed to improve our understanding of patients who will benefit from a restrictive or liberal fluid management strategy.

Acute respiratory distress syndrome (ARDS) is an acute inflammatory lung injury characterized by severe hypoxemic respiratory failure, bilateral opacities on chest imaging, and low lung compliance. ARDS is a heterogeneous syndrome that is the common end point of a wide variety of predisposing conditions, with complex pathophysiology and underlying mechanisms. Routine management of ARDS is centered on lung-protective ventilation strategies such as low tidal volume ventilation and targeting low airway pressures to avoid exacerbation of lung injury, as well as a conservative fluid management strategy.

Despite significant advances in understanding acute respiratory distress syndrome (ARDS), mortality rates remain high. The appropriate use of adjunctive therapies can improve outcomes, particularly for patients with moderate to severe hypoxia. In this review, the authors discuss the evidence basis behind prone positioning, recruitment maneuvers, neuromuscular blocking agents, corticosteroids, pulmonary vasodilators, and extracorporeal membrane oxygenation and considerations for their use in individual patients and specific clinical scenarios. Because the heterogeneity of ARDS poses challenges in finding universally effective treatments, an individualized approach and continued research efforts are crucial for optimizing the utilization of adjunctive therapies and improving patient outcomes.

to the prolonged mechanical ventilation patient population, are lacking. A structured and individualized approach developed by the multiprofessional team in discussion with the patient and their family is warranted.

Jonathan Taylor and Mary Elizabeth Wilcox

Recent research has brought renewed attention to the multifaceted physical and cognitive dysfunction that accompanies acute respiratory failure (ARF). This state-of-the-art review provides an overview of the evidence landscape encompassing ARF-associated neuromuscular and neurocognitive impairments. Risk factors, mechanisms, assessment tools, rehabilitation strategies, approaches to ventilator liberation, and interventions to minimize post–intensive care syndrome are emphasized. The complex interrelationship between physical disability, cognitive dysfunction, and long-term patient-centered outcomes is explored. This review highlights the need for comprehensive, multidisciplinary approaches to mitigate morbidity and accelerate recovery.

CRITICAL CARE CLINICS

SERIES OF RELATED INTEREST

Emergency Medicine Clinics
https://www.emed.theclinics.com/
Clinics in Chest Medicine
https://www.chestmed.theclinics.com/

THE CLINICS ARE AVAILABLE ONLINE!
Access your subscription at:
www.theclinics.com

Preface

Acute Respiratory Failure: Problems Solved and Unsolved

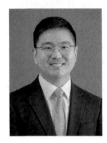 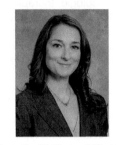

Philip Yang, MD, MSc   Annette M. Esper, MD, MSc
Editors

Acute respiratory failure (ARF) is a critical medical condition caused by various disease processes and is characterized by abnormal lung mechanics or function, impaired gas exchange, or disturbances in pulmonary circulation that results in the inability of the respiratory system to meet the oxygenation, ventilation, or metabolic demands of the body. This results in life-threatening metabolic and acid-base derangements, often leading to extrapulmonary organ failures and other complications. ARF is one of the most common conditions encountered in the intensive care unit (ICU), present in up to 56% to 69% of ICU admissions.[1] It also represents a significant burden on the health care system, accounting for 1.0 to 1.9 million hospitalizations and $30 to $54 billion in health care costs per year in the United States.[2]

Despite its clinical significance, ARF still remains a difficult condition to identify, understand, and properly manage. Prompt recognition and diagnosis of ARF is extremely difficult due to the rapid progression of ARF and the heterogeneity of potential causes and clinical presentation. In patients with acute respiratory distress syndrome (ARDS), the diagnosis is missed altogether in a substantial proportion of patients, leading to delays or omission of important interventions, such as lung-protective ventilation strategies and rescue therapies.[3] In addition, the management strategies for ARF consist largely of nonspecific supportive measures, and targeted or individualized treatment approaches still require further investigation. The increased availability of noninvasive positive pressure ventilation, high-flow nasal oxygen, and extracorporeal membrane oxygenation has provided clinicians with more management options for treating patients with ARF, but the optimal patient selection and clinical application of such therapies remain unclear. Furthermore, as outcomes from ARF improve and more patients survive their acute illness, increasing

Crit Care Clin 40 (2024) xiii–xv
https://doi.org/10.1016/j.ccc.2024.01.001
0749-0704/24/© 2024 Published by Elsevier Inc.

criticalcare.theclinics.com

attention has been focused on various complications and long-term impairments that may occur following the recovery from ARF.

While this issue of *Critical Care Clinics* is not meant to be a comprehensive review of all aspects of ARF, the topics were chosen to address many of the issues highlighted above. The first section of the issue covers the "core knowledge" of ARF, such as epidemiology, pathophysiology, diagnostic evaluation, and routine clinical management of ARF. This is followed by special considerations in ARF management, including invasive mechanical ventilation, pharmacologic therapies, and fluid management strategies. The next section covers ARDS, a complex subset within ARF, with detailed discussions of both routine and adjunctive treatments. The following section includes discussions of ARF in specific patient populations with unique clinical characteristics, such as pregnancy and severe acute brain injury. Finally, the last few articles discuss the postacute phase of ARF, including ventilator weaning and extubation strategies, as well as complications from ARF, such as prolonged respiratory failure, physical disability, and cognitive impairments.

We are both grateful and excited for the opportunity to collaborate with outstanding experts in this field and compile a review of important topics in ARF. We hope that this issue will not only highlight the recent advancements in ARF management but also stimulate discussion about the challenges that remain to be solved in future research for ARF.

DISCLOSURE

The Guest Editors have nothing to disclose.

Philip Yang, MD, MSc
Division of Pulmonary, Allergy
Critical Care, and Sleep Medicine
Emory University
Atlanta, GA, USA

6335 Hospital Parkway
Physician Plaza Suite 310
Johns Creek, GA 30097, USA

Annette M. Esper, MD, MSc
Division of Pulmonary, Allergy
Critical Care, and Sleep Medicine

Emory University
49 Jesse Hill Jr Drive Southeast
Faculty Office Building
Atlanta, GA 30303, USA

E-mail addresses:
philip.yang@emory.edu (P. Yang)
aesper@emory.edu (A.M. Esper)

REFERENCES

1. Vincent JL, Akça S, De Mendonça A, et al. The epidemiology of acute respiratory failure in critically ill patients. Chest 2002;121(5):1602–9.

2. Stefan MS, Shieh MS, Pekow PS, et al. Epidemiology and outcomes of acute respiratory failure in the United States, 2001 to 2009: a national survey. J Hosp Med 2013;8(2):76–82.
3. Bellani G, Laffey J, Pham T, et al. Epidemiology, patterns of care, and mortality for patients with acute respiratory distress syndrome in intensive care units in 50 countries. JAMA 2016;315(8):788–800.

Diagnosis and Epidemiology of Acute Respiratory Failure

Lingye Chen, MD*, Craig R. Rackley, MD

KEYWORDS

- Acute respiratory failure • Acute hypoxemic respiratory failure
- Acute hypercapnic respiratory failure • Diagnosis • Epidemiology

KEY POINTS

- Acute respiratory failure is a common clinical finding caused by insufficient oxygenation (hypoxemia) or ventilation (hypercapnia).
- Understanding the pathophysiology of acute respiratory failure can help to facilitate recognition, diagnosis, and treatment.
- The cause of acute respiratory failure can be identified through utilization of physical examination findings, laboratory analysis, and chest imaging.

INTRODUCTION

Acute respiratory failure is a broad term describing insufficient oxygenation (hypoxemia) or ventilation (hypercapnia). Acute hypoxemic and acute hypercapnic respiratory failure can happen in isolation or together. This is often dependent on the acuity of onset and any concurrent illness or chronic disease that may be present.

Understanding the pathophysiology of acute respiratory failure will facilitate recognition, diagnosis, and treatment. This review discusses the epidemiology of acute respiratory failure and also describes pathophysiologic principles to the diagnosis of acute respiratory failure. Using clinical evaluation, laboratory analysis, and chest imaging, the cause of acute respiratory failure can be identified. The authors divide most of the discussion between hypoxemic and hypercapnic respiratory failure.

DEFINITION AND EPIDEMIOLOGY

There is currently no consensus definition for acute respiratory failure. In some studies, acute respiratory failure is synonymous with the more specific acute respiratory distress

Funding support: None.
Division of Pulmonary, Allergy, and Critical Care Medicine, Department of Medicine, Duke University Medical Center, Durham, NC, USA
* Corresponding author. Division of Pulmonary, Allergy, and Critical Care Medicine, Duke University Medical Center, PO Box 102355, Durham, NC 27710.
E-mail address: lingye.chen@duke.edu

Crit Care Clin 40 (2024) 221–233
https://doi.org/10.1016/j.ccc.2023.12.001
0749-0704/24/© 2023 Elsevier Inc. All rights reserved.

syndrome (ARDS), whereas others use a broader definition. As such, the incidence of acute respiratory failure varies across studies. Studies in the 1990s defining respiratory failure as requiring intubation and mechanical ventilation found an incidence of 77.7 to 88.6 per 100,000 person-years in European countries[1,2] and 137.1 per 100,000 person-years in the United States.[3] However, because the definition of acute respiratory failure has expanded to include patients requiring noninvasive ventilation and high-flow nasal cannulas, respiratory failure is becoming an increasingly recognized diagnosis.[4] A longitudinal study demonstrated an increase in the diagnosis from 429 to 1275 cases per 100,000 adults per year between 2002 and 2017.[5]

In low-income countries, lower respiratory infections are the second leading cause of death. As the income of a country rises, the number of deaths caused by respiratory related illnesses decreases but remains a major cause of death.[6] In the United States, two of the top ten causes of death were chronic lower respiratory diseases (predominantly chronic obstructive pulmonary disease [COPD]) and lower respiratory infections.[7] Death from COPD is typically due to acute on chronic hypoxemic or hypercapnic respiratory failure, whereas death from acute lower respiratory infections is frequently due to acute hypoxemic $\pm$ hypercapnic respiratory failure and/or multiorgan failure due to complications of the infection.

Acute respiratory failure most often afflicts adults between 60 and 79 years of age and is typically associated with infection.[5,8] Although there has been an increase in the incidence of respiratory failure since the start of the twenty-first century, mortality has declined as critical care advanced.[5] For the purpose of this review, the authors simply define hypoxemia as a blood oxygen level lower than normal and hypercapnia as a blood carbon dioxide level higher than normal.

ETIOLOGY AND PATHOPHYSIOLOGY
Acute Hypoxemic Respiratory Failure

An understanding of oxygen transport and delivery is key to evaluating a patient with hypoxemia. The primary goal of oxygen transport is to deliver oxygen to the mitochondria where energy is generated to power the cellular processes vital to human life. The full benefit of oxygen is only realized when all of the steps from initial inspiration of oxygen through the nose and mouth to oxidative phosphorylation in the mitochondria are working effectively. After recognizing the patient may have an inadequate supply or utilization of oxygen, the clinician is faced with determining which process or processes are dysfunctional so that the most appropriate therapies can be deployed in a timely manner.

Evaluation of Hypoxemia

Hypoxemia is a commonly encountered clinical abnormality in both the inpatient hospital setting and the outpatient clinic. Clinicians must be able to quickly evaluate a patient to determine the etiology of hypoxemia and potentially mitigate the ill effects of this. Determining if a patient is hypoxemic can be done by directly measuring either the partial pressure of oxygen dissolved in blood (Pao_2) or the oxygen hemoglobin saturation (Sao_2). The Pao_2 can be directly measured via arterial blood sampling, but few places outside of hospitals have the ability to analyze blood gases. Furthermore, obtaining an arterial blood gas (ABG) sample requires a skilled practitioner and can be painful for the patient. Noninvasive pulse oximetry indirectly measures the percentage of oxygen bound to hemoglobin (Sao_2; when measured using pulse oximetry, it is reported as Spo_2). The measurement of Spo_2 requires far less training and is painless for the patient. The downside, however, is that pulse oximetry reports only hemoglobin saturation and cannot report dissolved O_2 and CO_2, which are often required to better define the etiology of hypoxemia.

Once a patient has been found to have hypoxemia, the etiology and severity of acute hypoxemic respiratory failure can be categorized by assessing the alveolar-arterial (A-a) oxygen gradient.[9–11] The A-a gradient is the difference in partial pressure of O_2 between the alveoli (P_{AO_2}) and the arterial blood (Pa_{O_2}). In other words, the A-a gradient is a measure of gas exchange and the ease with which oxygen transfers from the alveolar space across the alveolar–capillary membrane into the bloodstream.

To calculate the A-a gradient, we must calculate P_{AO_2} and measure Pa_{O_2}.

To calculate P_{AO_2}, we must know the atmospheric pressure (P_{atm}; 760 mm Hg at sea level), fraction of inhaled O_2 (Fi_{O_2}; 0.21 at room air), and arterial Pco_2 ($Paco_2$; in mm Hg):

$$P_{AO_2} = A = [P_{atm} - P_{H2O}] \times Fi_{O_2} - Paco_2/RQ$$

where

- P_{H2O} = partial pressure of water vapor at $37°C$ = 47 mm Hg
- RQ = respiratory quotient. It is a measure of metabolic activity and assumed to be 0.8.

Thus, at sea level and room air:

$$A = [760–47] \times 0.21 - Paco_2/0.8$$

$$A = 150 - Paco_2/0.8$$

As mentioned earlier Pa_{O_2} is measured via an arterial blood sample, which also measures $Paco_2$. Following arterial sampling, one can now calculate the A-a gradient of a person breathing room air:

$$\text{A-a gradient} = 150 - Paco_2/0.8 - Pa_{O_2}$$

A normal A-a gradient is between 5 and 25 mm Hg in adults, with a range reflecting the fact A-a gradient increases with age.

$$\text{Normal A-a gradient} = (age + 10)/4$$

The A-a gradient is helpful in determining whether hypoxemia is due to impairment in gas exchange or due to reduced alveolar ventilation. A low Pa_{O_2} with a normal A-a gradient implies that lung gas exchange is normal, but alveolar ventilation may be reduced, such as by central respiratory depression or obstruction of airflow. Reduced alveolar ventilation is accompanied by high $Paco_2$, which is easily detected on arterial blood sample. Low Pa_{O_2} with a normal A-a gradient also occurs when the partial pressure of inhaled O_2 (p_iO_2) is reduced, such as at extremely high altitudes. On the other hand, a low Pa_{O_2} with an elevated A-a gradient indicates poor gas exchange. This may be caused by edema, inflammation, fibrosis, damage to alveolar capillaries, an imbalance in ventilation to perfusion (V/Q), or right-to-left shunting. The authors discuss the evaluation of hypoxemia in patients with normal and abnormal A-a gradients and common associated diagnoses, as summarized in **Table 1**.

Hypoxemia with a normal alveolar-arterial gradient

When there is hypoxemia in the setting of a normal A-a gradient, the abnormality is not with the ability of the lungs to perform gas exchange but rather with external factors.

Table 1
Physiologic mechanisms of hypoxemia

Mechanisms of Hypoxemia	Chest X-Ray	Resolves with Supplemental O_2	Common Diagnoses
Normal A-a gradient			
Low inspired O_2 tension	Normal	Yes	High altitude
Hypoventilation	Normal	Yes	Opiate overdose Acute exacerbation of COPD or asthma
Elevated A-a gradient			
V/Q mismatch	Normal or abnormal	Yes	Pulmonary embolism Emphysema Right ventricular failure
Right-to-left shunt	Normal or abnormal	No	Consolidative pneumonia Large mucus plugging of central airway Intracardiac shunt
Diffusion impairment	Abnormal	Yes	Acute respiratory distress syndrome Aspiration Toxic inhalation Acute exacerbation of congestive heart failure

Hypoventilation. Hypoxemia from hypoventilation occurs when a patient's alveolar ventilation is inadequate to sufficiently clear CO_2 from the lungs. The elevated alveolar Pco_2 displaces some of the inspired oxygen, effectively lowering the alveolar oxygen tension. In other words, the presence of excess CO_2 leaves less room for O_2 to diffuse into the alveolus, and as a result, less oxygen diffuses into the capillaries and Pao_2 decreases. Hypoventilation can be seen in obstructive lung diseases (ie, chronic obstructive lung disease or asthma), use of certain medications or illicit drugs that can blunt the respiratory drive (ie, opiates, propofol, or benzodiazepines), neuromuscular disease, or obesity hypoventilation syndrome.

Low inhaled O_2 tension. The easiest example where p_iO_2 is low is at high altitude. At sea level, p_iO_2 is 150 mm Hg. At 8700 m in altitude (27,559 ft), near the peak of Mount Everest, p_iO_2 is 47 mm Hg. In 10 Mt Everest climbers who underwent ABG sampling at 8700 m, the mean Pao_2 was 24.6 mm Hg, which equated to a normal A-a gradient of 5 mm Hg.[12] Other examples include fire, where oxygen is being consumed, or mixed gases, such as improperly calibrated inhaled anesthetics used in the operating room. These problems should be readily apparent to the clinician based on the setting and rapidly improve with the administration of supplemental oxygen.

Hypoxemia with an elevated alveolar-arterial gradient

Acute hypoxemic respiratory failure more commonly occurs with an elevated A-a gradient or abnormality in the alveolar–capillary unit. The alveolar–capillary unit is the unit of gas exchange and is composed of a compartment of ventilation (alveolus), a compartment of perfusion (capillary), and the space that separates the two (interstitium). A defect in any of these three compartments leads to an impairment in gas exchange and hypoxemia.

Ventilation–perfusion mismatch. The term V/Q (ventilation/perfusion) refers to the amount of air entering the alveoli (V) relative to the capillary perfusion (Q) of those alveoli. Ideally, the flow of gas and blood are perfectly proportional to ensure maximal gas exchange. Such a scenario of equally matched ventilation and perfusion would have a V/Q ratio of 1.0, whereas a V/Q ratio of 2.0 indicates twice as much alveolar ventilation as alveolar capillary perfusion and ratio of 0.5 indicates half as much ventilation as perfusion.[8] Some degree of V/Q mismatching is present with most acute and chronic pulmonary diseases. Under most circumstances, hypoxemia secondary to V/Q mismatch can be overcome by administering supplemental oxygen.

A simple example of a condition leading to V/Q mismatch is a pulmonary embolus, where a segment of the lung is still ventilating normally, but the blood flow to that ventilated area is blocked by a clot. When there is only air movement but no perfusion, this is referred to as dead space ventilation, and this region of lung does not undergo gas exchange. Dead space exists as part of normal respiratory anatomy (anatomic dead space) and can be the result of pathology (pathologic or alveolar dead space). Anatomic dead space comprises the conducting airways and represents approximately 25% to 30% of the volume of inhaled air during normal breathing at rest. Any additional dead space is alveolar dead space.

Total dead space can be calculated as the fraction of the tidal volume that does not reach functioning alveoli: dead space fraction = (tidal volume – alveolar volume) / tidal volume

- Tidal volume = total volume of a single breath
- Alveolar volume = volume that reaches functional alveoli in a single breath

Whereas anatomic dead space is constant, the alveolar dead space is the most variable and relevant to disease states. High alveolar dead space increases V/Q mismatch. Alveolar dead space can be calculated using the Bohr equation and can be performed at the bedside if an end-tidal CO_2 monitor and ABG are available.

$$Alveolar\ dead\ space\ fraction = \frac{p_aCO_2 - p_{ET}CO_2}{p_aCO_2}$$

where $p_{ET}CO_2$ is the P_{CO_2} in exhaled air measured at the end of an exhaled breath. Increased alveolar dead space will increase the difference between Pa_{CO_2} and $p_{ET}CO_2$.

Right-to-left shunt. The inverse of a V/Q mismatch is the presence of perfusion in the absence of ventilation. Venous blood that directly enters arterial circulation without participating in gas exchange is called a shunt. This can occur due to anatomic intracardiac (eg, patent foramen ovale) or vascular abnormalities (eg, arteriovenous malformations) but most commonly occurs due to intrapulmonary shunting of blood through abnormal lung. An intrapulmonary shunt represents extreme V/Q mismatching with a V/Q ratio of 0 for a given segment of the lung. This can occur in the setting of atelectasis, pneumonia, or complete bronchial obstruction where pulmonary blood perfuses nonfunctional or non-ventilated alveoli. Regardless of the location or etiology of the shunt, venous blood does not come in contact with functional alveoli, resulting a hypoxemia that cannot be overcome by administering supplemental oxygen. In fact, a diagnosis of shunt can easily be made when there is little increase in Pa_{O_2} after having the patient inspire 100% oxygen. The most profound hypoxemia in patients with severe acute hypoxemic respiratory failure is typically due to significant intrapulmonary shunt fraction.

Intrapulmonary shunting occurs both normally and pathologically. Normally, approximately 2% to 5% of cardiac output perfuses the lungs to supply oxygen to the bronchial cells and pleura and returns to the left atrium without coming in contact with the alveolar capillaries. The calculation of total shunt fraction, defined as the ratio of shunted cardiac output to the total cardiac output, requires both an arterial and a mixed venous blood sample:

$$\frac{Shunted\ cardiac\ output = Q_S = C_{PC}O_2 - C_aO_2}{Total\ cardiac\ output = Q_T = C_{PC}O_2 - C_vO_2}$$

where

- $C_{PC}O_2$ = oxygen content of pulmonary capillary blood
- C_aO_2 = oxygen content of arterial blood, sampled from an artery in systemic circulation
- C_vO_2 = oxygen content of mixed venous blood, sampled from the pulmonary artery

Oxygen content of blood (C_xO_2) is calculated using the following equation:

$$C_xO_2 = (1.36 \times Hb \times S_xO_2) + (p_xO_2 \times 0.003)$$

- Hb = hemoglobin concentration
- x = location of blood sampled (ie, arterial, venous, or pulmonary capillary)

$C_{PC}O_2$ should have the highest O_2 content in the circulation, but it cannot be readily sampled. Therefore, for the purposes of calculating shunt fraction, it is assumed that the pulmonary capillary blood is 100% saturated and has a P_{O_2} of 101 mm Hg.

Impaired diffusion. We have thus far discussed abnormalities in ventilation and perfusion as etiologies of hypoxemic respiratory failure. The final compartment of the alveolar–capillary unit that can be compromised is the interstitium, a thin proteinaceous membrane that separates the alveolus and capillary. Conditions that increase the distance between alveolar gas and capillary blood lead to diffusion impairment. This can occur when the alveoli are partially filled with fluid, hyaline membranes, or other debris, which can be seen in infectious pneumonia or ARDS. Diffusion impairment also occurs in diseases that cause thickening of the interstitium and are broadly called interstitial lung diseases. Hypoxemia caused by diffusion impairment should be apparent on clinical examination and/or chest radiograph, and unlike a shunt, it can typically be overcome with supplemental oxygen. Although diffusion impairment affects the exchange of both O_2 and CO_2, as CO_2 diffuses more readily than O_2, hypoxemia results before hypercapnia.

The above five physiologic mechanisms of hypoxemia and examples of each are summarized in **Table 1**.

Acute Hypercapnic Respiratory Failure

Another mechanism of respiratory failure is inadequate ventilation, which results in abnormally high Pa_{CO_2} (normal Pa_{CO_2} 35–45 mm Hg) and respiratory acidosis. Of note, this article focuses on acute, not chronic, hypercapnic respiratory failure, the latter of which results in a much different clinical presentation. This section discusses the physiology and multiple etiologies of acute hypercapnic respiratory failure, as summarized in **Table 2**.

Decreased minute ventilation

In addition to transporting O_2 into the circulation to the cells, the other role of the lungs is exporting the byproduct of cellular respiration, CO_2, from the circulation. The

Table 2 Common diagnoses associated with acute hypercapnic respiratory failure	
Decreased minute ventilation	Can't breathe • Guillain–Barre syndrome • Myasthenia gravis • Critical illness myopathy Won't breathe • Brainstem stroke • Opiate overdose • General anesthetic
Increased dead space	Acute exacerbation of COPD or asthma Acute pulmonary embolism Acute respiratory distress syndrome

amount of CO_2 expired is determined by the size of the tidal breath (tidal volume) and frequency of breaths. Together, the product of these two variables is the minute ventilation (V_E).

$$V_E \text{ (L/min)} = \text{tidal volume (L/breath)} \times \text{respiratory rate (breaths/min)}$$

In normal healthy adults at rest, minute ventilation (5–8 L/min) perfectly balances out cellular respiration, resulting in a $Paco_2$ of 35 to 45 mm Hg. When minute ventilation is abnormally low, $Paco_2$ acutely increases and pH decreases. The corresponding decrease in pH arises from a shift in the equilibrium of the following equation mediated by carbonic anhydrase combining CO_2 and H_2O to ultimately produce hydrogen ions.

$$CO_2 + H_2O \leftrightarrow H_2CO_3 \leftrightarrow HCO_3^- + H^+$$

Decreased minute ventilation can be traced to two possible etiologies. The brainstem contains the pacemaker for the lungs, sending signals to the diaphragm and intercostal muscles to contract 12 to 15 times per minute at rest, higher during exercise. Disorders of the brainstem impair the ability of the patient to initiate breaths ("won't breathe"), and disorders of the peripheral nerves or respiratory muscles diminish the ability of the patient to generate adequate tidal volume ("can't breathe"). The former is seen most commonly in drugs that suppress the central nervous system, particularly opiates, but can also present following a stroke involving the brainstem. The latter is seen in morbid obesity (eg, obesity hypoventilation syndrome), neuromuscular disorders (eg, amyotrophic lateral sclerosis), or prolonged critical illness (eg, critical illness myopathy).

Increased dead space
Approximately 25% of a tidal breath is lost in normal, anatomic dead space—areas with air movement but absent of alveolar–capillary units necessary for gas exchange. These areas include the nose, mouth, posterior oropharynx, and the conducting airways. When pathologic dead space develops, such as with a pulmonary embolus, CO_2 cannot diffuse out of the capillaries and into the alveoli to be exhaled. This is the same concept of V/Q mismatch discussed earlier in this article. The presence of this pathologic dead space leads to not only acute hypoxemic but also acute hypercapnic respiratory failure.

Another common cause of increased dead space in the intensive care unit is ARDS, where dysregulation of the inflammatory and coagulation pathways, along with endothelial damage, lead to pulmonary microvascular injury and thrombus formation.[13,14] Patients can frequently have dead space fractions greater than 65%, requiring extremely high minute ventilation to adequately clear CO_2.[15] In fact, increased dead space fraction in ARDS is shown to be a predictor of mortality.[16]

DIAGNOSIS
Physical Examination

A diagnosis of acute respiratory failure can readily be made on initial bedside assessment, and a targeted examination can help guide the clinician to an accurate etiology. Pulse oximetry on room air will frequently show low SpO_2 in both acute hypoxemic and hypercapnic respiratory failure. In mild or early disease, SpO_2 may still be greater than 90% (normal SpO_2 95%–100%), but as disease severity progresses and SpO_2 continues to decrease less than 90%, patients may develop acrocyanosis, a bluish discoloration of the hands, feet, and areas around the lips.

In the absence of a depressed respiratory drive (eg, opiate overdose), patients will typically attempt to increase their ventilation to correct or compensate for their acute respiratory failure. This can manifest as marked respiratory distress, but frequently more subtle evidence of increased work of breathing is present. A common finding is breathing with higher tidal volumes at a slightly higher respiratory rate than normal, similar to a person performing light exercise. Patient position can also give clues to some degree of respiratory insufficiency. A patient positioned with the shoulders fixed (often in a tripod position) is better able to engage the accessory muscles of breathing, much like a runner who places their hands on their knees during heavy breathing after a sprint. As hypoxia and/or hypercapnia worsen, the patient may become confused, agitated, lethargic, or even comatose.

On pulmonary auscultation, there may be abnormal breath sounds such as wheezes, which indicate obstructive airway pathology, or rales (crackles), which indicate an alveolar disease. However, pulmonary auscultation can be normal in many of the causes of acute hypoxemic or hypercapnic respiratory failure that are not due to abnormal airways or lung parenchyma.

Finally, a thorough cardiac examination should be performed as certain abnormalities can indicate potential causes of acute respiratory failure, such as evidence of right heart strain (pulmonary emboli) or heart failure (pulmonary edema).

Laboratory Evaluation

Blood gases are the gold standard for diagnosing respiratory failure. Although these laboratories can be performed on arterial or venous blood, there are important differences between venous blood gas (VBG) and ABG. In general, a VBG will reflect more the byproduct of cellular respiration, whereas an ABG will reflect the effectiveness of gas exchange. Of the measurements on a blood gas, pH correlates most strongly between venous and arterial blood, with VBG pH lower than ABG pH by about 0.03.[17–19] Pco_2 is more variable with VBG Pco_2 higher than ABG Pco_2 by 5 to 7 mm Hg or significantly more in the presence of high oxygen consumption or low cardiac output.[17–19] On the other hand, there is no consistent correlation between Pao_2 and p_vO_2, and as such acute hypoxemic respiratory failure should be evaluated using only ABG or if not available, SpO_2.[19] In the case of acute hypoxemic respiratory failure, the ABG is useful in not only recognizing hypoxemia but also differentiating the etiology via the A-a gradient as discussed earlier.

Both VBG and ABG can be useful in not only recognizing hypercapnia but also determining whether the hypercapnic respiratory failure is acute or chronic. Because

CO_2 and H_2O become carbonic acid via carbonic anhydrase, an acute rise in CO_2 results in a low pH (ie, acute respiratory acidosis). For every 10 mm Hg rise in CO_2, pH will drop by 0.08. However, if elevated CO_2 is sustained, the kidneys begin to reabsorb bicarbonate in effort to normalize the pH, so for every 3 mm Hg rise in CO_2, there is a corresponding 1 mEq/L rise in serum bicarbonate.[20] Thus, acute hypercapnic respiratory failure can be identified by an elevated CO_2 and a low pH, whereas chronic compensated hypercapnic respiratory failure can be identified by elevated CO_2, normal or near-normal pH, and elevated serum bicarbonate.

Low P_{CO_2} can also be seen on blood gases, but unlike hypercapnia, hypercapnia does not general signify respiratory failure but rather can be present as compensation for metabolic acidosis. In a disorder of low serum bicarbonate such as renal failure, lactic acidosis, or diabetic ketoacidosis, pH falls. In effort to mitigate the acidemia, the respiratory center in the brainstem increases minute ventilation by increasing respiratory rate and tidal volume. The effect is the excessive expiration of CO_2.[20] The expected Pa_{CO_2} as the result of a given serum bicarbonate can be calculated using Winter's formula:

$$\text{Expected } Pa_{CO_2} = 1.5 \times [HCO_3^- \text{ mEq/L}] + 8 \pm 2$$

A measured Pa_{CO_2} greater than the expected Pa_{CO_2} suggests a concomitant respiratory acidosis (eg, respiratory muscle fatigue). A measured Pa_{CO_2} less than the expected Pa_{CO_2} suggests a concomitant respiratory alkalosis (eg, hyperventilation).

Imaging

Widely accessible, easily obtained, and interpretable by most physicians, chest x-ray is typically the first-line imaging modality used to evaluate respiratory failure. Chest x-ray can show gross airspace or interstitial abnormalities and pleural effusions. Common diagnoses that cause respiratory failure such as pneumonia and congestive heart failure can be readily made with a combination of physical examination and chest x-ray. However, chest x-rays are not sensitive nor are they effective at identifying pulmonary vascular disorders. When greater detail is required, cross-sectional imaging is preferred.

Of the imaging modalities, computed tomography (CT) of the chest provides the most anatomic information. CT with intravenous (IV) contrast informs of vascular abnormalities such as pulmonary emboli or vascular malformations. CT without IV contrast shows the pulmonary parenchyma, airways, and pleura—and their associated pathologies—in great detail. Whereas chest x-rays may limit a diagnosis to general parenchymal or pleural disease, a CT chest can greatly narrow the differential diagnosis of the parenchymal disease, show complex pleural effusions, and identify abnormalities within the airways. However, CT scans emit more radiation and are costlier compared with chest x-rays, and the IV contrast can worsen kidney function in patients with existing kidney disease.

For patients who are unable to obtain a contrasted CT scan (whether due to renal dysfunction or allergy to contrast) but with whom pulmonary embolism is suspected, a V/Q scan may be an alternative.[21] This nuclear medicine study uses a radiolabeled aerosol and an IV tracer to assess pulmonary ventilation and perfusion, respectively.[22] The presence of ventilation and absence of perfusion in the same region of the lung suggest presence of pulmonary embolism. However, given the abundance of other pulmonary abnormalities that produce similar pathophysiology, V/Q scan, while sensitive, is not specific for pulmonary embolism.[23]

The use of thoracic ultrasound in the diagnosis and monitoring of patient with acute respiratory failure is expanding as point-of-care ultrasound has become ubiquitous in the emergency department and critical care setting and an integral part of trainee education in these fields.[24] Clinicians have moved beyond simply using the ultrasound to guide placement of pleural catheters into pleural effusions to now rapidly diagnosing pneumothorax, pulmonary edema, consolidated lung, and diaphragmatic dysfunction.[25,26] Although ultrasound is one of the most convenient tools for diagnosing some life-threatening conditions with sensitivity comparable or superior to chest radiograph,[27,28] its sensitivity depends on operator skill and quality of ultrasound machine.[25]

Respiratory Fluid and Tissue Sampling

The most common need for sampling respiratory tract fluid is for the diagnosis of infection. Thus, the most common tests performed are microbiological, although the sensitivity in diagnosing bacterial pneumonia directly correlates with the quality of the specimen.[29] Outside of microbiological cultures, respiratory tract fluid may be sent for cytology, differential white blood cell count, or polymerase chain reaction testing to assist with the diagnosis of malignancy, interstitial lung disease, or other infections.

Expectorated sputum is the least invasive method for obtaining respiratory tract fluid samples. In instances where the patient cannot produce sputum, is immunocompromised, or has an atypical pneumonia or non-resolving pneumonia, bronchoscopy with bronchoalveolar lavage may be indicated to ensure an adequate lower respiratory tract sample.[30,31] Examination of the airway via bronchoscopy can also localize hemoptysis,[32] discover and remove mucus or other foreign bodies in the airway, and detect anatomic anomalies that may be contributing to respiratory failure. Bronchoscopy also offers a method of tissue sampling for centrally located lung masses.[33,34] Unsurprisingly, however, bronchoscopy comes with risks associated with invasive procedures, such as bleeding and pneumothorax, and with sedation, such as hemodynamic instability and worsening respiratory failure.

In cases of severe hypoxemic respiratory failure or ARDS of unknown etiology, tissue sampling must be approached with extreme caution and deliberation. Mortality following a surgical lung biopsy is 17% to 44% depending on the disease, and achieving a diagnosis that will change management is limited to 60% to 70%.[35,36]

SUMMARY

Acute respiratory failure is a commonly encountered clinical problem that broadly describes failure of oxygenation or ventilation. Acute hypoxemic and hypercapnic respiratory failure have numerous causes that can be differentiated with careful physical examination, blood gas analysis, and imaging assessment. Understanding the pathophysiology behind these diagnoses is extremely important in rapidly facilitating evaluation and treatment of acute respiratory failure.

CLINICS CARE POINTS

- Acute hypoxemic respiratory failure is the presence of low blood oxygen tension (low Pao_2) and is grouped in two broad categories: those with elevated alveolar-arterial oxygen gradient (more common) and those with normal alveolar-arterial oxygen gradient.
- Acute hypercapnic respiratory failure is the presence of excess dissolved carbon dioxide (high $Paco_2$) in the blood and is the result of poor ventilatory mechanics (can't breathe) or poor ventilatory drive (won't breathe).

- Acute hypoxemic and acute hypercapnic respiratory failures are not mutually exclusive and in fact can present together in diseases with both shunt and dead space physiology, such as acute respiratory distress syndrome or acute exacerbation of chronic obstructive pulmonary disease.
- The diagnosis respiratory failure can be made via arterial blood sampling and/or pulse oximetry.
- The etiology of respiratory failure can be identified through careful history, physical examination, and evaluation of chest imaging.

DISCLOSURE

Dr C.R. Rackley reports receiving consulting fees from Select Medical, Roche, and Inspira.

REFERENCES

1. Luhr OR, Antonsen K, Karlsson M, et al. Incidence and mortality after acute respiratory failure and acute respiratory distress syndrome in Sweden, Denmark, and Iceland. The ARF Study Group. Am J Respir Crit Care Med 1999;159:1849–61.
2. Lewandowski K, Metz J, Deutschmann C, et al. Incidence, severity, and mortality of acute respiratory failure in Berlin, Germany. Am J Respir Crit Care Med 1995; 151:1121–5.
3. Behrendt CE. Acute respiratory failure in the United States: incidence and 31-day survival. Chest 2000;118:1100–5.
4. Matthay MA, Arabi Y, Arroliga AC, et al. A new global definition of acute respiratory distress syndrome. Am J Respir Crit Care Med 2023. https://doi.org/10.1164/rccm.202303-0558WS.
5. Kempker JA, Abril MK, Chen Y, et al. The epidemiology of respiratory failure in the United States 2002-2017: a serial cross-sectional study. Crit Care Explor 2020;2: e0128.
6. W.H. Organization. The top 10 causes of death Available at: https://www.who.int/news-room/fact-sheets/detail/the-top-10-causes-of-death. Accessed 2023.
7. Deaths M Heron. Leading causes for 2019. Natl Vital Stat Rep 2021;70:1–114.
8. Vincent JL, Akça S, de Mendonça A, et al. The epidemiology of acute respiratory failure in critically ill patients(*). Chest 2002;121:1602–9.
9. All You ML. Really need to know to interpret arterial blood gases. Philadelphia: Lippencott Williams & Wilkins; 1999.
10. Stein PD, Goldhaber SZ, Henry JW. Alveolar-arterial oxygen gradient in the assessment of acute pulmonary embolism. Chest 1995;107:139–43.
11. Williams AJ. ABC of oxygen: assessing and interpreting arterial blood gases and acid-base balance. BMJ 1998;317:1213–6.
12. Grocott MP, Martin DS, Levett DZH, et al. Arterial blood gases and oxygen content in climbers on Mount Everest. N Engl J Med 2009;360:140–9.
13. Greene R. Pulmonary vascular obstruction in the adult respiratory distress syndrome. J Thorac Imaging 1986;1:31–8.
14. Tomashefski JF Jr, Davies P, Boggis C, et al. The pulmonary vascular lesions of the adult respiratory distress syndrome. Am J Pathol 1983;112:112–26.
15. Morales-Quinteros L, Schultz MJ, Bringué J, et al. Estimated dead space fraction and the ventilatory ratio are associated with mortality in early ARDS. Ann Intensive Care 2019;9:128.

16. Nuckton TJ, Alonso JA, Kallet RH, et al. Pulmonary dead-space fraction as a risk factor for death in the acute respiratory distress syndrome. N Engl J Med 2002; 346:1281–6.

17. Walkey AJ, Farber HW, O'Donnell C, et al. The accuracy of the central venous blood gas for acid-base monitoring. J Intensive Care Med 2010;25:104–10.

18. Phillips B, Peretz DI. A comparison of central venous and arterial blood gas values in the critically ill. Ann Intern Med 1969;70:745–9.

19. Zeserson E, Goodgame B, Hess JD, et al. Correlation of venous blood gas and pulse oximetry with arterial blood gas in the undifferentiated critically ill patient. J Intensive Care Med 2018;33:176–81.

20. Atkins EL. Assessment of acid-base disorders. A practical approach and review. Can Med Assoc J 1969;100:992–8.

21. Palm V, Rengier F, Rajiah P, et al. Acute pulmonary embolism: imaging techniques, findings, endovascular treatment and differential diagnoses. Röfo 2020; 192:38–49.

22. Mirza H, Hashmi MF. Lung ventilation perfusion scan (VQ Scan). Treasure Island (FL): StatPearls; 2023.

23. Investigators P. Value of the ventilation/perfusion scan in acute pulmonary embolism. Results of the prospective investigation of pulmonary embolism diagnosis (PIOPED). JAMA 1990;263:2753–9.

24. Mojoli F, Bouhemad B, Mongodi S, et al. Lung ultrasound for critically ill patients. Am J Respir Crit Care Med 2019;199:701–14.

25. Laursen CB, Clive A, Hallifax R, et al. European respiratory society statement on thoracic ultrasound. Eur Respir J 2021;57.

26. Hendin A, Koenig S, Millington SJ. Better with ultrasound: thoracic ultrasound. Chest 2020;158:2082–9.

27. Llamas-Alvarez AM, Tenza-Lozano EM, Latour-Perez J. Accuracy of lung ultrasonography in the diagnosis of pneumonia in adults: systematic review and meta-analysis. Chest 2017;151:374–82.

28. Xirouchaki N, Magkanas E, Vaporidi K, et al. Lung ultrasound in critically ill patients: comparison with bedside chest radiography. Intensive Care Med 2011; 37:1488–93.

29. Ogawa H, Kitsios GD, Iwata M, et al. Sputum gram stain for bacterial pathogen diagnosis in community-acquired pneumonia: a systematic review and bayesian meta-analysis of diagnostic accuracy and yield. Clin Infect Dis 2020;71: 499–513.

30. van der Eerden MM, Vlaspolder F, de Graaff CS, et al. Value of intensive diagnostic microbiological investigation in low- and high-risk patients with community-acquired pneumonia. Eur J Clin Microbiol Infect Dis 2005;24:241–9.

31. Feinsilver SH, Fein AM, Niederman MS, et al. Utility of fiberoptic bronchoscopy in nonresolving pneumonia. Chest 1990;98:1322–6.

32. Gong H Jr, Salvatierra C. Clinical efficacy of early and delayed fiberoptic bronchoscopy in patients with hemoptysis. Am Rev Respir Dis 1981;124:221–5.

33. Adams K, Shah PL, Edmonds L, et al. Test performance of endobronchial ultrasound and transbronchial needle aspiration biopsy for mediastinal staging in patients with lung cancer: systematic review and meta-analysis. Thorax 2009;64: 757–62.

34. Tan BB, Flaherty KR, Kazerooni EA, et al. The solitary pulmonary nodule. Chest 2003;123:89S–96S.

35. Almotairi A, Biswas S, Shahin J. The role of open lung biopsy in critically ill patients with hypoxic respiratory failure: a retrospective cohort study. Can Respir J 2016;2016:8715024.
36. Hutchinson JP, Fogarty AW, McKeever TM, et al. In-hospital mortality after surgical lung biopsy for interstitial lung disease in the United States. 2000 to 2011. Am J Respir Crit Care Med 2016;193:1161–7.

Diagnosis and Management of Acute Respiratory Failure

Madeline Lagina, MD, MPH[a], Thomas S. Valley, MD, MSc[a,b,c,d],*

KEYWORDS

- Hypoxemia • Hypercapnia • Respiratory failure • Diagnosis • Management

KEY POINTS

- Acute hypoxemic respiratory failure is defined by Pao_2 less than 60 mm Hg or SaO_2 less than 88% and may result from V/Q mismatch, shunt, hypoventilation, diffusion limitation, or low inspired oxygen tension.
- Acute hypercapnic respiratory failure is defined by $Paco_2 \geq$ 45 mm Hg and pH less than 7.35 and may result from alveolar hypoventilation, increased fraction of dead space, or increased production of carbon dioxide.
- Early diagnostic maneuvers, such as measurement of SpO_2 and arterial blood gas, can differentiate the type of respiratory failure and guide next steps in evaluation and management.
- Treatment should be directed at the primary derangement and targeted toward maintaining adequate tissue oxygenation and a normal pH with supportive modalities such as high-flow nasal cannula, noninvasive ventilation, or invasive mechanical ventilation.

INTRODUCTION

The lungs serve two primary functions: (1) to facilitate oxygen uptake and delivery to the vital organs and peripheral tissues and (2) to eliminate carbon dioxide and help maintain pH balance. When these primary functions fail, acute respiratory failure occurs. Management of acute respiratory failure depends on the etiology underlying the presentation; however, there is significant overlap in the stabilization and early treatment of patients with respiratory issues.

EARLY STABILIZATION OF THE PATIENT WITH ACUTE RESPIRATORY FAILURE

The first response to a critically ill patient should include immediate assessment and stabilization. This is accomplished by systematically identifying problems with circulation

[a] Division of Pulmonary and Critical Care, Department of Medicine, University of Michigan, Ann Arbor, MI, USA; [b] Center for Bioethics and Social Sciences in Medicine, University of Michigan Medical School, University of Michigan, Ann Arbor, MI, USA; [c] Institute for Healthcare Policy and Innovation, University of Michigan, Ann Arbor, MI, USA; [d] Department of Veterans Affairs, VA Ann Arbor Healthcare System, Ann Arbor, MI, USA
* Corresponding author. 2800 Plymouth Road, Building 16-G019W, Ann Arbor, MI 48109.
E-mail address: valleyt@med.umich.edu
Twitter: @maddielagina (M.L.); @tsvalley (T.S.V.)

Crit Care Clin 40 (2024) 235–253
https://doi.org/10.1016/j.ccc.2024.01.002
0749-0704/24/Published by Elsevier Inc.

criticalcare.theclinics.com

and breathing and simultaneously providing appropriate support. In 2010, the American Heart Association published new guidelines recommending an adjustment to the well-known mnemonic Airway, Breathing, and Circulation that prioritized circulatory support before respiratory support.[1] However, for the purposes of this review, the authors focus primarily on the parallel assessment and management of airway and breathing in patients with acute respiratory failure.

Airway and Breathing

Assessment of breathing pattern, frequency of respirations, and adequacy of oxygenation and ventilation should be performed simultaneously with the airway examination. The airway examination includes an evaluation of the patient's mental status as well as a focused examination of the oropharynx, chest wall, lungs, and heart. Obstruction of the airway should be addressed as soon as possible.

Oxygenation is often first assessed by pulse oximetry. Ventilation is typically evaluated through the measurement of the partial pressure of carbon dioxide (Pco_2) in arterial or venous blood. Noninvasive evaluation of Pco_2 can be achieved through the measurement of end-tidal CO_2 via capnometry or capnography. Capnometry delivers a numerical value alone. However, capnography also provides a waveform for the end-tidal CO_2 that is more reliable and allows for real-time evaluation of cardiac output and pulmonary blood flow.[2,3] Capnography is most frequently used to confirm placement of an endotracheal tube into the trachea, monitor adequacy of chest compressions during cardiopulmonary resuscitation (CPR), and evaluate for return of spontaneous circulation after cardiac arrest.[3,4] Early strategies to address issues with oxygenation or ventilation include chin tilt, jaw thrust, removal of foreign body, bag-valve-mask ventilation, insertion of a nasal or oral airway, endotracheal intubation, or tracheotomy.

IDENTIFYING THE TYPE OF ACUTE RESPIRATORY FAILURE

Early diagnostic maneuvers can help to distinguish between acute hypoxemic and hypercapnic respiratory failure. To start, the authors obtain oxygen saturation by pulse oximetry (SpO_2), oxygen saturation from arterial blood (SaO_2), partial pressure of oxygen in arterial blood (Pao_2), partial pressure of carbon dioxide in arterial blood ($Paco_2$), and hemoglobin level from a complete blood count.

Although arterial blood gas values remain the gold standard for evaluating the cause of acute respiratory failure, peripheral venous blood gas sampling has gained popularity for its ease of acquisition.[5,6] Several observational studies have demonstrated correlation of pH and Pco_2 between arterial and peripheral venous blood that justifies the use of the venous blood as a surrogate for arterial samples.[7,8] However, a meta-analysis published in 2014 identified wide variations between arterial and peripheral venous Pco_2 and Po_2 measurements and also noted clinically significant differences in diagnoses when venous blood gases were used to predict arterial values.[9] That said, pH was noted to correlate with reasonable accuracy in this study and has also demonstrated consistency when measured from peripheral venous blood gases in hypotensive patients.[7,9] Taken together, these data suggest that there is a role for venous blood sampling in the evaluation of an acutely ill patient, but the authors caution against the sole use of venous blood in lieu of arterial blood in the diagnosis of acute respiratory failure, particularly for acute hypoxemic respiratory failure.

ACUTE HYPOXEMIC RESPIRATORY FAILURE

Acute hypoxemic respiratory failure is defined by the inability of the respiratory system to maintain an adequate blood oxygen level to preserve normal organ function.

Clinically, oxygen saturation and Pao_2 are used as surrogate measures to assess adequate blood oxygen content. Hypoxemic respiratory failure is thus defined by a Pao_2 less than 60 mm Hg or SaO_2 less than 88%. There are five distinct but interconnected mechanisms that result in hypoxemia, which the authors detail later section. Clinical characteristics and disease-specific examples are included in **Table 1**.

CAUSES OF HYPOXEMIA

The causes of hypoxemia are understood through the pathophysiologic mechanisms that underlie them: ventilation/perfusion (V/Q) mismatch, shunt, diffusion limitation, hypoventilation, low inspired oxygen tension, oxygen delivery-consumption mismatch (see **Table 1**).

V/Q Mismatch

V/Q mismatch is the most common cause of hypoxemia in critically ill patients and is defined by a change to the typical ratio of ventilation and perfusion within the lung. Hypoxemia due to V/Q mismatch can be corrected with the addition of supplemental oxygen.[10]

Shunt

The most extreme example of reduced V/Q ratio is anatomic shunt, which occurs when there is complete impairment in ventilation despite adequate blood flow. Because the capillary blood is not exposed to ventilated lung units, hypoxemia due to shunt does not demonstrate the same improvement with supplemental oxygen as V/Q mismatch.[11] As the proportion of shunted blood, or shunt fraction, rises, progressive hypoxemia will become less responsive to supplemental oxygen. When the shunt fraction rises above 50%, Pao_2 is essentially independent of the fraction of inspired oxygen (Fio_2). At that point, supplemental oxygen therapy is typically ineffective.[12]

Diffusion Limitation

Diffusion limitation occurs when oxygen is unable to move across the alveolus into the capillary blood despite an unchanged V/Q ratio. Therefore, conditions that increase either membrane thickness (eg, interstitial lung disease or pulmonary hypertension) or rate of capillary blood flow (eg, increased cardiac output that can occur during exertion) can worsen diffusion and lead to hypoxemia.[11] Supplemental oxygen can correct hypoxemia generated by diffusion limitation.[13]

Hypoventilation

Hypoventilation can result in hypoxemia because of reduction in the partial pressure of oxygen in the alveolus (Pao_2) without concomitant changes in the ability of the capillary blood to extract oxygen.[11] Supplemental oxygen will improve hypoxemia from hypoventilation but does not improve hypercapnia.

Low Inspired Oxygen Tension

With reductions in PiO_2 at high altitude (including on aircrafts), hypoxemia is caused by the resulting low Pao_2 and is improved with the addition of supplemental oxygen.[11]

Oxygen Delivery–Consumption Mismatch

When oxygen demand by the peripheral tissues is exceeded by supply—as in states of hypermetabolism, low cardiac output, low oxygen carrying capacity—hypoxemia can result. In these cases, provision of supplemental oxygen and treatment

Table 1
Mechanisms of hypoxemia

Mechanism of Hypoxemia	Clinical Characteristics	Examples
V/Q mismatch	• Widened A-a gradient • Improves with O_2 • Limited impact on $Paco_2$ unless >30% dead space fraction	• Alveolar filling (pneumonia, pulmonary edema, pulmonary hemorrhage, and malignancy) • Atelectasis
Shunt	• Widened A-a gradient • Does not improve significantly with O_2 • When shunt fraction >50%, Pao_2 is independent of Fio_2	• Intracardiac shunt (ASD, PFO) • Intrapulmonary shunt (pulmonary AVM, hepatopulmonary syndrome) • Massive PE • Atelectasis, pneumonia, pulmonary edema, ARDS • Central airway occlusion • Severe small airways disease/asthma exacerbation
Diffusion limitation	• Widened A-a gradient • Improves with O_2	• Interstitial lung disease • Emphysema • Pulmonary vascular disease
Hypoventilation	• Normal A-a gradient • Improves with O_2	• Neuromuscular disease • Chest wall disorders • Central neurologic disorders • Sedating medications • Obstructive lung disease
Low inspired Fio_2	• Normal A-a gradient • Improves with O_2	• Altitude • Air travel
Oxygen delivery-consumption imbalance	• Widened A-a gradient	• Anemia • Hypermetabolic states • Low cardiac output

Abbreviations: ASD, atrial septal defect; PE, pulmonary embolism.

targeted toward correcting the underlying supply-demand mismatch will improve hypoxemia.

EVALUATION OF ACUTE HYPOXEMIC RESPIRATORY FAILURE

The authors begin the evaluation for acute hypoxemic respiratory failure by checking peripheral oxygen saturation (SpO$_2$) to determine if hypoxemia is present. If the SpO$_2$ is abnormal or the SpO$_2$ is normal, but the patient demonstrates clinical evidence of respiratory failure (eg, dyspnea, increased work of breathing), the authors perform an arterial blood gas for evaluation of arterial oxygen saturation (SaO$_2$). If the SaO$_2$ is low, the authors calculate the A-a gradient.

The A-a gradient is the difference between the P$_{AO_2}$ and the P$_{aO_2}$. The P$_{AO_2}$ is calculated using the alveolar gas equation (**Fig. 1**), and the P$_{aO_2}$ is measured from arterial blood. This equation allows for identification of abnormalities in oxygen absorption in the lung. Because the lung demonstrates variable ventilation/perfusion ratios in the normal state, a small difference in P$_{AO_2}$ and P$_{aO_2}$ is expected. A calculation of the normal A-a gradient for a person breathing room air at sea level is demonstrated in **Fig. 2**. The normal A-a gradient also increases with age. The age-adjustment equation for the normal A-a gradient is shown in **Fig. 3**.

If the A-a gradient is wider than expected, the etiology of hypoxemia can be narrowed to V/Q mismatch, shunt, or diffusion limitation. To delineate further, the authors begin with a chest x-ray to evaluate for pneumothorax, alveolar filling, or interstitial process. In select populations, cross-sectional imaging of the chest may be warranted in follow-up to the chest x-ray or as the initial imaging method. Computed tomography (CT) can assist with the diagnosis of infectious etiologies, particularly fungal infections, interstitial disease or inflammatory disorders impacting the lung, and for pulmonary embolism via angiography.[14] Specifically, the authors proceed with CT of the chest, instead of chest x-ray, in immunocompromised patients or when there is high suspicion of the previously mentioned conditions. If there is clinical concern for shunt, as demonstrated by limited response to supplemental oxygen, CT angiography of the chest or cardiac ultrasound with shunt study can be pursued. Contribution from an oxygen supply-demand mismatch can also be measured from a central venous oxygen saturation. If the central venous oxygen saturation is low, oxygen consumption by peripheral tissues exceeds delivery, which is indicative of hypermetabolic states, impaired cardiac output, or anemia.

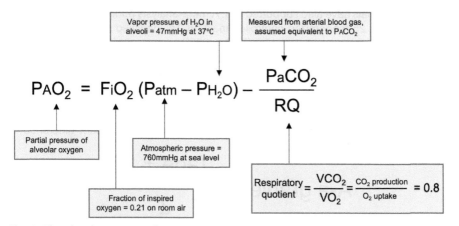

Fig. 1. The alveolar gas equation.

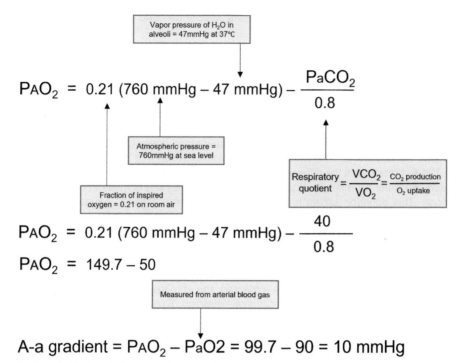

Fig. 2. Calculation of the normal A-a gradient.

MANAGEMENT OF ACUTE HYPOXEMIC RESPIRATORY FAILURE

Although the management of hypoxemia is focused primarily on treatment of the underlying disorder, all hypoxemic patients should be provided with supplemental oxygen therapy to maintain adequate oxygen delivery to tissues. The optimal oxygen target is still under investigation. Many sources argue for a conservative oxygen approach, targeting Pa_{O_2} between 55 and 80 mm Hg.[15]

Conservative approaches have theoretic basis, as hyperoxemia may result in tissue injury involving multiple systems including the lungs and central nervous system.[16] Some clinical trials have also supported this. A meta-analysis published in 2018 examining data from 25 randomized controlled trials (RCTs) identified an increased risk of mortality with liberal oxygen strategies ($SpO_2 > 96\%$) compared with conservative strategies.[17] On the other hand, other data have demonstrated a signal for increased mesenteric ischemia and 90-day mortality with conservative oxygen strategies (SpO_2 88%–92%) in patients with severe acute respiratory distress syndrome (ARDS), suggesting a possible benefit to targeting an intermediate oxygen saturation (SpO_2 92%–96%).[18] More recent data on this topic have been conflicting, as a large RCT examining liberal, intermediate, and conservative oxygen strategies found no significant difference in

$$\text{A-a gradient} = \frac{(\text{age} + 10)}{4}$$

Fig. 3. Age-adjusted A-a gradient equation.

ventilator-free days between groups and no increased signal for harm in any group, supporting the conclusion that an SpO_2 between 90% and 98% may be safe.[19]

Monitoring for hypoxemia is complicated further by recent studies that have identified limitations in noninvasive oxygen monitoring. Pulse oximetry has been criticized for both inaccuracy and systematic bias based on skin tone.[20–23] A large 2020 multicenter study identified occult hypoxemia (defined by having a SpO_2 92%–96% on pulse oximetry but a $SaO_2 < 88\%$ in the arterial blood) in 11.4% of Black patients compared with 3.6% of White patients.[23]

Given this concern, early arterial blood sampling for patients in whom respiratory failure is suspected based on clinical examination, but not by SpO_2 measurement, should be performed to evaluate the arterial oxygen saturation.[21,23] Taking into account the emerging data suggesting that higher oxygen targets may not result in harm for patients receiving mechanical ventilation, one might consider using higher SpO_2 thresholds in patients at risk for pulse oximeter inaccuracy (ie, individuals with darker skin tone).[17,19,23]

Based on these data, the authors generally believe that a SpO_2 within a range of 90% to 98% is likely to be safe, and the authors consider using a more liberal strategy (eg, 92%–98%) in patients with darker skin tones in whom SaO_2 or Pao_2 have not or cannot be measured.

Oxygen Delivery Modalities

Treatment of hypoxemic respiratory failure can be achieved via multiple different modalities. The most accessible of these devices is conventional oxygen therapy, which can be delivered via standard nasal cannula or facemask at flow rates up to 6 L of oxygen per minute. For each liter of oxygen per minute delivered by standard nasal cannula, the expected Fio_2 that is delivered increases by approximately 4% above the Fio_2 of room air (ie, 21%).[24] **Table 2** provides further breakdown of oxygen delivery devices and estimated Fio_2.

Critically ill patients sometimes increase their minute ventilation above the oxygen delivery rates achieved by standard nasal cannulas or simple facemasks (ie, > 6 liters per minute [LPM]). This results in a dilution of the administered oxygen supply with additional room air. To overcome this problem in hypoxemic patients, high-flow nasal cannulas (HFNC) were developed with flow rates of supplemental oxygen up to 60 L per minute. Non-rebreather masks with oxygen reservoirs can also serve to maximally concentrate Fio_2 to prevent dilution by room air.

The COVID-19 pandemic magnified the intensity of research devoted to respiratory support devices such as HFNC and noninvasive ventilation (NIV) in hypoxemic

Table 2 Oxygen delivery devices		
Oxygen Delivery Device	**Deliverable Flow Rates ($L \cdot min^{-1}$)**	**Estimated Fio_2 (%)**
Nasal cannula	1–2	24–28
	3–4	20–35
	5–6	38–44
Simple face mask	5–10	35–55
Venturi mask[a]	5–15	24–50
Non-rebreather mask[a]	10–15	80–95
High-flow nasal cannula[a]	Up to 60	30–100

[a] High-flow oxygen delivery modalities.

patients. However, this research was met with mixed results.[25–27] A trial of patients with COVID-19 that compared HFNC to NIV via helmet interface found that NIV may reduce the risk of mechanical ventilation without impacting mortality.[26] Although interpretation can be challenging, some have raised the possibility that patients who received NIV and eventually required mechanical ventilation may have experienced self-inflicted lung injury from large tidal volumes that resulted from the use of NIV.[28] Despite this, a subsequent trial comparing NIV through continuous positive airway pressure (CPAP) or HFNC with conventional oxygen therapy in patients with COVID-19 found a mortality reduction with CPAP compared with conventional oxygen (36% vs 44%, respectively) but no difference in mortality between HFNC and conventional oxygen.[25]

Despite this, the American College of Physicians published a clinical practice guideline in 2021 that recommended HFNC over NIV for all individuals with acute hypoxemic respiratory failure.[30] This recommendation was based largely on a 2015 RCT that demonstrated mortality benefit with the use of HFNC over NIV.[31] The study included roughly 200 patients with acute hypoxemic respiratory failure due to multiple etiologies and documented an absolute risk reduction of mortality of nearly 16% (mortality rates of 12.4% vs 28.2%, respectively), an increase in ventilator-free days, and a reduced risk of hospital-acquired pneumonia in patients receiving HFNC compared with NIV.[30,31] Evidence also suggests improvement in patient dyspnea with HFNC compared with conventional oxygen therapy, suggesting that some increase in work of breathing may be appropriately addressed by HFNC alone.[30] Further cited benefits of HFNC include improved patient comfort and less interface displacement, thus fewer interruptions to ventilatory support, when compared with NIV.[32]

Accordingly, the authors use conventional oxygen therapy to patients with hypoxemia but normal work of breathing. In patients with persistent hypoxemia that requires greater than 6 LPM of supplemental oxygen (or approximately 40% Fio_2), the authors use HFNC. For patients with acute hypoxemic respiratory failure, dyspnea, or elevated work of breathing, the authors use HFNC. If there is persistently elevated work of breathing despite improvement in hypoxemia in patients with COVID-19, the authors consider a trial of NIV before intubation and mechanical ventilation.[25,26]

In certain cases, the authors consider NIV as the initial treatment. In patients presenting with acute cardiogenic pulmonary edema, the use of NIV (including CPAP) has been shown to improve respiratory distress (defined by symptoms of dyspnea and derangements in physiologic parameters like heart and respiratory rate) when compared with standard oxygen therapy.[33] Further studies have identified reduced in-hospital mortality with use of NIV in this population.[34] NIV for patients with obstructive lung disease has also been well-studied. Robust data from research spanning more than 3 decades have substantiated the use of NIV for respiratory failure resulting from acute exacerbations of chronic obstructive pulmonary disease (COPD).[35] As a result, the European Respiratory Society/American Thoracic Society guideline for management of COPD exacerbations issued a strong recommendation for the use of NIV in 2017.[36] The authors initiate NIV as first-line treatment for hypoxemia in patients with acute cardiogenic pulmonary edema or acute exacerbations of COPD, whereas disease-specific interventions are begun. In patients who demonstrate inadequate response to the above therapies or exhibit signs of hemodynamic instability, endotracheal intubation and mechanical ventilation are necessary.

Indications for Intubation

Despite its importance to critical care, the threshold at which to intubate a patient for acute hypoxic respiratory failure remains uncertain.[37–39] Some support an early intubation strategy to limit exposure to injuriously large tidal volumes that may result from severe dyspnea and ventilatory support mechanisms such as HFNC and NIV.[40] Recent data, including those that emerged from the COVID-19 pandemic, have afforded little clarity. Several observational studies have correlated pre-intubation HFNC use with elevated mortality possibly due to delay of intubation and mechanical ventilation.[41,42] However, a 2021 meta-analysis of 12 studies evaluating outcomes associated with the timing of intubation (early [ie, within 24 hours] vs late intubation) in patients with acute hypoxic respiratory failure due to COVID-19 did not reveal significant differences in all-cause mortality between groups.[29] Conversely, a more recent observational study examining a historical cohort of patients with COVID-19 identified an increase in mortality associated with a pre-intubation HFNC trial lasting more than 48 hours.[43] Further data are warranted to determine the safety of proceeding with HFNC past 48 hours for patients with acute hypoxic respiratory failure.

Given the equipoise, the authors tend not to use a standardized time limit on HFNC or NIV trial before intubation for all-comers with acute hypoxic respiratory failure. Rather, the authors implement a case-by-case trial with close monitoring to determine whether and when to move to invasive mechanical ventilation. In general, when HFNC or NIV fail to adequately manage a patient's respiratory failure or markers of tissue hypoperfusion become evident, the authors proceed with endotracheal intubation and invasive mechanical ventilation. Of course, in every case, the decision to initiate mechanical ventilation should be weighed carefully with a patient's preferences, the risks of endotracheal intubation, and the risks of mechanical ventilation.[38]

Patients with acute hypoxemic respiratory failure are challenging in the peri-intubation period. Acute hypoxemic respiratory failure has been described as one of several conditions that present a "physiologically difficult airway."[44–46] Patients who are hypoxemic, regardless of the mechanism, are at high risk of developing worsening oxygenation during rapid sequence induction (RSI) due to the cessation of respiratory function with neuromuscular blockade. This process makes intubation more likely to be associated with downstream complications, such as arrhythmia, hemodynamic instability, or cardiac arrest.[45,47,48]

One of the most important interventions for patients with hypoxemia is adequate preoxygenation, which the Society for Airway Management recommends should last for at least 3 minutes before intubation and be delivered either through HFNC or NIV. Adequate preoxygenation can provide more time between initiation of RSI and first desaturation by creating a large alveolar oxygen reserve, which has been shown to increase the chance of first-pass success for intubation.[45,49]

Apneic oxygenation (ie, continued delivery of oxygen during the period of apnea that follows neuromuscular blockade but precedes intubation during RSI) has received attention as a possible method by which to prevent desaturation in the peri-intubation period, though data have been mixed. In observational studies, passive apneic oxygenation is associated with fewer desaturations and more first-pass success.[50–52] However, a 2016 RCT evaluating the role of passive apneic oxygenation found no significant difference in oxygen saturations between patients receiving 15 L passive apneic oxygenation by high-flow nasal cannula compared with those who did not.[53] More robust evidence supports the use of bag-valve-mask ventilation for prevention of hypoxemia during the apneic period without evidence of increased risk for aspiration.[54] Given possible benefit and limited evidence of harm, the authors use apneic oxygenation via bag-valve-mask ventilation when available in patients with acute hypoxic respiratory failure undergoing RSI.[49–52] If available, video laryngoscopy should be considered as the primary method for endotracheal intubation over direct laryngoscopy, as data suggest that its use substantially increases first-pass success in critically ill patients.[55] In patients with refractory hypoxemia, inhaled pulmonary vasodilators or awake fiberoptic intubations could be considered to reduce harms associated with RSI.[44,45]

In patients exhibiting signs of circulatory collapse and respiratory failure, resuscitation and RSI should be considered simultaneously, though resuscitation should not delay intubation if needed.[56] In a trial of roughly 1000 patients in intensive care units undergoing endotracheal intubation, fluid bolus of 500 mL of crystalloid during RSI had no significant impact on reducing hypotension (defined by drop in systolic blood pressure < 65 mm Hg or increased dose of vasopressors).[56] For those patients who demonstrate hemodynamic instability and respiratory failure, vasopressor therapy should be used to maintain blood pressure targets during intubation. Fluid resuscitation should be aimed at treating hypovolemia if present.[56,57]

ACUTE HYPERCAPNIC RESPIRATORY FAILURE

Hypercapnia occurs when the lungs are unable to eliminate carbon dioxide (CO_2) to keep levels at or below 45 mm Hg. Once hypercapnia has been identified, it is important to understand whether the source is a primary respiratory or neurologic dysfunction or whether the elevated $Paco_2$ is compensatory, in response to a primary metabolic alkalosis.

An arterial blood gas and a blood chemistry panel, along with clinical history and physical examination, are essential in identifying the presence of acute hypercapnic respiratory failure. Acute hypercapnic respiratory failure is diagnosed when the $Paco_2$ is $\geq$ 45 mm Hg and the blood pH is acidic, defined by a pH less than 7.35. Chronic hypercapnic respiratory failure is diagnosed when the $Paco_2$ is $\geq$ 45 mm Hg, the increase in the $Paco_2$ is not compensatory for a primary metabolic alkalosis, and the blood pH is normal or near normal. **Table 3** provides the expected changes in pH and $Paco_2$ in acute and chronic hypercapnic respiratory failure.

Causes of Hypercapnia

Hypercapnic respiratory failure results from alveolar hypoventilation, increased fraction of dead space, increased production of carbon dioxide, or a combination thereof. CO_2 production can also sometimes overwhelm elimination, usually in patients with compromised baseline pulmonary reserve, which can result in elevations in $Paco_2$ in the absence of a new pulmonary problem.[58] The mechanisms of hypercapnia can be understood through the mnemonic "won't breathe, can't breathe, can't breathe enough."

"Won't breathe" causes of hypercapnia include central disorders of hypoventilation which result in reduced respiratory drive and subsequent alveolar hypoventilation. Common causes of central hypoventilation include stroke, use of sedative medications, central and obstructive sleep apnea, obesity hypoventilation, and hypothyroidism.[59] These disorders are characterized by a normal A-a gradient, indicating a reduction in alveolar ventilation.

"Can't breathe" disorders result from limited ventilatory capacity of the lungs, including advanced obstructive lung disease, diseases of the chest wall, or neuromuscular disease

Table 3
Expected changes in pH and $Paco_2$ in acute and chronic hypercapnic respiratory failure

	Increase in $Paco_2$	Increase in HCO_3	Decrease in pH
Acute hypercapnia	10 mm Hg	1 mEq/L	0.08
Chronic hypercapnia	10 mm Hg	3.5 mEq/L	0.03

that prevent the adequate functioning of respiratory muscles without impairing central respiratory drive. Clinical history and examination are essential in distinguishing these disorders and could include review of prior pulmonary function testing or imaging.

Finally, "can't breathe enough" disorders result from an overproduction of CO_2 that overwhelms lung function or new elevations in the proportion of dead space ventilation that cannot be overcome by compensatory increases in minute ventilation.[59] A more complete list of the disorders causing hypercapnia, stratified by category, is included in **Table 4**.

EVALUATION OF ACUTE HYPERCAPNIC RESPIRATORY FAILURE

To evaluate for the presence of acute hypercapnic respiratory failure, the authors obtain pulse oximetry, an arterial blood gas measurement, and a full blood chemistry panel. Evaluation of the arterial blood gas should be performed to identify acute, chronic, or acute on chronic hypercapnic respiratory failure. Pulse oximetry measurement or SaO_2 measurement can identify patients with mixed hypoxemic and hypercapnic respiratory failure. Calculation of the A-a gradient should be performed regardless of the presence of hypoxemia as a normal A-a gradient in a patient with hypercapnic respiratory failure signifies alveolar hypoventilation or increased CO_2 production.

Patients with hypercapnia may report symptoms of shortness of breath, headache, somnolence, or they may demonstrate increased work of breathing, agitation, or anxiety.[60] As $Paco_2$ rises and pH decreases, multiple organ systems may be impacted. Cardiac and diaphragmatic contractility are reduced, resulting in increased risk for arrhythmia, circulatory collapse, and further perpetuating CO_2 retention.[58,61] Acute hypercapnia can result in depressed mentation and decreased respiratory drive, typically occurring when $Paco_2$ rises above 75 mm Hg in normally eucapnic individuals.[60] Cerebral blood flow is increased as a result of elevated $Paco_2$, which can result in elevated intracranial pressures, seizures, and coma in severe cases.[60]

The initial clinical evaluation is aimed at identifying the mechanism of hypercapnia. In all patients with hypercapnic respiratory failure, in addition to early stabilization and assessment of airway, breathing, circulation, the authors perform a neurologic examination that includes evaluation for focal neurologic deficit (cranial nerve examination, speech evaluation, muscle strength testing) as well as an assessment of global mental status. From there, further examination and evaluation can be guided by the patient's breathing pattern.

If there are signs of reduced respiratory drive (ie, low respiratory rate) in the setting of hypercapnia, the authors consider central, "won't breathe" etiologies. If accompanying neurologic findings are consistent with acute stroke (eg, facial droop, dysarthria, muscle weakness, sensation changes), the authors pursue immediate imaging and expert consultation. In addition, the authors perform a simultaneous medication review, focused history, or drug screen to identify medications or substances that may blunt the respiratory drive and result in global mental status changes including narcotics, benzodiazepines, barbiturates, or alcohol. If history or laboratory testing indicate exposure to respiratory depressants, appropriate reversal agents should be administered.

If there are signs of increased respiratory effort (ie, tachypnea) in the setting of hypercapnia, the authors consider "can't breathe" or "can't breathe enough" etiologies. The authors quickly review the patient's medical history for neuromuscular disorders, chest wall disease, pleural disease, or obstructive lung disease which may result in impairment of respiratory efficiency and increased dead space ventilation. The

Table 4
Mechanisms of hypercapnia

Mechanism of Hypercapnia	Category	Pathophysiology	Examples
Hypoventilation	"Won't breathe"	Decreased central respiratory drive	• Sedatives (alcohol, benzodiazepines, opiates) • Central disorders (encephalitis, stroke, medullary tumors, obesity hypoventilation)
Hypoventilation	"Can't breathe"	Impaired function of respiratory muscles due to altered neuromuscular function	• Myasthenia gravis, ALS, GBS, spinal cord injury • Toxins: botulism, organophosphates • Thyroid disorders
Hypoventilation	"Can't breathe"	Chest wall disorders and pleural disease	• Kyphoscoliosis, large pleural effusions, diaphragmatic paralysis, prior sternotomy/chest wall surgery, obesity
Increased proportion of dead space	"Can't breathe"	Airway obstruction resulting in elevated V/Q ratios	• Emphysema, hyperinflation, severe asthma, central airway obstruction
Increased proportion of dead space	"Can't breathe"	Pulmonary vascular disease resulting in elevated V/Q ratios	• Severe pulmonary embolism, pulmonary vascular disease, interstitial lung disease, ARDS
Increased CO_2 production	"Can't breathe enough"	CO_2 production overwhelms pulmonary CO_2 elimination	• Fever, exercise, sepsis, hyperalimentation, thyrotoxicosis

Abbreviations: ALS, amyotrophic lateral sclerosis; GBS, Guillain Barre syndrome.

authors also perform a focused physical examination with attention to breathe sounds (eg, degree of air movement and character of breath sounds) and chest wall findings to help differentiate between obstructive lung disease and neuromuscular causes of hypercapnia. Because low cardiac output can increase dead space fraction and hypercapnia by the way of reduced pulmonary perfusion and increased thoracic gas volume, careful assessment and treatment for concomitant shock is paramount.[62]

MANAGEMENT OF ACUTE HYPERCAPNIC RESPIRATORY FAILURE

The primary goal of management for patients with acute hypercapnic respiratory failure is to provide respiratory support to increase work of breathing. For patients who are candidates, NIV is typically the first-line therapy. The authors select patients for NIV based on several criteria. First, patients receiving NIV must be spontaneously breathing. Second, patients must demonstrate the ability to protect their airway and remove the NIV mask in the event of emesis as aspiration of gastric secretions presents a major risk to those receiving NIV. There are situations that arise in which patients who do not meet these criteria may be trialed on NIV, but these individuals should be monitored closely, ideally in a critical care setting.

Emerging evidence has suggested that HFNC can be safely used in patients with hypercapnic respiratory failure who cannot tolerate or are not candidates for NIV. One meta-analysis published in 2020 concluded that HFNC was non-inferior to NIV in preventing intubation in patients with mild to moderate hypercapnia and cited no significant differences in blood gas analysis or respiratory rate between support mechanisms in the included studies.[63] Further attention is being directed toward the use of HFNC in the treatment of COPD and chronic hypercapnia with promising early results.[64] Given this, the authors consider the use of HFNC for patients with acute hypercapnic respiratory failure who are not candidates for NIV.

However, targeting normal or higher oxygen saturation ranges has the potential to result in an alteration of physiologic hypoxic vasoconstriction in individuals with COPD which could conversely worsen dead space ventilation and hypercapnia. Oxygen saturations of 93% or greater have been correlated with elevated mortality in hospitalized patients with acute exacerbations of COPD.[65] In addition, treatment of hypoventilation alone can improve oxygenation in patients with hypercapnic respiratory failure.[66] Thus, the authors target the SpO_2 range of 88% to 92% in this population and careful monitor HFNC or NIV trials.

SpO_2, SaO_2, $Paco_2$, and clinical status should be serially evaluated during any trial of NIV or HFNC. End-tidal CO_2 monitoring can be used in these circumstances but caution should be taken when interpreting the results. End-tidal CO_2 measurement is impacted not just by minute ventilation but also by other physiologic parameters including cardiac output and ventilation/perfusion matching. Thus, it can at times be an unreliable surrogate for $Paco_2$ in patients with alterations to normal respiratory and cardiac function.[67,68] Monitoring the difference between the end-tidal CO_2 and the $Paco_2$, or CO_2 gradient, to assess for adequacy of ventilatory support during NIV trial has been proposed but has not been sufficiently studied.[69] Given this, the authors do not routinely use end-tidal CO2 to estimate $Paco_2$ in the setting of hypercapnic respiratory failure. Although transcutaneous CO_2 monitoring seems to have better accuracy in estimating $Paco_2$ when compared with end-tidal CO_2 and could be considered for monitoring response to ventilatory support over time, the authors favor serial blood gas collection for pH and $Paco_2$ assessment over noninvasive monitoring at this time.[70]

If during a trial of NIV or HFNC, the pH does not normalize, the $Paco_2$ does not improve, or the patient's clinical status worsens despite adequate ventilatory support (which includes ensuring mask fit, minute ventilation, and adjusting NIV settings), then intubation and invasive mechanical ventilation are indicated.[71] The appropriate length of NIV trial before intubation for patients with hypercapnic respiratory failure is unknown. It is estimated that benefit from initiation of NIV in the setting of acute exacerbation of COPD should be seen within 1 to 4 hours.[72] Further, a relatively small retrospective cohort study published in 2021 documented increased 30-day mortality and increased ventilator dependence for patients who failed a trial of NIV or HFNC after more than 6 hours compared with those who failed in fewer than 6 hours.[73] Given these data, the authors generally restrict trials of NIV support for hypercapnic respiratory failure to 4 hours and proceed with intubation and mechanical ventilation if no benefit is observed within this timeframe.

Intubation for Hypercapnic Respiratory Failure

Severe pH derangements from hypercapnic respiratory failure tend to correct quickly with restoration of alveolar ventilation.[44] During RSI for endotracheal intubation, attention should be paid to the impact of apnea on worsening acidemia, which could result in complications.[44,46] In these cases, one might consider avoiding neuromuscular blockade entirely by using alternate sedative agents or pursuing awake fiberoptic intubation.[46,74,75]

In most cases, the authors continue ventilation with NIV with a respiratory rate or bag-valve-mask during the apneic period of RSI.[54] Advanced surgical airways should be considered in select patients with hypercapnia due to upper airway obstruction for whom endotracheal intubation is not feasible. This is optimally performed with a multidisciplinary approach that involves critical care, anesthesia, and surgical teams.

MANAGEMENT OF MIXED HYPOXEMIC AND HYPERCAPNIC RESPIRATORY FAILURE

Given the overlap between mechanisms causing hypoxemia and hypercapnia, some patients present with both derangements. Although treatment should always be aimed toward addressing the primary or most severe dysfunction, it may be difficult to

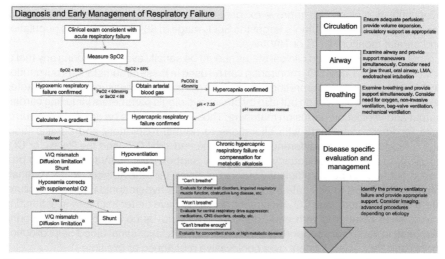

Fig. 4. Diagnosis and early management of respiratory failure. [a]Specific to hypoxic respiratory failure.

differentiate the type of respiratory failure in the initial stabilization period. Some have proposed that NIV, when used in the wrong patient populations, could cause harm by generating self-inflicted lung injury.[30,40] Although there may be some conceptual basis for this, there is limited evidence to suggest a clinically meaningful signal for harm. Furthermore, data borne out of COVID-19 argue that the use of NIV may result in fewer intubations without increasing mortality.[25,26] In patients with increased work of breathing and concern for hypercapnic respiratory failure, the authors initiate NIV. If concomitant hypoxemia is identified, the authors initiate supplemental oxygen to maintain Pao_2 greater than 60 mm Hg with SaO_2 88% to 92%, given the potential for hyperoxemia to worsen hypercapnia in select populations.

SUMMARY

Fig. 4 describes our algorithm for diagnosis and early management of acute respiratory failure. It is imperative that the diagnosis and early management of acute respiratory failure happen in parallel. Early stabilization can be achieved by implementing an organized approach to assessment and management. Further stratification of disease is based on clinical history, physical examination, and rapid laboratory assessment. Calculation of the A-a gradient can help clarify the underlying disease pathology for both hypoxemia and hypercapnia. Treatment of acute respiratory failure varies based on the underlying the presentation. However, oxygen and ventilatory support mechanisms, such as HFNC, NIV, or invasive mechanical ventilation, should aim to maintain a Pao_2 greater than 60 mm Hg, SaO_2 greater than 88%, normal pH, and reduced dyspnea.

CLINICS CARE POINTS

- The initial approach to the patient with acute respiratory failure depends on the extent to which hypoxemia or hypercapnia are present and should consist of parallel assessment of and support for airway, breathing, and oxygen delivery to the tissues.
- Treatment should be directed toward reversing the primary respiratory derangement.
- Supportive respiratory technology, such as high-flow nasal cannula, noninvasive ventilation, or invasive mechanical ventilation, are critical to ensuring adequate oxygenation and ventilation for the critically ill patient.

DISCLOSURE

The authors have nothing to disclose. Funding provided through NHLBI K23 HL140165 and NHLBI R01 HL157361. This manuscript does not necessarily represent the view of the US Government or the Department of Veterans Affairs.

REFERENCES

1. Field JM, Hazinski MF, Sayre MR, et al. Part 1: executive summary: 2010 American heart association guidelines for cardiopulmonary resuscitation and emergency cardiovascular care. Circulation. Nov 2 2010;122(18 Suppl 3):S640–56.
2. Deakin CD, Morrison LJ, Morley PT, et al. Part 8: advanced life support: 2010 International Consensus on cardiopulmonary resuscitation and emergency cardiovascular care science with treatment recommendations. Resuscitation 2010; 81(Suppl 1):e93–174.

3. Brian KW, David NC, Ruben DR. Capnography/capnometry during mechanical ventilation: 2011. Respir Care 2011;56(4):503.
4. Lecompte-Osorio P, Pearson SD, Pieroni CH, et al. Bedside estimates of dead space using end-tidal CO(2) are independently associated with mortality in ARDS. Crit Care 2021;25(1):333.
5. Davis MD, Walsh BK, Sittig SE, et al. AARC clinical practice guideline: blood gas analysis and hemoximetry: 2013. Respir Care 2013;58(10):1694–703.
6. Rowling SC, Fløjstrup M, Henriksen DP, et al. Arterial blood gas analysis: as safe as we think? A multicentre historical cohort study. ERJ Open Res 2022;8(1).
7. Prasad H, Vempalli N, Agrawal N, et al. Correlation and agreement between arterial and venous blood gas analysis in patients with hypotension-an emergency department-based cross-sectional study. Int J Emerg Med 2023;16(1):18.
8. Arnold TDW, Miller M, van Wessem KP, et al. Base deficit from the first peripheral venous sample: a surrogate for arterial Base deficit in the trauma Bay. J Trauma Acute Care Surg 2011;71(4).
9. Byrne AL, Bennett M, Chatterji R, et al. Peripheral venous and arterial blood gas analysis in adults: are they comparable? A systematic review and meta-analysis. Respirology 2014;19(2):168–75.
10. Sarkar M, Niranjan N, Banyal PK. Mechanisms of hypoxemia. Lung India 2017; 34(1):47–60.
11. Johan P, Robb WG. Gas exchange and ventilation–perfusion relationships in the lung. Eur Respir J 2014;44(4):1023.
12. Marino PL. Hypoxemia and hypercapnia. Marino's: the ICU Book. 4th edition. Philadelphia, PA: Wolters Kluwer Health/Lippincott Williams & Wilkins; 2014. chap 20.
13. Pittman RN. Chapter 4, Oxygen Transport. Regulation of tissue oxygenation, . Morgan & Claypool Life Sciences. San Rafael, CA; 2011.
14. Washington L, Khan A, Mohammed TL, et al. ACR Appropriateness Criteria on acute respiratory illness. J Am Coll Radiol 2009;6(10):675–80.
15. Brower RG, Matthay MA, Morris A, et al. Ventilation with lower tidal volumes as compared with traditional tidal volumes for acute lung injury and the acute respiratory distress syndrome. N Engl J Med 2000;342(18):1301–8.
16. Hafner S, Beloncle F, Koch A, et al. Hyperoxia in intensive care, emergency, and peri-operative medicine: Dr. Jekyll or Mr. Hyde? A 2015 update. Ann Intensive Care 2015;5(1):42.
17. Chu DK, Kim LH, Young PJ, et al. Mortality and morbidity in acutely ill adults treated with liberal versus conservative oxygen therapy (IOTA): a systematic review and meta-analysis. Lancet 2018;391(10131):1693–705.
18. Barrot L, Asfar P, Mauny F, et al. Liberal or conservative oxygen therapy for acute respiratory distress syndrome. N Engl J Med 2020;382(11):999–1008.
19. Semler MW, Casey JD, Lloyd BD, et al. Oxygen-saturation targets for critically ill adults receiving mechanical ventilation. N Engl J Med 2022;387(19):1759–69.
20. Van Meter A, Williams U, Zavala A, et al. Beat to Beat: a measured Look at the history of pulse oximetry. Journal of Anesthesia History 2017;3(1):24–6.
21. Bickler PE, Feiner JR, Severinghaus JW. Effects of skin pigmentation on pulse oximeter accuracy at low saturation. Anesthesiology 2005;102(4):715–9.
22. Gupta S, Medikayala S, Singh B, et al. Leukocytosis and Spurious hypoxemia. Cureus. Jun 2021;13(6):e15942.
23. Sjoding MW, Dickson RP, Iwashyna TJ, et al. Racial bias in pulse oximetry measurement. N Engl J Med 2020;383(25):2477–8.

24. Hardavella G, Karampinis I, Frille A, et al. Oxygen devices and delivery systems. Breathe (Sheff) 2019;15(3):e108–16.
25. Perkins GD, Ji C, Connolly BA, et al. Effect of noninvasive respiratory strategies on intubation or mortality among patients with acute hypoxemic respiratory failure and COVID-19: the RECOVERY-RS randomized clinical trial. JAMA 2022;327(6): 546–58. https://doi.org/10.1001/jama.2022.0028.
26. Grieco DL, Menga LS, Cesarano M, et al. Effect of helmet noninvasive ventilation vs high-flow nasal oxygen on Days free of respiratory support in patients with COVID-19 and moderate to severe hypoxemic respiratory failure: the HENIVOT randomized clinical trial. JAMA 2021;325(17):1731–43.
27. Ospina-Tascón GA, Calderón-Tapia LE, García AF, et al. Effect of high-flow oxygen therapy vs conventional oxygen therapy on invasive mechanical ventilation and clinical Recovery in patients with severe COVID-19: a randomized clinical trial. JAMA 2021;326(21):2161–71.
28. Battaglini D, Robba C, Ball L, et al. Noninvasive respiratory support and patient self-inflicted lung injury in COVID-19: a narrative review. Br J Anaesth 2021; 127(3):353–64.
29. Papoutsi E, Giannakoulis VG, Xourgia E, et al. Effect of timing of intubation on clinical outcomes of critically ill patients with COVID-19: a systematic review and meta-analysis of non-randomized cohort studies. Crit Care 2021;25(1):121.
30. Qaseem A, Etxeandia-Ikobaltzeta I, Fitterman N, et al. Appropriate Use of high-flow nasal oxygen in hospitalized patients for initial or Postextubation management of acute respiratory failure: a clinical guideline from the American College of Physicians. Ann Intern Med 2021;174(7):977–84.
31. Frat JP, Thille AW, Mercat A, et al. High-flow oxygen through nasal cannula in acute hypoxemic respiratory failure. N Engl J Med 2015;372(23):2185–96.
32. Papazian L, Corley A, Hess D, et al. Use of high-flow nasal cannula oxygenation in ICU adults: a narrative review. Intensive Care Med 2016;42(9):1336–49.
33. Gray A, Goodacre S, Newby DE, et al. Noninvasive ventilation in acute cardiogenic pulmonary edema. N Engl J Med 2008;359(2):142–51.
34. Mariani J, Macchia A, Belziti C, et al. Noninvasive ventilation in acute cardiogenic pulmonary edema: a meta-analysis of randomized controlled trials. J Card Fail 2011;17(10):850–9.
35. Shah NM, D'Cruz RF, Murphy PB. Update: non-invasive ventilation in chronic obstructive pulmonary disease. J Thorac Dis 2018;10(Suppl 1):S71–9.
36. Wedzicha JAEC-C, Miravitlles M, Hurst JR, et al. Management of COPD exacerbations: a European respiratory Society/American thoracic Society guideline. Eur Respir J 2017;49(3).
37. Pisano A, Yavorovskiy A, Verniero L, et al. Indications for tracheal intubation in patients with Coronavirus disease 2019 (COVID-19). J Cardiothorac Vasc Anesth 2021;35(5):1276–80.
38. Cabrini L, Ghislanzoni L, Severgnini P, et al. Early versus late tracheal intubation in COVID-19 patients: a "pros/cons" debate also considering heart-lung interactions. Minerva Cardiol Angiol 2021;69(5):596–605.
39. Tobin MJ, Laghi F, Jubran A. Caution about early intubation and mechanical ventilation in COVID-19. Ann Intensive Care 2020;10(1):78.
40. Grieco DL, Menga LS, Eleuteri D, et al. Patient self-inflicted lung injury: implications for acute hypoxemic respiratory failure and ARDS patients on non-invasive support. Minerva Anestesiol 2019;85(9):1014–23.
41. Kang BJ, Koh Y, Lim CM, et al. Failure of high-flow nasal cannula therapy may delay intubation and increase mortality. Intensive Care Med 2015;41(4):623–32.

42. Miller DC, Pu J, Kukafka D, et al. Failure of high flow nasal cannula and subsequent intubation is associated with increased mortality as compared to failure of non-invasive ventilation and mechanical ventilation alone: a real-World retrospective analysis. J Intensive Care Med 2022;37(1):41–5.

43. López-Ramírez VY, Sanabria-Rodríguez OO, Bottia-Córdoba S, et al. Delayed mechanical ventilation with prolonged high-flow nasal cannula exposure time as a risk factor for mortality in acute respiratory distress syndrome due to SARS-CoV-2. Intern Emerg Med 2023;18(2):429–37.

44. Mosier JM. Physiologically difficult airway in critically ill patients: winning the race between haemoglobin desaturation and tracheal intubation. Br J Anaesth 2020; 125(1):e1–4.

45. Kornas RL, Owyang CG, Sakles JC, et al. Evaluation and management of the physiologically difficult airway: Consensus recommendations from Society for airway management. Anesth Analg 2021;132(2):395–405.

46. Mosier JM, Joshi R, Hypes C, et al. The physiologically difficult airway. West J Emerg Med 2015;16(7):1109–17.

47. Mort TC. The incidence and risk factors for cardiac arrest during emergency tracheal intubation: a justification for incorporating the ASA Guidelines in the remote location. J Clin Anesth 2004;16(7):508–16.

48. Russotto V, Myatra SN, Laffey JG, et al. Intubation practices and Adverse peri-intubation events in critically ill patients from 29 Countries. JAMA 2021;325(12): 1164–72.

49. Davis DP, Lemieux J, Serra J, et al. Preoxygenation reduces desaturation events and improves intubation success. Air Med J 2015;34(2):82–5.

50. Wimalasena Y, Burns B, Reid C, et al. Apneic oxygenation was associated with decreased desaturation rates during rapid sequence intubation by an Australian helicopter emergency medicine service. Ann Emerg Med 2015;65(4):371–6.

51. Sakles JC, Mosier JM, Patanwala AE, et al. First pass success without hypoxemia is increased with the Use of apneic oxygenation during rapid sequence intubation in the emergency department. Acad Emerg Med 2016;23(6):703–10.

52. Sakles JC. Maintenance of oxygenation during rapid sequence intubation in the emergency department. Acad Emerg Med 2017;24(11):1395–404.

53. Semler MW, Janz DR, Lentz RJ, et al. Randomized trial of apneic oxygenation during endotracheal intubation of the critically ill. Am J Respir Crit Care Med 2016;193(3):273–80.

54. Casey JD, Janz DR, Russell DW, et al. Bag-mask ventilation during tracheal intubation of critically ill adults. N Engl J Med 2019;380(9):811–21.

55. Prekker ME, Driver BE, Trent SA, et al. Video versus direct laryngoscopy for tracheal intubation of critically ill adults. N Engl J Med 2023;389(5):418–29.

56. Russell DW, Casey JD, Gibbs KW, et al. Effect of fluid bolus Administration on cardiovascular collapse among critically ill patients undergoing tracheal intubation: a randomized clinical trial. JAMA 2022;328(3):270–9.

57. Janz DR, Casey JD, Semler MW, et al. Effect of a fluid bolus on cardiovascular collapse among critically ill adults undergoing tracheal intubation (PrePARE): a randomised controlled trial. Lancet Respir Med 2019;7(12):1039–47.

58. Juan G, Calverley P, Talamo C, et al. Effect of carbon dioxide on diaphragmatic function in human beings. N Engl J Med 1984;310(14):874–9.

59. Feller-Kopman DJ, Schwartzstein, Richard M. The evaluation, diagnosis, and treatment of the adult patient with acute hypercapnic respiratory failure. In: Stoller JK, Finlay, Geraldine, ed. UpToDate. Wolters Kluwer; 2022 https://www.uptodate.

com/contents/the-evaluation-diagnosis-and-treatment-of-the-adult-patient-with-acute-hypercapnic-respiratory-failure. Accessed June 6, 2023.

60. Drechsler M, Morris J. Carbon dioxide Narcosis. St. Petersburg, FL: StatPearls. StatPearls Publishing Copyright © 2023, StatPearls Publishing LLC.; 2023.

61. Price HL. Effects of carbon dioxide on the cardiovascular system. Anesthesiology 1960;21:652–63.

62. Bayat S, Albu G, Layachi S, et al. Acute hemorrhagic shock decreases airway resistance in anesthetized rat. J Appl Physiol 2011;111(2):458–64.

63. Huang Y, Lei W, Zhang W, et al. High-flow nasal cannula in hypercapnic respiratory failure: a systematic review and meta-analysis. Can Respir J 2020;2020: 7406457.

64. Pitre T, Abbasi S, Su J, et al. Home high flow nasal cannula for chronic hypercapnic respiratory failure in COPD: a systematic review and meta-analysis. Respir Med 2023;219:107420.

65. Echevarria C, Steer J, Wason J, et al. Oxygen therapy and inpatient mortality in COPD exacerbation. Emerg Med J 2021;38(3):170–7.

66. Hanson CW 3rd, Marshall BE, Frasch HF, et al. Causes of hypercarbia with oxygen therapy in patients with chronic obstructive pulmonary disease. Crit Care Med 1996;24(1):23–8.

67. Jabre P, Jacob L, Auger H, et al. Capnography monitoring in nonintubated patients with respiratory distress. Am J Emerg Med 2009;27(9):1056–9.

68. Campion EM, Robinson CK, Brant N, et al. End-tidal carbon dioxide underestimates plasma carbon dioxide during emergent trauma laparotomy leading to hypoventilation and misguided resuscitation: a Western Trauma Association Multicenter Study. J Trauma Acute Care Surg 2019;87(5):1119–24.

69. Defilippis V, D'Antini D, Cinnella G, et al. End-tidal arterial CO2 partial pressure gradient in patients with severe hypercapnia undergoing noninvasive ventilation. Open Access Emerg Med 2013;5:1–7.

70. Lermuzeaux M, Meric H, Sauneuf B, et al. Superiority of transcutaneous CO2 over end-tidal CO2 measurement for monitoring respiratory failure in nonintubated patients: a pilot study. J Crit Care 2016;31(1):150–6.

71. Davidson AC, Banham S, Elliott M, et al. BTS/ICS guideline for the ventilatory management of acute hypercapnic respiratory failure in adults. Thorax 2016; 71(Suppl 2):ii1–35.

72. Plant PK, Owen JL, Elliott MW. Non-invasive ventilation in acute exacerbations of chronic obstructive pulmonary disease: long term survival and predictors of in-hospital outcome. Thorax 2001;56(9):708–12.

73. Nishikimi M, Nishida K, Shindo Y, et al. Failure of non-invasive respiratory support after 6 hours from initiation is associated with ICU mortality. PLoS One 2021;16(4): e0251030.

74. Merelman AH, Perlmutter MC, Strayer RJ. Alternatives to rapid sequence intubation: Contemporary airway management with Ketamine. West J Emerg Med 2019; 20(3):466–71.

75. Lentz S, Grossman A, Koyfman A, et al. High-risk airway management in the emergency department. Part I: diseases and approaches. J Emerg Med 2020; 59(1):84–95.

Invasive Mechanical Ventilation

Jennifer C. Szafran, MD*, Bhakti K. Patel, MD

KEYWORDS

- Mechanical ventilation • Assist control • Respiratory mechanics • Plateau pressure
- Tidal volume • Positive end-expiratory pressure (PEEP)

KEY POINTS

- Invasive mechanical ventilation allows clinicians to support gas exchange and work of breathing in patients with respiratory failure. However, there is also potential for iatrogenesis.
- By understanding the benefits and limitations of different modes of ventilation and goals for gas exchange, clinicians can choose a strategy that provides appropriate support while minimizing harm.
- The ventilator can also provide crucial diagnostic information in the form of respiratory mechanics. These, and the mechanical ventilation strategy, should be regularly reassessed.

INTRODUCTION

Invasive mechanical ventilation may be indicated in cases of severe gas exchange abnormalities or an absence of airway protection. The precise indications vary, and the method of mechanical ventilation should be adapted to the cause of respiratory failure and the individual patient's physiology. The goals of mechanical ventilation are to maintain sufficient gas exchange and to minimize iatrogenic harm while allowing time for lung recovery.

INTUBATION

In cases of acute respiratory failure, intubations are often emergent with minimal time for preparation. In this context, many factors can influence the intubation strategy, with rapid sequence intubation techniques often used to maximize speed of intubation and minimize aspiration risk.[1,2] In certain cases, including anticipated difficult airways, high aspiration risks, and severe physiologic derangements that may prevent the patient from tolerating apnea or induction medications, awake intubations can be

Department of Medicine, Section of Pulmonary and Critical Care, University of Chicago, 5841 South Maryland Avenue, Chicago, IL 60637, USA
* Corresponding author.
E-mail address: Jennifer.Szafran@uchicagomedicine.org

Crit Care Clin 40 (2024) 255–273
https://doi.org/10.1016/j.ccc.2024.01.003   criticalcare.theclinics.com
0749-0704/24/© 2024 Elsevier Inc. All rights reserved.

considered. Regardless of the technique, consideration should be given to a backup plan before an initial attempt. The 2022 American Society of Anesthesiologists Practice Guidelines for Management of the Difficult Airway provide an algorithm to aid in identifying patients in whom to perform an awake intubation and in troubleshooting difficult airways.[3]

Recent emerging data surrounding intubation have focused on strategies for oxygen delivery and hemodynamic support. In critically ill adults, bag valve mask ventilation after induction and before laryngoscopy, as compared with no bag valve mask ventilation, has been associated with a lower incidence of periintubation severe hypoxemia without a significant increase in operator-reported or imaging-identified aspiration.[4] Two trials have demonstrated no effect of a routine preintubation fluid bolus in critically ill adults on the incidence of periintubation cardiovascular collapse.[5,6] (**Table 1** for summaries of key randomized control trials pertinent to mechanical ventilation.)

Once the patient is intubated, the initial medication strategy should focus on analgesia to treat any pain with sedation as a supplement to treat any residual agitation. Of note, if the paralytic used during intubation is not reversed, the patient must be deeply sedated for the duration of the paralytic. The 2018 Prevention and Management of Pain, Agitation/Sedation, Delirium, Immobility, and Sleep Disruption Guidelines include key principles that can guide the initial sedation strategy. For example, for critically ill adults, propofol or dexmedetomidine is recommended over benzodiazepines (conditional, low-quality evidence).[7]

MODES OF MECHANICAL VENTILATION

Modes of mechanical ventilation can be distinguished based on breath initiation and breath delivery. (**Table 2** highlights key differences in ventilator modes.) Breaths can be initiated by the ventilator, the patient, or a combination of the two. A key dichotomy in many modes of ventilation is whether breaths are delivered with a set amount of volume or a set amount of pressure. In either case, the other (dependent) variable reflects the compliance of the respiratory system (C_{rs}) and can thus provide critical information about pathophysiology.

C_{rs} = change in volume/change in pressure

In other words, if volume is set on the ventilator, pressure is the dependent variable monitored to understand compliance. If pressure is set on the ventilator, volume is the dependent variable monitored to understand compliance.

Assist Control

Assist control (AC) methods are common forms of invasive mechanical ventilation in the medical intensive care unit (ICU). In these modes, the ventilator guarantees a minimum number of breaths (the set respiratory rate) and a set amount of volume (assist control volume [AC/V]) or pressure (assist control pressure [AC/P]) delivered for each breath. If the patient breathes over this set rate, the breaths delivered will be identical to those breaths initiated by the ventilator. This is in contrast to a control mode of ventilation, in which the ventilator will not deliver any breaths triggered by the patient. (However, in clinical practice, few make this distinction as AC is typically used.)

Additional variables set by the provider include fraction of inspired oxygen (Fio_2), which is set in all modes of ventilation, and positive end-expiratory pressure (PEEP). In AC/V, both a peak flow and a flow pattern can be set. These, in combination with the set tidal volume, determine the inspiratory and expiratory time. In AC/P, an inspiratory time or an inspiratory:expiratory ratio can be set.

Table 1
Key randomized control trials for ventilator management

Trial/Title	Citation	Key Finding(s)
Intubation		
PreVent "Bag-Mask Ventilation during Tracheal Intubation of Critically Ill Adults"	Casey et al,[4] 2019	Critically ill adults who received bag valve mask ventilation after induction and before tracheal intubation had higher median nadir oxygen saturations and a lower incidence of severe hypoxemia (saturation <80%) than those who did not receive bag mask ventilation
PrePARE "Effect of a Fluid Bolus on Cardiovascular Collapse among Critically Ill Adults Undergoing Tracheal Intubation (PrePARE): a Randomised Controlled Trial"	Janz et al,[5] 2019	There was no significant difference in the incidence of cardiovascular collapse (significant hypotension, cardiac arrest, and death) in critically ill adults who received or did not receive a preintubation bolus
PREPARE II "Effect of Fluid Bolus Administration on Cardiovascular Collapse Among Critically Ill Patients Undergoing Tracheal Intubation A Randomized Clinical Trial"	Russell et al,[6] 2022	In critically ill adults receiving noninvasive positive pressure ventilation or bag mask ventilation before intubation, there was no significant difference in the incidence of cardiovascular collapse (significant hypotension, cardiac arrest, and death) between those who received or did not receive a preintubation bolus
Modes of ventilation		
OSCILLATE "High-Frequency Oscillation in Early Acute Respiratory Distress Syndrome"	Ferguson et al,[19] 2013	In adults with moderate to severe ARDS, patients who received HFOV demonstrated increased in-hospital mortality compared with those who received a low tidal volume high PEEP strategy
OSCAR "High-Frequency Oscillation for Acute Respiratory Distress Syndrome"	Young et al,[18] 2013	In adults with moderate to severe ARDS, patients who received HFOV demonstrated no difference in 30-d mortality as compared with those who received usual care
Oxygen targets		

(continued on next page)

Table 1
(continued)

Trial/Title	Citation	Key Finding(s)
Oxygen-ICU "Effect of Conservative vs Conventional Oxygen Therapy on Mortality Among Patients in an Intensive Care Unit: The Oxygen-ICU Randomized Clinical Trial"	Girardis et al,[24] 2016	In medical-surgical ICU patients at a single center, patients who received conservative oxygen therapy demonstrated lower ICU mortality than those receiving conventional care
ICU-ROX "Conservative Oxygen Therapy during Mechanical Ventilation in the ICU"	Mackle et al,[25] 2020	In mechanically ventilated adults, patients who received conservative-oxygen therapy did not demonstrate a difference in ventilator-free days as compared to those who received usual oxygen therapy
LOCO$_2$ "Liberal or Conservative Oxygen Therapy for Acute Respiratory Distress Syndrome"	Barrot et al,[26] 2020	In patients with ARDS, patients who received a conservative-oxygenation strategy demonstrated no difference in 28-d mortality but a signal for increased 90-d mortality as compared with those who received a liberal oxygen strategy
HOT-ICU "Lower or Higher Oxygenation Targets for Acute Hypoxemic Respiratory Failure"	Schjørring et al,[27] 2021	In ICU patients with acute hypoxic respiratory failure, patients who received a lower-oxygenation strategy did not demonstrate a difference in 90-d mortality as compared with those who received a higher oxygenation strategy
Tidal Volume		
ARMA "Ventilation with Lower Tidal Volumes as Compared with Traditional Tidal Volumes for Acute Lung Injury and the Acute Respiratory Distress Syndrome"	Brower et al,[28] 2000	In patients with acute lung injury and ARDS, a lower tidal volume strategy (initial volume of 6 mL/kg PBW and P_{plat} of 30 cm H_2O or less) when compared with traditional therapy (initial volume of 12 mL/kg PBW with a P_{plat} of 50 cm H_2O or less) resulted in decreased mortality and increased ventilator-free days
IMPROVE "A Trial of Intraoperative Low-Tidal-Volume Ventilation in Abdominal Surgery"	Futier et al,[29] 2013	In patients undergoing abdominal surgery with at least intermediate risk of pulmonary complications, patients who received a lung protective ventilation strategy (tidal volume of 6–8 mL/kg PBW, PEEP of 6-8 cm H_2O, recruitment maneuvers) compared with those who received a nonprotective strategy (tidal volume of 10–12 mL/kg PBW, no PEEP, no recruitment maneuvers) demonstrated decreased incidence of a composite complications outcome

Study	Description
PReVENT "Effect of a Low vs Intermediate Tidal Volume Strategy on Ventilator-Free Days in Intensive Care Unit Patients Without ARDS: A Randomized Clinical Trial" Simonis et al,[30] 2018	In mechanically ventilated ICU patients without ARDS, those who received a low tidal volume strategy (initial volume of 6 mL/kg PBW) vs those who received an intermediate tidal volume strategy (initial volume of 10 mL/kg PBW) did not demonstrate a difference in ventilator-free days
PEEP	
"Higher versus Lower Positive End-Expiratory Pressures in Patients with the Acute Respiratory Distress Syndrome" Brower et al,[31] 2004	In patients with acute lung injury and ARDS receiving a lung protective ventilation strategy, those who received a low PEEP strategy did not demonstrate a difference in hospital mortality or ventilator-free days as compared with those who received a high PEEP strategy
"Ventilation Strategy Using Low Tidal Volumes, Recruitment Maneuvers, and High Positive End-expiratory Pressure for Acute Lung Injury and Acute Respiratory Distress Syndrome: a Randomized Controlled Trial" Meade et al,[32] 2008	In patients with acute lung injury and ARDS, patients who received a ventilator strategy that included low tidal volumes, high PEEP, and recruitment maneuvers did not demonstrate a difference in hospital mortality or barotrauma as compared with patients who received traditional lung-protective ventilation
"Positive End-Expiratory Pressure Setting in Adults With Acute Lung Injury and Acute Respiratory Distress Syndrome: A Randomized Controlled Trial" Mercat et al,[33] 2008	In patients with acute lung injury receiving low tidal volume ventilation, patients who received an increased recruitment strategy (goal P_{plat} of 28–30 cm H_2O) as compared with patients who received a moderate PEEP strategy (5–9 cm H_2O) did not demonstrate reduced 28-d mortality but did demonstrate reduced duration of mechanical ventilation and organ failure
ART "Effect of Lung Recruitment and Titrated Positive End-Expiratory Pressure (PEEP) vs Low PEEP on Mortality in Patients With Acute Respiratory Distress Syndrome: A Randomized Clinical Trial" Cavalcanti et al,[34] 2017	In patients with moderate to severe ARDS, those who received a PEEP strategy that included lung recruitment maneuvers demonstrated increased 28-d mortality as compared with those who received a low PEEP strategy

Table 2
Modes of mechanical ventilation

Mode of Ventilation	Breath Initiation (Trigger)	Breath Delivery (Limit)	Breath Termination (Cycle)	Set Variables	C_{rs}-dependent Variable	PROS	CONS
AC/V	Patient or ventilator	Set tidal volume	Tidal volume	RR, T_w PEEP, Fio_2, and flow	Pressure	Well studied for ARDS. Easy to obtain multiple useful lung mechanics. Can guarantee a minimum minute ventilation	Some issues with patient dyssynchrony can arise
AC/P	Patient or ventilator	Set pressure	Time	RR, P_c, PEEP, Fio_2, and inspiratory time	Volume	Sometimes assists with ventilator dyssynchrony	Increased risk of autoPEEP compared with AC/V given generally longer inspiratory time
PSV	Patient	Set pressure	Flow (breath terminates after a predetermined decrease in flow)	Ps, PEEP, Fio_2	Volume	Can be a more comfortable breathing pattern for patients	Energy expenditure/ metabolic demand. No guaranteed breaths other than backup mode
SIMV	Patient or ventilator	Set tidal volume for prespecified number of breaths. Additional efforts by patient pressure supported	Variable depending on breath	RR, T_w PEEP, Fio_2, flow, P_s for additional patient-initiated breaths	Volume or pressure (depending on breath)	Potential for some diaphragmatic exercise while maintaining control over more variables than pressure support	Less successful than some other weaning strategies

	Patient or ventilator				Pressure required to achieve target volume	Ventilator adjusts to patient changes	Provider may miss changes in compliance that are clinically important. Higher risk of autoPEEP
PRVC	Patient or ventilator	Pressure adjusted to achieve target tidal volume	Time	RR, target T_w max pressure, PEEP, Fio_2, and inspiratory time	Pressure required to achieve target volume	Ventilator adjusts to patient changes	Provider may miss changes in compliance that are clinically important. Higher risk of autoPEEP
APRV	Patient	Unsupported breaths (± tube compensation) or pressure supported breaths above a P_{high} or P_{low}	Flow for each individual breath (set time spent at P_{high} and P_{low})	P_{high}, P_{low}, T_{high}, T_{low} and Fio_2	Volume	Alveolar recruitment, possible rescue method for severe hypoxia	Limited feedback from ventilator. Metabolic demand of spontaneous breathing. High intrathoracic pressure. Trend toward higher mortality in pediatric population
High HFOV	Ventilator	Amplitude (change in pressure)	Time	Frequency, amplitude, mean airway pressure, flow, I:E ratio, and Fio_2		Possible minimization of volutrauma	Mortality same to worse as with standard modes. Limited feedback from ventilator

Note: A ventilator-triggered breath is determined by time (to guarantee a respiratory rate). A patient-triggered breath can be initiated (depending on settings) by either a specified change in flow or pressure.

Abbreviations: Fio_2, Fraction of inhaled oxygen; P_c, Pressure control; P_{high}, High PEEP; P_{low}, low PEEP; P_s, pressure support; RR, respiratory rate; T_{high}, Duration of high PEEP; T_{low}, Duration of low PEEP; flow can refer to both peak flow and flow pattern; T_w, Tidal volume.

As described in the "Respiratory Mechanics" section, AC/V is particularly useful for obtaining and interpreting respiratory mechanics. It is well studied in acute respiratory distress syndrome (ARDS) with resultant evidence-based parameters. Additionally, because both tidal volume and minimum respiratory rate are set by the provider, a minimum minute ventilation can be guaranteed. However, particularly with low tidal volume strategies, ventilator dyssychrony can result. AC/P may result in a more natural flow pattern and thus improved work of breathing[8] and ventilator synchrony in some cases. However, in general, compared with AC/V, a longer inspiratory time is needed to deliver the same volume of breath in AC/P. This increased inspiratory time results in an increased risk of autoPEEP. Additionally, because tidal volume is a dependent variable not set by the operator in AC/P, minute ventilation cannot be guaranteed. Therefore, close monitoring is required to ensure consistent ventilation.

Pressure Support

Support modes of ventilation rely on respiratory effort from the patient. In pressure support ventilation (PSV), the provider sets the PEEP and the pressure support (P_s), which is the pressure provided in addition to the PEEP during inspiration. An increased P_s without a change in PEEP will result in an increased driving pressure and thus, typically, an increased tidal volume. In AC/P, during inspiration, patients receive the chosen pressure for a set amount of time. In contrast, in PSV, patients receive the set amount of pressure until there is a prespecified change in their inspiratory effort (based on a change in flow). Although there is a backup mode of ventilation set in case of emergencies, in PSV, all breaths must be initiated by the patient. This makes PSV a good choice of mode in a patient who has normal lung function and a normal respiratory drive but is intubated for airway protection, allowing them diaphragmatic exercise and potentially less analgesia/sedation. In fact, some sedation strategies are not compatible with PSV if they significantly decrease the respiratory drive. However, the effort/energy expenditure required for the patient to control all the breaths in PSV may not be desired depending on the nature of the patient's critical illness.

Synchronized Intermittent Mandatory Ventilation

Synchronized intermittent mandatory ventilation (SIMV) combines AC modes of ventilation with PSV. The provider sets a certain number of breaths to be delivered by volume control (intermittent modes using pressure control also exist). Any additional patient-initiated breaths are delivered as pressure-supported breaths. Because of these pressure-supported breaths, SIMV was originally assumed to have exercise benefits for weaning. However, it may actually prolong time to extubation when compared with some other methods, including intermittent spontaneous breathing trials and PSV, depending on the criteria used.[9,10]

Pressure Regulated Volume Control

Pressure regulated volume control (PRVC) is a pressure control mode of ventilation that automatically adjusts to meet a target tidal volume. The provider sets a rate, target tidal volume, PEEP, and maximum pressure control. During inspiration, the machine delivers a level of pressure and then adjusts future breaths based on the observed tidal volume. For example, if the observed tidal volume is less than the set target tidal volume, during the next inhalation, the ventilator will deliver more pressure. If the observed tidal volume is more than the set target tidal volume, during the next inhalation, the ventilator will deliver less pressure. The benefit of this mode is that it can adapt to a patient's evolving physiology. However, this is also a significant potential downside. Because the machine adjusts automatically, a provider may not be alerted/notice if an important physiologic change has taken place (eg, if more pressure is needed to maintain the same tidal volume). Additionally, the machine may have trouble successfully adjusting if there is significant ventilator dyssynchrony. Finally, as with AC/P, there is often increased risk of autoPEEP due to longer time to deliver breaths when compared with AC/V.

Airway Pressure Release Ventilation

Airway pressure release ventilation (APRV) is sometimes considered in patients that are very difficult to oxygenate. The goal of APRV is to maximize lung recruitment while minimizing potential ventilator-associated lung injury due to repeated opening and closing of alveolar units. To achieve this, the mode allows for spontaneous breathing at a high PEEP (P_{high}) for time T_{high} alternating with a relatively short period of exhalation (T_{low}) at a low PEEP (P_{low}). Risks include those associated with long periods of elevated intrathoracic pressures (including decreased venous return) and a risk of autoPEEP. There is much heterogeneity in the ARDS and trauma literature regarding APRV, making it difficult to form a definitive conclusion regarding its efficacy compared with other modes of ventilation[11–15,16–22] with some demonstration of increased ventilator-free days in adults with ARDS[14] but one study demonstrating a trend toward increased mortality in a pediatric ARDS population.[17]

High-Frequency Modes of Ventilation

High-frequency modes of ventilation are rarely used in adults as an attempted rescue therapy for patients who are unable to achieve adequate gas exchange with conventional modes of ventilation. As the name implies, this mode delivers breaths at very high rates (multiples above physiologic respiratory rates) and very low tidal volumes with a set mean airway pressure. Due to the low tidal volumes, one potential benefit is the minimization of volutrauma. The most studied mode in this category is high-frequency oscillatory ventilation (HFOV), in which the provider selects a frequency (rate), amplitude, mean airway pressure, flow, I:E ratio, and Fio_2. However, HFOV has been demonstrated to result in no difference[18] or an increase[19] in mortality as compared with more standard methods of ventilation in patients with moderate or severe ARDS and should thus be used with caution.

RESPIRATORY MECHANICS

Although there are many modes of mechanical ventilation available, using diagnostics within one consistent mode allows for minute-to-minute understanding of a patient's evolving pathophysiology. Respiratory mechanics are measurements of pressure, volume, and/or flow that provide information about the function of the respiratory system. They are traditionally measured in AC/V mode with a square waveform (flow is either zero or a constant rate, as opposed to a decelerating waveform).

In AC/V, the volume and flow are selected by the provider, and thus, the pressure is the dependent variable that is measured. The peak airway pressure (P_{peak}) is the highest pressure in a respiratory cycle, reached at the end of inspiration. It is the sum of resistive pressure (P_{res}), elastic pressure (P_{el}), and PEEP.[20]

$$P_{peak} = P_{res} + P_{el} + PEEP$$

P_{res} is proportional to flow and resistance of the respiratory system (R_{rs}) and is thus elevated, for example, in obstructive lung diseases.

$$P_{res} = Flow \times R_{rs}$$

P_{el} is inversely proportional to C_{rs} and is thus elevated, for example, in restrictive lung diseases and obesity. Of note, the C_{rs} includes the compliance of both the lung and the chest wall.

$$P_{el} = V_t/C_{rs}$$

P_{el} can be calculated by measuring a plateau pressure (P_{plat}). P_{plat} is the sum of P_{el} and PEEP. It is determined at the bedside via an inspiratory hold (**Fig. 1**). At the end of inspiration, the provider stops the flow of air. At this time, the pressure, with some limitations, should be representative of the pressure at the alveoli.

$$P_{plat} = P_{el} + PEEP = V_t/C_{rs} + PEEP$$

If the provider has measured P_{peak}, P_{plat}, and PEEP (set by provider), the P_{res} and P_{el} can be calculated. A normal value for P_{res} is about 10 cm H_2O or less. If abnormal, these values can be helpful in determining whether the patient has obstructive or restrictive pathophysiology on initial mechanical ventilation. Importantly, serial measurements at stable tidal volumes and flow can help to diagnose new problems that develop (**Fig. 2**).

Sample Patient Case

Respiratory mechanics were measured for Patient A during mechanical ventilation on AC/V with a square flow waveform. The following values were obtained: P_{peak} of 25 cm

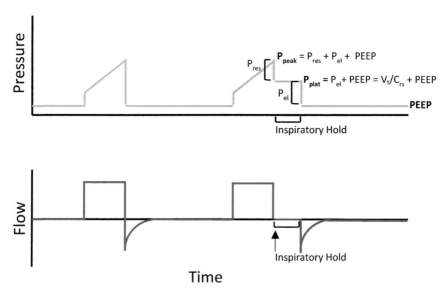

Fig. 1. Inspiratory hold maneuver and lung mechanics measurements. An inspiratory hold is conducted by holding the flow at zero at the end of inspiration. Demonstrated here in AC/V ventilation. Three pressures are measured: peak airway pressure (P_{peak}), plateau pressure (P_{plat}), and positive end-expiratory pressure (PEEP). P_{peak} is the pressure reached at the end of inspiration, immediately before the inspiratory hold, and thus the highest pressure in a respiratory cycle. It is the sum of the P_{res}, the P_{el}, and the PEEP. P_{plat} is the pressure measured during the inspiratory hold and thus representative of the pressure at the alveoli. It is the sum of P_{el} and PEEP. C_{rs}, compliance of the respiratory system; V_t, tidal volume.

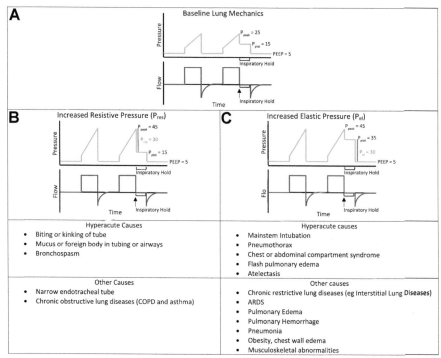

Fig. 2. Interpreting a change in lung mechanics. (A) Baseline lung mechanics measured with an inspiratory hold in AC/V ventilation. P_{peak}, peak airway pressure; P_{plat}, plateau pressure; PEEP, positive end-expiratory pressure. The same patient depicted in (A) has different changes in lung mechanics represented in (B) and (C). If the P_{peak} increases without a proportional change in P_{plat} (B), then the resistive pressure (P_{res}) has increased, and the problem is due to an impediment to airflow. If the P_{peak} increases with a similar change in P_{plat} (C), then elastic pressure (P_{el}) has increased, and the problem is due to worsening respiratory system compliance.

H_2O, P_{plat} of 15 cm H_2O, and a PEEP of 5 cm H_2O (see **Fig. 2A**). Later in the day, the provider is called to the patient's bedside because the P_{peak} suddenly increased to 45 cm H_2O. There have been no changes to the settings on the ventilator. The provider remeasures the pressures.

If the P_{peak} has increased but the P_{plat} has not, then there is a new issue with airways resistance or flow. In this case, the numbers measured for Patient A are P_{peak} = 45 cm H_2O, P_{plat} = 15 cm H_2O, and PEEP = 5 cm H_2O. The calculated P_{res} has dramatically increased (from 10 cm H_2O to 30 cm H_2O), suggesting an issue with airways resistance or flow (see **Fig. 2B**). When developing a differential, a good strategy is to think through (and assess at bedside) the circuit starting at the mouth to identify potential sources of resistance to flow. Examples include patient biting on tubing or kinking of the tubing, mucus in tubing, and bronchospasm.

If the peak airway pressure has increased, and the P_{plat} has increased similarly, there is a new issue with respiratory system compliance. In this case, the numbers measured for Patient A are P_{peak} = 45 cm H_2O, P_{plat} = 35 cm H_2O, and PEEP = 5 cm H_2O. The calculated P_{el} has dramatically increased (from 10 cm H_2O to 30 cm H_2O), suggesting an issue with respiratory system compliance (see **Fig. 2C**). Examples that happen in the acute setting include the movement of the endotracheal tube into one lung (and thus

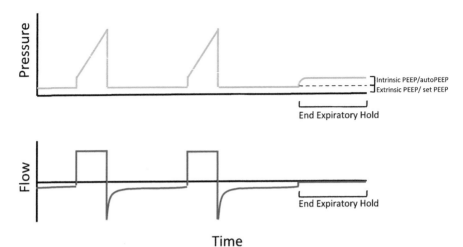

Fig. 3. End expiratory hold maneuver demonstrating autoPEEP. AC/V pressure and flow waveforms. The flow during exhalation does not return to zero between breaths, suggesting incomplete exhalation and the potential for autoPEEP. This is confirmed with an end expiratory hold. At the end of exhalation, the flow is held at zero. If there is no autoPEEP, the pressure waveform should match the set PEEP on the ventilator. If there is intrinsic PEEP, here autoPEEP from incomplete exhalation, the additional pressure above the set PEEP is the autoPEEP.

new single lung ventilation), pneumothorax, flash pulmonary edema, large mucus plugging causing significant atelectasis, and compartment syndrome in the abdomen or chest.

End Expiratory Pressure

Another important measurement on the ventilator is the end expiratory pressure (**Fig. 3**). This is measured by performing an end expiratory hold at the end of exhalation (holding flow at zero). This measured pressure should match the PEEP that the provider set on the ventilator. If the pressure measured during and end expiratory hold is higher than the PEEP, this indicates a level of intrinsic PEEP. This can result from the autoPEEP due to a patient repeatedly being unable to fully exhale before the next breath (eg, in the case of status asthmaticus). Significant autoPEEP is important to identify because it can result in decreased gas exchange, shock, and circulatory arrest from decreased venous return.

SPECIAL GOALS

Although many general principles can be applied to all patients with respiratory failure undergoing mechanical ventilation, there are some conditions that require a tailored approach.

Acute Respiratory Distress Syndrome

Mechanical ventilation strategies in ARDS have been frequently studied. As a result, ARDS is the only type of acute respiratory failure with multiple guidelines[21,22] outlining evidence-based strategies for mechanical ventilation. Patients with ARDS are at particularly high risk of volutrauma and barotrauma, consistent with the characteristic diffuse alveolar damage and subsequent worsening lung compliance. In this context, there is significant potential for iatrogenesis during mechanical ventilation. As a result, a lung-protective ventilation strategy that includes low tidal volumes (4–8 mL/kg predicted body weight [PBW]) and a target P_{plat} of 30 cm H_2O or less is used.

Obstructive Lung Disease

Exacerbations of asthma and chronic obstructive pulmonary disease (COPD) can be particularly difficult to manage on the ventilator. Patients often require a significantly increased expiratory time to fully exhale. Failure to fully exhale can result in autoPEEP. This can result in decreased gas exchange, shock, and even circulatory arrest from decreased venous return. To avoid this, inspiratory time should be minimized so that expiratory time can be maximized. The most effective strategy to accomplish this is reducing the respiratory rate. Due to patient tachypnea, achieving this reduction in respiratory rate sometimes requires deep sedation and even paralysis to achieve. In AC/V, increasing peak flow rate and selecting a square flow waveform will minimize inspiratory time (and predictably increase peak airway pressures). In AC/P, an inspiratory time can be selected by the physician. Acutely, if autoPEEP results in hemodynamic compromise, the patient should be disconnected from the ventilator, brief pressure should be applied to the chest to minimize any remaining volume, and the patient should be reconnected to the ventilator with new settings that decrease the inspiratory:expiratory ratio. If the hemodynamic compromise was indeed from auto-PEEP, the improvements should be instantaneous but this maneuver may need to be repeated if the hemodynamic changes recur.

VARIABLES TO MANIPULATE

Before adjusting variables on the ventilator, it is important to understand our goals. These goals can include target values for dependent variables, as well as lung protection.

Targets

Minute ventilation is a product of tidal volume and respiratory rate. Therefore, these 2 variables influence partial pressure of CO_2 (P_{CO_2}) and thus pH. In contrast, PEEP and Fio_2 primarily influence partial pressure of oxygen (Po_2) and oxygen saturation (SpO_2). Therefore, targets for pH and Po_2 help guide titration of these variables on the ventilator.

pH

In part because patients may have varying levels of baseline P_{CO_2}, a pH target (rather than a P_{CO_2} target) is generally used to guide ventilation. A relatively normal pH is a reasonable target when possible in the context of lung protective ventilation. However, permissive hypercapnia and the resulting respiratory acidosis are generally well tolerated if needed.[23] This is often required in cases of ARDS or severe exacerbations of reactive airways disease. Though there is not a consensus as to the lower limit of tolerated pH, pH $\geq$ 7.2 is a reasonable goal. It is similarly important to avoid severe alkalosis, which can have consequences that include arrhythmias and seizures. Alkalosis can also decrease or eliminate respiratory drive, which can decrease success with spontaneous breathing trials.

Pao₂/Oxygen Saturation

Oxygenation targets remain a topic of controversy. Although initial single-center data of medical-surgical ICU patients suggested that a conservative oxygen strategy (partial pressure of oxygen in arterial blood [Pao_2] between 70 mm Hg and 100 mm Hg or

SpO$_2$ between 94% and 98%) resulted in lower ICU mortality as compared with controls,[24] subsequent trials (using different O$_2$ targets) in mechanically ventilated patients,[25] patients with ARDS,[26] and ICU patients with acute hypoxic respiratory failure[27] have not demonstrated a consistent difference in outcomes. This remains an area of active investigation.

Tidal Volume

A low tidal volume strategy (4–8 mL/kg PBW) has been demonstrated to decrease mortality and increase ventilator free days when compared with a high tidal volume strategy (initially 12 mL/kg PBW) in ARDS[28] and is recommended by multiple ARDS guidelines.[16,17] This strategy is often extrapolated to the management of mechanically ventilated patients with other pathology. This is supported by some data. For example, data from surgical patients demonstrated that, even in the intraoperative period, lung protective ventilation resulted in a decreased incidence of clinical complications.[29] A benefit of a low tidal volume strategy versus an intermediate tidal volume strategy has not been demonstrated. In the PReVENT trial of mechanically ventilated patients without ARDS, those receiving a low tidal volume strategy (initial volume of 6 mL/kg PBW) as compared with those receiving an intermediate tidal volume strategy (initial volume of 10 mL/kg PBW) did not demonstrate increased ventilator-free days.[30] In patients with severe obstructive lung disease exacerbations that require very low respiratory rates or in patients with severe metabolic acidosis, a more liberal tidal volume strategy (8–10 mL/kg of PBW) may be required to maintain a safe pH.

Respiratory Rate

Mechanically ventilated patients with respiratory failure can have a variety of factors that lead to an increased required minute ventilation (eg, increased metabolic demand and increased dead space) and thus an increased required respiratory rate. Additionally, a lung protective tidal volume strategy usually results in tidal volumes lower than that of the typical spontaneous breath in a healthy person. As a result, a high respiratory rate is often required. This is particularly true in ARDS (low tidal volume strategy, increased dead space) and patients with shock (the ventilator must often compensate for increased metabolic acidosis.) Whenever a set respiratory rate on the ventilator is increased, the provider should ensure no autoPEEP results. This is particularly true in patients with obstructive lung disease, who might require very low respiratory rates to prevent autoPEEP. When respiratory alkalosis is identified, the provider should ensure it is not iatrogenic (ie, the patient is breathing at the set rate and tidal volume, which have been set too high, resulting in too high of a minute ventilation). If the alkalosis is not iatrogenic (ie, the patient is breathing over the set respiratory rate), the cause of the tachypnea should be identified and addressed.

Positive End-Expiratory Pressure

Goals of PEEP include recruiting alveoli and preventing ventilator-associated lung injury due to repeated alveolar collapse. Although an active area of investigation for many years, there is no consensus regarding the best strategy for choosing PEEP.[31–33] However, generally, a lung-protective ventilation strategy includes a goal P$_{plat}$ of less than 30 cm H$_2$O. Additionally, evidence suggests strategies that include recruitment maneuvers that use very high levels of PEEP (25–45 cm H$_2$O) result in increased mortality.[34]

Other strategies for PEEP adjustment currently under investigation include targeting lower driving pressures (calculated equivalently to P$_{el}$ as P$_{plat}$ − PEEP)[35–38] with one reasonable target less than 15 cm H$_2$O. Esophageal monitoring can be used to measure transpulmonary pressures and has been implemented with mixed results.[39,40]

The idea behind this strategy is to account for situations, such as decreased chest wall compliance due to obesity, when plateau pressures may not be an accurate representation of transpulmonary pressures. Other potential considerations requiring more investigation include pressure–volume curves, stress index, and electrical impedance tomography.[41]

Fraction of Inspired Oxygen

Very high levels of Fio_2 raise concern for toxicity related to reactive oxygen species. For this reason, the goal is using the lowest Fio_2 needed to achieve a set SpO_2 or P_aO_2 target, with Fio_2 of 60% or less preferred when possible.[42]

Flow

Both peak inspiratory flow rate and flow waveforms can be set. These rarely need to be manipulated. However, flow does contribute to peak airway pressures, so it should remain constant between serial measurements of respiratory mechanics. Similarly, respiratory mechanics are traditionally calculated with a square flow waveform (flow is either zero or a constant value) on AC/V. One condition that may benefit from manipulation of flow is an obstructive lung disease exacerbation. These patients may benefit from an increase in flow (with monitoring of resulting airway pressures) to decrease the inspiratory:expiratory ratio and allow longer time to exhale.

Trigger

The provider can set the ventilator to allow a patient to trigger a breath by generating either a certain flow or a certain pressure. This does not often have to be manipulated from standard settings. Patients with respiratory muscle weakness (especially when on a support mode of ventilation) may require adjustments to trigger settings to make it easier to trigger a breath. In contrast, if trigger threshold is set too low (based on absolute value), breaths could be triggered by nonrespiratory stimuli (cardiac pulsation, condensation in the tubing, myoclonus, and so forth).

VENTILATOR DYSSYNCHRONY

Even when ventilator settings are carefully chosen based on the considerations listed above, if a patient maintains a respiratory drive, the "desired" breathing pattern may differ significantly from the ventilator settings. This can result in perturbations to the expected delivered breath referred to as ventilator dyssynchrony. Ventilator dyssynchrony puts the patient at additional risk of ventilator-associated lung injury (including volutrauma and barotrauma). Perhaps for this reason, in observational studies, high ventilator dyssynchrony has been associated with longer duration of mechanical ventilation[43,44] and higher mortality.[45] Increases in sedation are not always effective at reducing ventilator dyssynchrony and have been shown to be less effective than making adjustments to ventilator settings.[46] Therefore, initial efforts should focus on ventilator adjustments. There are many types of ventilator dyssynchrony. Three important, intervenable examples are listed as follows.

Breath Stacking

Breath stacking, or double triggering, results from a patient triggering a second breath before exhalation on a first breath is completed. This can result in increased tidal volumes and pressures. Strategies to improve this can include changing ventilator modes, with PSV often highlighted.[47] However, caution should be used when switching to a spontaneous mode of ventilation to ensure that patients are still taking lung-protective breaths. High respiratory drive, even in patients who are not mechanically ventilated, can contribute to an injurious breathing pattern with associated patient self-inflicted lung injury.[48] Another strategy to reduce breath stacking is to increase inspiratory time. In AC/V, this can be done by adding an inspiratory pause, changing flow (decreased flow will prolong inspiratory time, although some dyssynchrony results from insufficient flow), or increasing tidal volume (which may also decrease the patient's sensation of "air hunger"). Any increase in inspiratory time will result in a decrease in expiratory time, so after these changes, the provider must confirm that no auto-PEEP has developed.

Ineffective Triggering

When a patient creates a respiratory effort (identified as a change in pressure and flow) that does not trigger a full breath on the ventilator, this is referred to as ineffective triggering. This can occur when the trigger threshold is not set at a level to detect the patient efforts or in the case of intrinsic PEEP.[36] Therefore, it can often be improved with adjustments to the trigger threshold or, in the case of intrinsic PEEP, adjustments to the ventilator to reduce auto-PEEP or increase extrinsic PEEP.

Autocycling

Occasionally, dyssynchrony is not the result of respiratory efforts from the patient. In autocycling, the ventilator may detect a breath trigger resulting from a change outside of the patient's respiratory muscles, including moving condensation in the ventilator tubing, myoclonus, or cardiac oscillations.[49] A high index of suspicion is needed to identify this issue. The erroneous trigger should be eliminated if possible (eg, tubing exchanged). Adjusting the trigger threshold can be used if needed.

EXTUBATION

Because of the potential harms associated with mechanical ventilation, as soon as a patient is intubated, regular consideration should be given to when the patient can appropriately be extubated. This decision is based on a variety of factors, as reviewed in another article of this collection. Regardless of the cause of respiratory failure, it is important to assess at least daily, and often more frequently, whether the patient is appropriate for liberation.

SUMMARY

Invasive mechanical ventilation allows clinicians to support the gas exchange and work of breathing of patients with respiratory failure. Although mechanical ventilation provides a potential bridge to lung recovery, there is also potential for iatrogenesis. Understanding modes of ventilation and the variables that can be manipulated in each facilitates the goals of sufficient gas exchange and avoiding harm. Ventilators also provide crucial diagnostic information that should be regularly reassessed throughout the duration of mechanical ventilation.

CLINICS CARE POINTS

- Modes of mechanical ventilation can be distinguished based on breath initiation and breath delivery.
- Whether ventilator modes use a set volume or a set pressure, the dependent variable provides important information about respiratory system compliance.

- In AC/volume, the P_{peak} is the highest pressure in a respiratory cycle and is the sum of the P_{res}, P_{el}, and the positive end-expiratory pressure. Regularly determining these pressures provides important information about a patient's evolving physiology.

- When determining a mode and settings for mechanical ventilation, it is important to understand the limitations and potential risks of different modes, determine goals for gas exchange, and choose settings to minimize iatrogenesis.

DISCLOSURES

J.C. Szafran has nothing to disclose. B.K. Patel receives funding from the NIH, United States/NHLBI (K23 HL148387) and the SECURED grant.

REFERENCES

1. Stept WJ, Safar P. Rapid induction-intubation for prevention of gastric-content aspiration. Anesth Analg 1970;49(4):633–6.
2. El-Orbany M, Connolly LA. Rapid sequence induction and intubation: current controversy. Anesth Analg 2010;110(5):1318–25.
3. Apfelbaum JL, Hagberg CA, Connis RT, et al. American Society of Anesthesiologists practice guidelines for management of the difficult airway. Anesthesiology 2022;136(1):31–81.
4. Casey JD, Janz DR, Russell DW, et al. Bag-mask ventilation during tracheal intubation of critically ill adults. N Engl J Med 2019;380(9):811–21.
5. Janz DR, Casey JD, Semler MW, et al. Effect of a fluid bolus on cardiovascular collapse among critically ill adults undergoing tracheal intubation (PrePARE): a randomised controlled trial. Lancet Respir Med 2019;7(12):1039–47.
6. Russell DW, Casey JD, Gibbs KW, et al. Effect of fluid bolus administration on cardiovascular collapse among critically ill patients undergoing tracheal intubation: a randomized clinical trial. JAMA 2022;328(3):270–9.
7. Devlin JW, Skrobik Y, Gélinas C, et al. Clinical practice guidelines for the prevention and management of pain, agitation/sedation, delirium, immobility, and sleep disruption in adult patients in the ICU. Crit Care Med 2018;46(9):e825–73.
8. Cinnella G, Conti G, Lofaso F, et al. Effects of assisted ventilation on the work of breathing: volume-controlled versus pressure-controlled ventilation. Am J Respir Crit Care Med 1996;153(3):1025–33.
9. Brochard L, Rauss A, Benito S, et al. Comparison of three methods of gradual withdrawal from ventilatory support during weaning from mechanical ventilation. Am J Respir Crit Care Med 1994;150(4):896–903.
10. Esteban A, Frutos F, Tobin MJ, et al. A comparison of four methods of weaning patients from mechanical ventilation. Spanish Lung Failure Collaborative Group. N Engl J Med 1995;332(6):345–50.
11. Varpula T, Valta P, Niemi R, et al. Airway pressure release ventilation as a primary ventilatory mode in acute respiratory distress syndrome. Acta Anaesthesiol Scand 2004;48(6):722–31.
12. Maxwell RA, Green JM, Waldrop J, et al. A randomized prospective trial of airway pressure release ventilation and low tidal volume ventilation in adult trauma patients with acute respiratory failure. J Trauma 2010;69(3):501–10.
13. Maung AA, Schuster KM, Kaplan LJ, et al. Compared to conventional ventilation, airway pressure release ventilation may increase ventilator days in trauma patients. J Trauma Acute Care Surg 2012;73(2):507–10.

14. Zhou Y, Jin X, Lv Y, et al. Early application of airway pressure release ventilation may reduce the duration of mechanical ventilation in acute respiratory distress syndrome. Intensive Care Med 2017;43(11):1648–59.

15. Hirshberg EL, Lanspa MJ, Peterson J, et al. Randomized feasibility trial of a low tidal volume-airway pressure release ventilation protocol compared with traditional airway pressure release ventilation and volume control ventilation protocols. Crit Care Med 2018;46(12):1943–52.

16. Putensen C, Zech S, Wrigge H, et al. Long-term effects of spontaneous breathing during ventilatory support in patients with acute lung injury. Am J Respir Crit Care Med 2001;164(1):43–9.

17. Lalgudi Ganesan S, Jayashree M, Chandra Singhi S, et al. Airway pressure Release ventilation in pediatric acute respiratory distress syndrome. A randomized controlled trial. Am J Respir Crit Care Med 2018;198(9):1199–207.

18. Young D, Lamb SE, Shah S, et al. High-frequency oscillation for acute respiratory distress syndrome. N Engl J Med 2013;368(9):806–13.

19. Ferguson ND, Cook DJ, Guyatt GH, et al. High-frequency oscillation in early acute respiratory distress syndrome. N Engl J Med 2013;368(9):795–805.

20. Giani M, Bronco A, Bellani G. How to measure respiratory mechanics during controlled mechanical ventilation. AboutOpen 2019;6(1):86–9.

21. Fan E, Del Sorbo L, Goligher EC, et al. An Official American Thoracic Society/European Society of Intensive Care Medicine/Society of Critical Care Medicine clinical practice guideline: mechanical ventilation in adult patients with acute respiratory distress syndrome. Am J Respir Crit Care Med 2017;195(9):1253–63.

22. Grasselli G, Calfee CS, Camporota L, et al. ESICM guidelines on acute respiratory distress syndrome: definition, phenotyping and respiratory support strategies. Intensive Care Med 2023;49(7):727–59.

23. Bidani A, Tzouanakis AE, Cardenas VJ Jr, et al. Permissive hypercapnia in acute respiratory failure. JAMA 1994;272(12):957–62.

24. Girardis M, Busani S, Damiani E, et al. Effect of conservative vs conventional oxygen therapy on mortality among patients in an intensive care Unit: the oxygen-ICU randomized clinical trial. JAMA 2016;316(15):1583–9.

25. Mackle D, Bellomo R, Bailey M, et al. Conservative oxygen therapy during mechanical ventilation in the ICU. N Engl J Med 2020;382(11):989–98.

26. Barrot L, Asfar P, Mauny F, et al. Liberal or conservative oxygen therapy for acute respiratory distress syndrome. N Engl J Med 2020;382(11):999–1008.

27. Schjørring OL, Klitgaard TL, Perner A, et al. Lower or higher oxygenation targets for acute hypoxemic respiratory failure. N Engl J Med 2021;384(14):1301–11.

28. Brower RG, Matthay MA, Morris A, et al. Ventilation with lower tidal volumes as compared with traditional tidal volumes for acute lung injury and the acute respiratory distress syndrome. N Engl J Med 2000;342(18):1301–8.

29. Futier E, Constantin JM, Paugam-Burtz C, et al. A trial of intraoperative low-tidal-volume ventilation in abdominal surgery. N Engl J Med 2013;369(5):428–37.

30. Simonis FD, Serpa Neto A, Binnekade JM, et al. Effect of a low vs intermediate tidal volume strategy on ventilator-free days in intensive care unit patients without ARDS: a randomized clinical trial. JAMA 2018;320(18):1872–80.

31. Brower RG, Lanken PN, MacIntyre N, et al. Higher versus lower positive end-expiratory pressures in patients with the acute respiratory distress syndrome. N Engl J Med 2004;351(4):327–36.

32. Meade MO, Cook DJ, Guyatt GH, et al. Ventilation strategy using low tidal volumes, recruitment maneuvers, and high positive end-expiratory pressure for

acute lung injury and acute respiratory distress syndrome: a randomized controlled trial. JAMA 2008;299(6):637–45.

33. Mercat A, Richard JC, Vielle B, et al. Positive end-expiratory pressure setting in adults with acute lung injury and acute respiratory distress syndrome: a randomized controlled trial. JAMA 2008;299(6):646–55.

34. Cavalcanti AB, Suzumura ÉA, Laranjeira LN, et al. Effect of lung recruitment and titrated positive end-expiratory pressure (PEEP) vs low PEEP on mortality in patients with acute respiratory distress syndrome: a randomized clinical trial. JAMA 2017;318(14):1335–45.

35. Amato MB, Meade MO, Slutsky AS, et al. Driving pressure and survival in the acute respiratory distress syndrome. N Engl J Med 2015 Feb 19;372(8):747–55.

36. Bellani G, Laffey JG, Pham T, et al. Epidemiology, patterns of care, and mortality for patients with acute respiratory distress syndrome in intensive care units in 50 countries. JAMA 2016;315(8):788–800.

37. Bellani G, Grassi A, Sosio S, et al. Driving pressure is associated with outcome during assisted ventilation in acute respiratory distress syndrome. Anesthesiology 2019 Sep;131(3):594–604.

38. Goligher EC, Costa ELV, Yarnell CJ, et al. Effect of lowering Vt on mortality in acute respiratory distress syndrome varies with respiratory system elastance. Am J Respir Crit Care Med 2021 Jun 1;203(11):1378–85.

39. Talmor D, Sarge T, Malhotra A, et al. Mechanical ventilation guided by esophageal pressure in acute lung injury. N Engl J Med 2008;359(20):2095–104.

40. Beitler JR, Sarge T, Banner-Goodspeed VM, et al. Effect of titrating positive end-expiratory pressure (PEEP) with an esophageal pressure-guided strategy vs an empirical high PEEP-Fio2 strategy on death and days free from mechanical ventilation among patients with acute respiratory distress syndrome: a randomized clinical trial. JAMA 2019 Mar 5;321(9):846–57.

41. Dugan K, Patel B. Precision in mechanical ventilation. In: Gomez JL, Himes BE, Kaminski N, editors. Precision in pulmonary, critical care, and sleep medicine. Springer Nature Switzerland AG; 2020. p. 355–67.

42. Kallet RH, Matthay MA. Hyperoxic acute lung injury. Respir Care 2013 Jan;58(1): 123–41.

43. Thille AW, Rodriguez P, Cabello B, et al. Patient-ventilator asynchrony during assisted mechanical ventilation. Intensive Care Med 2006;32(10):1515–22.

44. de Wit M, Miller KB, Green DA, et al. Ineffective triggering predicts increased duration of mechanical ventilation. Crit Care Med 2009;37(10):2740–5.

45. Blanch L, Villagra A, Sales B, et al. Asynchronies during mechanical ventilation are associated with mortality. Intensive Care Med 2015;41(4):633–41.

46. Chanques G, Kress JP, Pohlman A, et al. Impact of ventilator adjustment and sedation-analgesia practices on severe asynchrony in patients ventilated in assist-control mode. Crit Care Med 2013;41(9):2177–87.

47. De Oliveira B, Aljaberi N, Taha A, et al. Patient-ventilator dyssynchrony in critically ill patients. J Clin Med 2021;10(19):4550.

48. Brochard L, Slutsky A, Pesenti A. Mechanical ventilation to minimize progression of lung injury in acute respiratory failure. Am J Respir Crit Care Med 2017;195(4): 438–42.

49. Arbour R. Cardiogenic oscillation and ventilator autotriggering in brain-dead patients: a case series. Am J Crit Care 2009;18(5):488–95, 496.

Pharmacologic Treatments in Acute Respiratory Failure

Elizabeth Levy, MD, John P. Reilly, MD, MSCE*

KEYWORDS

- Acute respiratory distress syndrome • Acute respiratory failure • Pharmacotherapy
- COVID-19 • Corticosteroids • Neuromuscular blockade

KEY POINTS

- Despite decades of research, there are limited effective pharmacotherapies for acute respiratory failure and acute respiratory distress syndrome.
- Corticosteroids, neuromuscular blockade and pulmonary vasodilators are the most commonly used adjunctive pharmacotherapies for acute respiratory distress syndrome.
- Recent evidence suggests that endotypes and/or subphenotypes of acute respiratory failure exist and may benefit from a precision approach rather than "one size fits all."

INTRODUCTION

Acute respiratory failure is a complex and heterogenous clinical entity of which there are multiple etiologies including infection, trauma, and shock. The management of acute respiratory failure relies on supportive care with the use of non-invasive and invasive oxygen delivery and ventilatory support. Pharmacotherapeutic options depend on the etiology of respiratory failure and focus on reversing the underlying issue, such as antibiotics for infection. Pharmacologic therapies for the most severe form of respiratory failure, acute respiratory distress syndrome (ARDS), target mechanisms of lung injury and alveolar capillary barrier dysfunction and will be the focus of this review.

Since its advent over 50 years ago, there remains no effective ARDS pharmacotherapy targeting specific pathologic mechanisms; however, several pharmacotherapies have been studied with varying success.[1,2] Multiple mechanisms contribute to dysregulated inflammation in ARDS leading to endothelial and epithelial barrier permeability and, ultimately, pulmonary edema. The predominant mechanism varies between individuals and this heterogeneity makes identification of a successful

Division of Pulmonary, Allergy and Critical Care Medicine, Department of Medicine, University of Pennsylvania, Perelman School of Medicine, 3400 Spruce Street, Philadelphia, PA 19146, USA
* Corresponding author. Division of Pulmonary, Allergy and Critical Care Medicine, Department of Medicine, University of Pennsylvania, Perelman School of Medicine, 3400 Spruce Street, Philadelphia, PA 19146.
E-mail address: John.Reilly@pennmedicine.upenn.edu

Crit Care Clin 40 (2024) 275–289
https://doi.org/10.1016/j.ccc.2023.12.002
0749-0704/24/© 2023 Elsevier Inc. All rights reserved.

pharmacologic treatment challenging[3] (**Fig. 1**, **Table 1**). At present, clinicians rely primarily on supportive measures that minimize lung overdistension, through lung protective ventilation and prone positioning.[4] Potential therapeutic options will be discussed, highlighting that a "one size fits all" approach may not always be appropriate.

Corticosteroids

The utility of corticosteroids as a treatment option for ARDS has been debated for almost as long as ARDS has been recognized.[1] Following a primary insult, inflammatory mediators such as Interleukin (IL)-1β and IL-6 are released into the systemic circulation, reaching the alveolar capillary interface. An inflammatory alveolar exudate develops and causes hypoxemic respiratory failure.[5] Corticosteroids are agonists that bind to glucocorticoid receptors leading to inhibition of pro-inflammatory cytokines and chemokines and a non-specific anti-inflammatory effect. Recently, evidence has grown for the use of corticosteroids in overlapping critically ill populations, including community acquired pneumonia and septic shock. The use of steroids in ARDS is growing with observational data suggesting that 20% of patients with ARDS receive corticosteroids, with usage doubling in patients with moderate-severe ARDS.[6,7] Despite theoretic benefits, corticosteroids have potential downsides including secondary infections, delirium, hyperglycemia, and long-term neuromuscular weakness.

Studies assessing the benefit of corticosteroids have evaluated varying doses, formulations, and durations, with inconsistent results. Most ARDS trials have studied hydrocortisone, methylprednisolone, or dexamethasone, each with their own distinct pharmacokinetic profiles and mineralocorticoid activity (**Table 2**). Initial studies of high-dose corticosteroids failed to show improvement in survival[8–11]; however, a

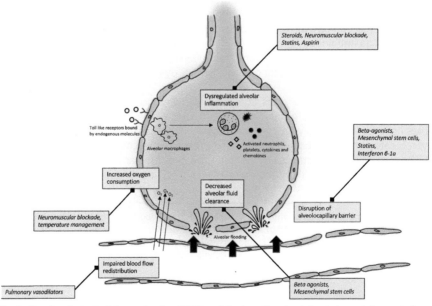

Fig. 1. Previously tested therapies for ARDS and their pathophysiologic targets in acute lung injury and alveolar capillary barrier dysfunction.

Table 1
Pathophysiologic mechanisms of ARDS and select previously tested therapies

Mechanism[2]	Pharmacotherapies[a] and Non-pharmacologic Treatments
Dysregulated inflammation Endogenous molecules bind to Toll-like receptors on lung epithelium and alveolar macrophages lead to accumulation of inflammatory cells	Steroids[8–16] Neuromuscular blockade[28,29] Statins[66,75] Aspirin[76] Tocilizumab[b,51–54] Baricitinib[b,55,56,77]
Disruption of alveolocapillary barrier Increased inflammatory cells destabilize tight junctions increasing lung endothelial and epithelial permeability leading to pulmonary edema	Beta-agonists[78,79] Mesenchymal stem cells[41–44] Imatinib[b,80] Statins[66,75] Interferon β-1a[81]
Decreased alveolar fluid clearance (AFC) Ion channels function inefficiently in hypoxemic environment, biomechanical stress reduces AFC, proinflammatory cytokines reduce AFC	Beta agonists[78,79] Mesenchymal stem cells[41–44] Low tidal volume ventilation, limiting inspiratory pressures[c,82]
Impaired blood flow redistribution Loss of compensatory hypoxemic vasoconstriction leads to intrapulmonary shunting	Pulmonary vasodilators[33–38,83] Prone positioning[c,84]
Increased oxygen consumption Increased work of breathing and ventilator dyssynchrony after lung injury	Neuromuscular blockade[28,29] Temperature management[c,85]

[a] Drugs are pleiotropic with many other actions.
[b] Studied in COVID-ARDS.
[c] Non-pharmacologic interventions.

subsequent trial assessing moderate dose of steroids (2 mg/kg methylprednisolone for 32 days) showed benefit. Albeit a small study, methylprednisolone was associated with decreased mortality and improvements in lung injury score, oxygenation, and organ dysfunction.[12] This finding was duplicated in a subsequent trial (91 patients)

Table 2
Steroids studied in ARDS

Corticosteroid	Strength[a]	Daily Dose (mg)[5,a]	Mineralocorticoid Activity[86]	Considerations/ General Use
Hydrocortisone	Low Moderate High	<400–500 500–1500 >1500	High	Septic shock, adrenal insufficiency
Methylprednisolone	Low Moderate High	<80–100 100–300 >300	Minimal	First steroid studied in ARDS, known rapid distribution into lungs[14]
Dexamethasone	Low Moderate High	<15–18 18–56 >56	Minimal	Long half-life limits need for taper[14]

[a] No clear definition for the quantification of glucocorticoid doses used in critical illness, most critical care studies use this strength breakdown.[5]

assessing lower dose steroids (methylprednisolone 1 mg/kg) at ARDS onset.[13] More recently, Villar and colleagues conducted a randomized controlled trial comparing moderate to high dose dexamethasone for 10 days (20 mg then 10 mg for 5 days each) to placebo in patients with moderate-severe ARDS with P:F less than 200. This trial revealed a reduction in ventilator free days by 4.8 days and a 15% absolute risk reduction in 60-day mortality (21% vs 36%); however, the trial had several potential limitations including a lack of blinding and difficult accrual over 5 years. Additionally, most patients had other indications for steroids, including sepsis and pneumonia.[14] Systematic reviews have concluded that steroids probably provide a benefit by lowering mortality and reducing duration of mechanical ventilation, and consistent effects are seen with different corticosteroid types and dosages.[15,16]

The timing of corticosteroid administration in ARDS also matters. Early administration of moderate dose steroids has shown potential benefit. Late administration of steroids in ARDS was evaluated in the Late Steroid Rescue Study (LaSRS), a randomized controlled trial evaluating moderate-dose methylprednisolone in patients with persistent ARDS.[17] Patients with moderate-severe ARDS were enrolled 7 to 28 days after the onset of ARDS and treated with 2 mg/kg/day methylprednisolone for 14 days. No difference was found in mortality between treatment and control groups. Most importantly, patients treated with steroids 14 days or more after ARDS onset had increased mortality. This trial demonstrated that use of steroids after 14 days of ARDS onset is harmful.

The evidence for steroids in attenuating lung inflammation has also been evaluated in severe community acquired pneumonia (CAP). CAPE-COD, a European multicenter, double blind, randomized controlled trial, compared hydrocortisone administered within 24 hours of hospital presentation (200 mg daily for 4 or 8 days determined by clinical improvement, then a taper) to placebo. Patients treated with hydrocortisone demonstrated a statistically significant decrease in the risk of death at 28 days (6.2% vs 11.9%).[18] Importantly, 45% of subjects had respiratory failure at enrollment requiring invasive or non-invasive ventilation suggesting that steroids in severe CAP may be of benefit, specifically in patients with acute respiratory failure regardless of whether a patient has ARDS. Another trial published around the same time showed discrepant results. ESCAPE, a double-blind randomized, placebo-controlled trial, enrolled patients with CAP 72 to 96 hours after hospital presentation and randomized to placebo or methylprednisolone (40 mg/day for 7 days and a 20-day taper).[19] No difference was found in 60-day mortality between groups. Differences in trial design help explain these conflicting results. Timing of initiation of glucocorticoids differed between the 2 studies. Administration of steroids at 72 to 96 hours in the ESCAPE trial may have missed the therapeutic window. Additionally, the majority of patients in CAPE-COD had an identified bacterial pathogen and an elevated C-reactive protein (CRP) level, suggesting active inflammation.[20] Meta analyses have concluded that corticosteroid use in CAP is associated with lower risk of progression to invasive mechanical ventilation and may improve mortality without increasing adverse events such as gastrointestinal bleeding and healthcare-associated infection.[21,22]

The cumulative evidence suggests that corticosteroids likely provide benefit for patients with ARDS when administered early. The most recent Society of Critical Care Medicine and the European Society of Intensive Care Medicine conditionally recommend methylprednisolone in patients with early ARDS (up to 7 days of onset; P:F < 200) at a dose of 1 mg/kg/day and late persistent ARDS (after 6 days) at a dose of 2 mg/kg/day based on moderate quality evidence.[23] While this is a reasonable approach, more research is needed to better understand which patients with ARDS may benefit from steroids, and what dose and duration provide the most benefit while minimizing risk. Long term effects of corticosteroids also remain unknown. Individual participant-level data meta-analyses could help answer these important questions.

Neuromuscular Blockade

Neuromuscular blockade agents (NMBA) decrease oxygen consumption, improve gas exchange, and decrease plateau pressures and inflammation, all of which have a theoretic benefit in instances of acute respiratory failure and ARDS.[24-27] Therefore, various NMBA have been used to promote ventilator synchrony and improve oxygenation in moderate to severe hypoxemic respiratory failure; however, their use has been associated with prolonged neuromuscular weakness. Two large, randomized trials have evaluated the use of NMBA in patients with ARDS.

ARDS et Curarisation Systemique trial (ACURASYS) assigned patients with severe ARDS to receive 48 hours of continuous infusion of cisatracurium or placebo.[28] Cisatracurium was chosen as it is metabolized by Hoffman degradation and does not rely on normal renal or hepatic function. Patients in the cisatracurium group had a 90-day mortality of 31.6% compared to 40.7% in the placebo group. An important criticism of this trial is that to ensure blinding, both arms received deep sedation–an intervention that is potentially harmful to patients. Additionally, NMBA was administered over the first 48 hours of the patient's illness, yet the survival curves did not separate until day 18.

The question of NMBA was reexamined in the Reevaluation of Systemic Early Neuromuscular Blockade (ROSE) trial.[29] This multicenter, unblinded, trial randomized patients with moderate-severe ARDS and compared early continuous cisatracurium with concomitant heavy sedation compared to usual care with lighter sedation targets. Importantly, this trial was stopped at the second interim analysis for futility. No difference was found in 90-day mortality, with a mortality rate of 42.5% in the intervention and 42.8% in the control group. No differences were seen in secondary outcomes including incidence of barotrauma and days free of ventilation. One explanation for the starkly different results of the ROSE and ACURASYS trial is the difference in sedation strategies used in each trial's control group.

The results of ACURASYS and ROSE suggest NMBA should not be used routinely in all patients with severe ARDS. However, it is possible that NMBA may be beneficial in select patients, such as those with severe ventilator dyssynchrony or to facilitate placing patients in the prone position.

Pulmonary Vasodilators

Severe hypoxemia is common in ARDS and other forms of acute respiratory failure. In ARDS, alveolar obstruction from pulmonary edema and atelectasis lead to hypoxemia. In normal lungs, hypoxemic vasoconstriction results in redistribution of perfusion (Q) to areas with better ventilation (V) and improves V/Q matching. In ARDS, the lung's ability to redistribute blood flow is severely impaired leading to areas of intrapulmonary shunting (high perfusion with low ventilation) as well as dead space ventilation (high ventilation with low perfusion).[30] Impaired blood flow redistribution leads to worsening hypoxemia. Given this, targeting the pulmonary vasculature to improve ventilation-perfusion matching and rebalance pulmonary vascular tone has been of interest.

Inhaled pulmonary vasodilators, such as nitric oxide and prostacyclins, act on the pulmonary vasculature causing vascular smooth muscle relaxation. Nitric oxide leads to smooth muscle relaxation through activation of soluble guanylyl cyclase, activating cyclic GMP-dependent protein kinases (cGKI). cGKIs decrease sensitivity of myosin to calcium-induced contraction and inhibits release of calcium.[31] Inhaled prostaglandins, such as epoprostenol, activate G-protein leading to increased intracellular cAMP and activation of protein kinase A, leading to relaxation of smooth muscle and vasodilation of pulmonary arteries.[30] Inhaled prostaglandins also have anti-inflammatory and anti-platelet properties, an added potential benefit in ARDS.[32]

Two early single-center trials of inhaled nitric oxide demonstrated improved oxygenation in ARDS but no difference in clinical outcomes.[33,34] Following these initial trials, multiple multicenter trials have reproduced these results.[35,36] Systematic analyses have concluded that while inhaled nitric oxide improves oxygenation and pulmonary pressures, it does not improve mortality even in patients with severe ARDS.[37] Additionally, patients treated with inhaled nitric oxide had an increased risk of renal failure, thus its use is not without risk. Inhaled prostaglandins are less well studied, and most data are observational. The data for inhaled prostaglandins demonstrate similar results to nitric oxide, although, a recent randomized trial in Germany failed to show improvements in oxygenation or mortality in patients treated with inhaled prostacyclin.[38]

Although supported by physiologic rationale, there has been no conclusive evidence that inhaled pulmonary vasodilators improve outcomes in patients with ARDS. Despite the lack of evidence, physicians use pulmonary vasodilators in up to 12% of patients with severe ARDS.[7] Pulmonary vasodilators improve oxygenation, thus their use may be helpful in situations of refractory hypoxemia when planning the next intervention, such as prone positioning or ECMO cannulation. It is unknown if inhaled vasodilators improve other patient-centered outcomes beyond mortality, such as long-term neurocognitive impairment.

Investigational Therapies

Multiple other therapies are being studied in ARDS and acute respiratory failure, including statins, macrolide antibiotics, mesenchymal stem cells, and aspirin. Bone marrow-derived mesenchymal stem/stromal cells (MSCs) release paracrine soluble factors that decrease inflammation and increase alveolar capillary repair.[39,40] Following promising preclinical studies, safety and tolerability have been evaluated in Phase 1 and 2 clinical trials. There are several studies showing safety of MSCs in patients with non-COVID and COVID ARDS.[41-44] While not powered for evaluation of clinical outcomes, the MUST-ARDS trial revealed decreased mortality and increase in intensive care unit (ICU) and ventilator free days in the treatment group,[43] a finding that requires further evaluation in large phase III/IV trials. Cell-based therapy for ARDS has therapeutic potential but more evidence is needed before translating to clinical practice.

COVID-19 Specific Therapies

From the beginning of the COVID-19 pandemic, the need for effective pharmacotherapy for ARDS was highlighted. The pandemic provided tremendous inertia for ARDS clinical trials and testing of various pharmacotherapies for severe respiratory failure due to severe acute respiratory virus COVID-2019 (SARS-CoV-2). Some trials focused on pathogen-specific aspects of the virus,[45] while others focused on dysregulated inflammation that follows acute infection. Many trials targeting inflammation-mediated lung injury showed promise in patients with severe respiratory failure and provide biological plausibility for future studies in non-COVID-19 ARDS.

Like other viral infections such as SARS and influenza, host immune response to SARS-CoV-2 infection plays a role in the development of organ failure. The RECOVERY Collaborative Group, and other adaptive trial designs, such as REMAP-CAP, evaluated the effects of multiple potential treatments for COVID-19. Given the evidence for steroid therapy in non-COVID ARDS, and inflammatory injury in patients with COVID-19, corticosteroids were one of the first therapeutic strategies employed for treatment of severe COVID-19. The RECOVERY trial randomized patients to standard of care alone or standard of care plus dexamethasone 6 mg for 10 days.[46] This trial showed a significant reduction in 28-day mortality in the dexamethasone group (22.9% vs 25.7%). Additionally, the absolute risk reduction in 28-day mortality for patients who received dexamethasone was 12.3% in patients on invasive mechanical ventilation, suggesting this population particularly benefited. A meta-analysis concluded that treatment with systemic corticosteroids was associated with lower 28-day all-cause mortality in patients with severe COVID-19.[47] Dexamethasone was one of the first therapeutic options available for COVID-19 and was immediately incorporated into major societal treatment guidelines.[48,49]

The benefit of corticosteroids in COVID-19 supported the hypothesis that host-response to infection played a significant role in subsequent organ dysfunction. Interleukin-6 (IL-6), a pleiotropic cytokine with a significant role in inflammation had previously been identified as a potential target for ARDS and was found to be elevated in COVID-19.[50] Expediently, trials began to evaluate efficacy of IL-6 pathway targets with IL6 receptor monoclonal antibodies (tocilizumab and sarilumab) and JAK inhibitors (baricitinib).

A Study to Evaluate the Safety and Efficacy of Tocilizumab in Patients With Severe COVID-19 Pneumonia (COVACTA), a multicenter placebo-controlled trial, randomized patients with severe COVID-19 to receive either placebo or a single intravenous dose of tocilizumab (followed by an additional dose based on clinical trajectory).[51] This trial found no difference between treatment and control groups in the primary outcome of clinical status at day 28. Additionally, they found no difference in serious adverse events or 28-day morality between groups. Two additional studies, REMAP-CAP and RECOVERY found more promising results.[52,53] In REMAP-CAP, patients with COVID-19 admitted to an ICU receiving either respiratory support (invasive and non-invasive ventilation or high flow nasal cannula), or cardiovascular support (vasopressors or inotropes) were randomized to receive either tocilizumab, sarilumab or control.[52] Patients treated with tocilizumab or sarilumab had a greater number of organ support-free days (OR 1.64 for tocilizumab and OR 1.76 for sarilumab). In the pooled analysis of both IL6-R antagonists, there was an increased odds for in-hospital survival (OR 1.64). The RECOVERY trial evaluated effects of tocilizumab in patients with COVID-19 with hypoxia and systemic inflammation.[53] RECOVERY found that the tocilizumab group had reduced 28-day mortality and increased probability of discharge at 28 days. In addition, patients without invasive ventilation at study entry had a reduced probability of progression to mechanical ventilation or death. In a meta-analysis, treatment with IL-6 antagonists for patients with COVID-19 was associated with lower 28-day all-cause mortality.[54]

Baracitinib, a Janus kinase inhibitor, inhibits intracellular signaling pathways of multiple cytokines implicated in the pathogenesis of severe COVID-19 infection. In ACTT-2 (Adaptive COVID-19 Treatment Trial), patients with COVID-19 and oxygen saturation <94% on room air were randomized to receive remdesivir and baracitinib or remdesivir and placebo.[55] Patients in the remdesivir plus baracitinib group recovered a median of 1 day faster than patients in the placebo group. Patients receiving noninvasive ventilation or high-flow oxygen had an even faster time to recovery (rate ratio 1.51). Importantly, patients without the need for baseline oxygen support did not receive additional benefit from baracitinib. COV-BARRIER provided additional evidence of benefit with baracitinib.[56] Eligible patients included those with active COVID-19 infection, at least one elevated inflammatory marker and need for baseline oxygen support. This study did not find a reduction in the primary composite endpoint of disease progression but did have a 38.2% relative reduction in 28-day mortality, which was maintained at 60 days. The results of these 2 trials led baracitinib to be approved by the Food and Drug Administration in June 2022 for treatment of COVID-19.[57]

The benefits of corticosteroids and immunomodulators such as IL6-R antagonists in COVID-19 have important implications for future research in non-COVID ARDS. Both corticosteroids and IL6 pathway targets showed benefit in those patients already receiving respiratory support suggesting that once respiratory failure develops, the illness may be dominated by a hyperinflammatory host response to infection with SARS-CoV2.[46] While results of COVID-19 cohorts cannot be generalized to the entire ARDS population, specific subphenotypes of ARDS may receive benefit with the immunomodulatory therapies used for COVID-19. This is an important area requiring more investigation.

Precision Medicine and Future Directions

ARDS has been recognized as a heterogeneous syndrome; however, most previous trials applied a "one size fits all" approach to ARDS therapeutics or, alternatively, selected subjects based on severity of hypoxemia. More recent evidence suggests that endotypes and/or subphenotypes of ARDS exist that may benefit from a precision approach.[58,59] While no specific therapies have been proven to be effective in biologically defined subtypes of disease, 2 approaches attempting to identify these populations have been used. The first approach employs unsupervised clustering methods based on clinical and biological characteristics to derive subphenotypes of ARDS. Calfee and colleagues have identified and validated 2 distinct subphenotypes of ARDS using a statistical method, latent class analysis (LCA), applied to clinical and plasma protein biomarker data. The phenotypes are termed hyperinflammatory and hypoinflammatory.[60,61] LCA applied to trial cohorts and observational data have consistently identified this 2-phenotype model. Approximately 30% of patients are characterized as hyperinflammatory and 70% fit a hypoinflammatory phenotype.[60–64] Interestingly, neither severity of hypoxemia nor severity of illness distinguish these 2 phenotypes. The hyperinflammatory phenotype experiences consistently worse outcomes, with a 60-day mortality that is twice as high as the hypoinflammatory phenotype.[65]

In addition to identifying these 2 distinct phenotypes, Calfee and colleagues have identified significant heterogeneity of treatment effects by subphenotype by re-evaluating prior RCTs using LCA and demonstrating that these subphenotypes respond differently to specific pharmacotherapies. The HARP-2 trial (Hydroxymethyl-glutaryl-CoA Reductase Inhibition with Simvastatin in Acute Lung Injury to Reduce Pulmonary Dysfunction-2[66]) investigated simvastatin for treatment of ARDS. While, simvastatin did not increase the number of ventilator-free days or improve clinical outcomes in the trial, a secondary analysis of HARP-2 found that patients in the hyperinflammatory subphenotype had improved outcomes with simvastatin compared to placebo.[64] The original trial found no difference in 28-day morality between treatment with simvastatin and placebo, but in the secondary analysis, patients with the hyperinflammatory subphenotype treated with simvastatin had significantly improved 28-day survival (32% vs 45%, P = .008) and 90-day survival. This trial highlights the importance of identification of ARDS subphenotypes and suggests that targeting distinct phenotypes is crucial for future pharmacotherapies in ARDS.

Evidence of differential treatment effect in ARDS subphenotypes has also been shown with non-pharmacologic interventions. The ALVEOLI trial compared different positive end expiratory pressure (PEEP) strategies and found no difference between groups.[67] When subphenotypes were investigated, a differential effect of PEEP strategy on mortality between phenotypes was found.[60] High PEEP appeared beneficial in the hyperinflammatory phenotype but harmful in the hypoinflammatory phenotype. These results require confirmation in a prospective trial before they are utilized at the bedside; however, they provide further support of heterogeneity of treatment effect within ARDS.

A second approach used to identify endotypes or subphenotypes of ARDS employs knowledge of a biological pathway, markers indicating disruption of that pathway, and potential therapeutic targets within the pathway. Meyer and colleagues employed this method in sepsis, a syndrome with substantial overlap with acute respiratory failure, to identify heterogeneous treatment effect of recombinant interleukin-1 receptor antagonist (rhIL1RA) based on plasma biomarkers of the IL-1 axis. Patients with plasma IL1RA above a specific threshold treated with rhIL1RA had a reduction in adjusted mortality from 45.4% to 34.3% whereas those below the IL1RA threshold treated with rhIL1RA had no change in mortality,[68] resulting in an overall treatment effect that did not cross the statical threshold for efficacy. This same therapeutic was leveraged as a potential treatment of COVID-19 given its efficacy in disease entities with hyperinflammation.[69–71] A systematic review and individual patient-level meta-analysis found that rhIL1RA was most effective at lowering mortality in patients with COVID-19 with elevated CRP levels,[72] adding to the body of literature supporting precision medicine in subphenotypes of otherwise heterogeneous populations of critically ill patients.

Biological phenotyping in critical care, and specifically ARDS, has made significant progress over the last decade, but no prospective evaluations of ARDS subphenotypes have been conducted yet. This is largely due to difficulty of translating the current models to the bedside. The existing retrospectively validated ARDS LCA models include 20 to 30 variables, which are impractical for prospective use. A prospective bedside classification of phenotypes in a small cohort of patients with COVID-19 ARDS showed proof-of-concept.[73] An ongoing study, Phenotypes in the Acute Respiratory Distress Syndrome, aims to prospectively identify hyperinflammatory and hypoinflammatory phenotypes of ARDS using a point-of-care assay (NCT04009330). Results of this study have the potential to allow for bedside identification of biological phenotypes and ultimately, incorporate phenotyping into clinical trials.[65] The ability to provide precision medicine at the bedside relies on successfully characterizing patients according to predicted treatment response in real-time. Given the heterogeneity of ARDS, the future of successful therapeutics lies in a precision medicine approach, as we strive to match the right therapy to the right patient at the right time.[65,74] Experts agree that advancement of precision medicine in acute respiratory failure remains essential in the path to improve morbidity and mortality in ARDS.[74]

SUMMARY

Despite decades of research, there are limited effective pharmacotherapies for acute respiratory failure and ARDS. Pharmacologic treatments have attempted to target biological pathways that are dysregulated in ARDS. Identifying effective pharmacotherapy for ARDS remains a research area of utmost importance. When deciding on potential therapeutics for patients with ARDS, a "one size fits all" approach may not be most appropriate. Carefully selected patients may benefit more than others from specific therapies, a concept that is supported by evidence of significant heterogeneity within ARDS. The key to finding effective pharmacotherapies for ARDS requires a deeper understanding of ARDS pathophysiology and the ability to identify subphenotypes of ARDS at the bedside.

CLINICS CARE POINTS

- Consensus recommendations for acute respiratory distress syndrome management include lung protective ventilation utilizing low tidal volume ventilation (4-8 mL/predicted body weight) and limiting inspiratory pressures (plateau pressures <30 cm H_2O). Prone positioning for patients with moderate-severe ARDS (P:F < 150) is also recommended.[4]
- Steroids may be beneficial for patients with ARDS but the exact dose, formulation and duration of therapy is unknown. Steroids used late in the course of ARDS are harmful.
- Neuromuscular blockade should not be used routinely in all patients with severe ARDS but may be beneficial in patients with severe ventilator dyssynchrony and high inspiratory pressures. In patients managed with neuromuscular blockade, continued use should be reevaluated daily.

DISCLOSURE

Dr E. Levy reports funding from the National Institutes of Health, United States (T32-HL098054). Dr J. Reilly reports funding from the National Institutes of Health (R01-HL155159, U01-HL168419) and the Department of Defense, United States (W81XWH2010432).

REFERENCES

1. Meyer NJ, Gattinoni L, Calfee CS. Acute respiratory distress syndrome. Lancet 2021;398(10300):622–37.
2. Huppert LA, Matthay MA, Ware LB. Pathogenesis of acute respiratory distress syndrome. Semin Respir Crit Care Med 2019;40(1):31–9.
3. Matthay MA, McAuley DF, Ware LB. Clinical trials in acute respiratory distress syndrome: challenges and opportunities. Lancet Respir Med 2017;5(6):524–34.
4. Fan E, Del Sorbo L, Goligher EC, et al. An official american thoracic society/european society of intensive care medicine/society of critical care medicine clinical practice guideline: mechanical ventilation in adult patients with acute respiratory distress syndrome. Am J Respir Crit Care Med 2017;195(9):1253–63.
5. Meduri GU, Annane D, Confalonieri M, et al. Pharmacological principles guiding prolonged glucocorticoid treatment in ARDS. Intensive Care Med 2020;46(12):2284–96.
6. Bellani G, Laffey JG, Pham T, et al. Epidemiology, patterns of care, and mortality for patients with acute respiratory distress syndrome in intensive care units in 50 countries. JAMA 2016;315(8):788–800.
7. Qadir N, Bartz RR, Cooter ML, et al. Variation in early management practices in moderate-to-severe ARDS in the United States: the severe ARDS: generating evidence study. Chest 2021;160(4):1304–15.
8. Bernard GR, Luce JM, Sprung CL, et al. High-dose corticosteroids in patients with the adult respiratory distress syndrome. N Engl J Med 1987;317(25):1565–70.
9. Bone RC, Fisher CJ, Clemmer TP, et al. Early methylprednisolone treatment for septic syndrome and the adult respiratory distress syndrome. Chest 1987;92(6):1032–6.
10. Luce JM, Montgomery AB, Marks JD, et al. Ineffectiveness of high-dose methylprednisolone in preventing parenchymal lung injury and improving mortality in patients with septic shock. Am Rev Respir Dis 1988;138(1):62–8.

11. Weigelt JA, Norcross JF, Borman KR, et al. Early steroid therapy for respiratory failure. Arch Surg 1985;120(5):536–40.
12. Meduri GU, Headley AS, Golden E, et al. Effect of prolonged methylprednisolone therapy in unresolving acute respiratory distress syndrome: a randomized controlled trial. JAMA 1998;280(2):159–65.
13. Meduri GU, Golden E, Freire AX, et al. Methylprednisolone infusion in early severe ARDS: results of a randomized controlled trial. Chest 2007;131(4):954–63.
14. Villar J, Ferrando C, Martínez D, et al. Dexamethasone treatment for the acute respiratory distress syndrome: a multicentre, randomised controlled trial. Lancet Respir Med 2020;8(3):267–76.
15. Lewis SR, Pritchard MW, Thomas CM, et al. Pharmacological agents for adults with acute respiratory distress syndrome. Cochrane Database Syst Rev 2019; 7(7):CD004477.
16. Chaudhuri D, Sasaki K, Karkar A, et al. Corticosteroids in COVID-19 and non-COVID-19 ARDS: a systematic review and meta-analysis. Intensive Care Med 2021;47(5):521–37.
17. Steinberg KP, Hudson LD, Goodman RB, et al. Efficacy and safety of corticosteroids for persistent acute respiratory distress syndrome. N Engl J Med 2006; 354(16):1671–84.
18. Dequin PF, Meziani F, Quenot JP, et al. Hydrocortisone in severe community-acquired pneumonia. N Engl J Med 2023;388(21):1931–41.
19. Meduri GU, Shih MC, Bridges L, et al. Low-dose methylprednisolone treatment in critically ill patients with severe community-acquired pneumonia. Intensive Care Med 2022;48(8):1009–23.
20. Metlay JP, Waterer GW. Time to treat severe community-acquired pneumonia with steroids? N Engl J Med 2023;388(21):2001–2.
21. Wu JY, Tsai YW, Hsu WH, et al. Efficacy and safety of adjunctive corticosteroids in the treatment of severe community-acquired pneumonia: a systematic review and meta-analysis of randomized controlled trials. Crit Care 2023;27(1):274.
22. Saleem N, Kulkarni A, Snow TAC, et al. Effect of corticosteroids on mortality and clinical cure in community-acquired pneumonia: a systematic review, meta-analysis, and meta-regression of randomized control trials. Chest 2023;163(3): 484–97.
23. Annane D, Pastores SM, Rochwerg B, et al. Guidelines for the diagnosis and management of critical illness-related corticosteroid insufficiency (CIRCI) in critically ill patients (Part I): society of Critical Care Medicine (SCCM) and European Society of Intensive Care Medicine (ESICM) 2017. Intensive Care Med 2017; 43(12):1751–63.
24. Gainnier M, Roch A, Forel JM, et al. Effect of neuromuscular blocking agents on gas exchange in patients presenting with acute respiratory distress syndrome. Crit Care Med 2004;32(1):113–9.
25. Forel JM, Roch A, Marin V, et al. Neuromuscular blocking agents decrease inflammatory response in patients presenting with acute respiratory distress syndrome. Crit Care Med 2006;34(11):2749–57.
26. Guervilly C, Bisbal M, Forel JM, et al. Effects of neuromuscular blockers on trans-pulmonary pressures in moderate to severe acute respiratory distress syndrome. Intensive Care Med 2017;43(3):408–18.
27. Slutsky AS. Neuromuscular blocking agents in ARDS. N Engl J Med 2010; 363(12):1176–80.
28. Papazian L, Forel JM, Gacouin A, et al. Neuromuscular blockers in early acute respiratory distress syndrome. N Engl J Med 2010;363(12):1107–16.

29. Moss M, Ulysse CA, Angus DC, et al. Early neuromuscular blockade in the acute respiratory distress syndrome. reply. N Engl J Med 2019;381(8):787–8.
30. Gierhardt M, Pak O, Walmrath D, et al. Impairment of hypoxic pulmonary vaso-constriction in acute respiratory distress syndrome. Eur Respir Rev 2021; 30(161):210059.
31. Griffiths MJ, Evans TW. Inhaled nitric oxide therapy in adults. N Engl J Med 2005; 353(25):2683–95.
32. Fuller BM, Mohr NM, Skrupky L, et al. The use of inhaled prostaglandins in patients with ARDS: a systematic review and meta-analysis. Chest 2015;147(6): 1510–22.
33. Michael JR, Barton RG, Saffle JR, et al. Inhaled nitric oxide versus conventional therapy: effect on oxygenation in ARDS. Am J Respir Crit Care Med 1998;157(5 Pt 1):1372–80.
34. Troncy E, Collet JP, Shapiro S, et al. Inhaled nitric oxide in acute respiratory distress syndrome: a pilot randomized controlled study. Am J Respir Crit Care Med 1998;157(5 Pt 1):1483–8.
35. Lundin S, Mang H, Smithies M, et al. Inhalation of nitric oxide in acute lung injury: results of a European multicentre study. The European Study Group of Inhaled Nitric Oxide. Intensive Care Med 1999;25(9):911–9.
36. Taylor RW, Zimmerman JL, Dellinger RP, et al. Low-dose inhaled nitric oxide in patients with acute lung injury: a randomized controlled trial. JAMA 2004;291(13): 1603–9.
37. Adhikari NK, Dellinger RP, Lundin S, et al. Inhaled nitric oxide does not reduce mortality in patients with acute respiratory distress syndrome regardless of severity: systematic review and meta-analysis. Crit Care Med 2014;42(2):404–12.
38. Haeberle HA, Calov S, Martus P, et al. Inhaled prostacyclin therapy in the acute respiratory distress syndrome: a randomized controlled multicenter trial. Respir Res 2023;24(1):58.
39. Matthay MA. Therapeutic potential of mesenchymal stromal cells for acute respiratory distress syndrome. Ann Am Thorac Soc 2015;12(Suppl 1):S54–7.
40. Han J, Liu Y, Liu H, et al. Genetically modified mesenchymal stem cell therapy for acute respiratory distress syndrome. Stem Cell Res Ther 2019;10(1):386.
41. Matthay MA, Calfee CS, Zhuo H, et al. Treatment with allogeneic mesenchymal stromal cells for moderate to severe acute respiratory distress syndrome (START study): a randomised phase 2a safety trial. Lancet Respir Med 2019;7(2):154–62.
42. Gorman E, Shankar-Hari M, Hopkins P, et al. Repair of acute respiratory distress syndrome by stromal cell administration (REALIST) trial: a phase 1 trial. EClinical-Medicine 2021;41:101167.
43. Bellingan G, Jacono F, Bannard-Smith J, et al. Safety and efficacy of multipotent adult progenitor cells in acute respiratory distress syndrome (MUST-ARDS): a multicentre, randomised, double-blind, placebo-controlled phase 1/2 trial. Intensive Care Med 2022;48(1):36–44.
44. Whittaker Brown SA, Iancu-Rubin C, Aboelela A, et al. Mesenchymal stromal cell therapy for acute respiratory distress syndrome due to coronavirus disease 2019. Cytotherapy 2022;24(8):835–40.
45. Beigel JH, Tomashek KM, Dodd LE, et al. Remdesivir for the treatment of Covid-19 - final report. N Engl J Med 2020;383(19):1813–26.
46. Horby P, Lim WS, Emberson JR, et al. Dexamethasone in Hospitalized Patients with Covid-19. N Engl J Med 2021;384(8):693–704.

47. Sterne JAC, Murthy S, Diaz JV, et al. Association Between Administration of Systemic Corticosteroids and Mortality Among Critically Ill Patients With COVID-19: A Meta-analysis. JAMA 2020;324(13):1330–41.
48. COVID-19 Treatment Guidelines Panel. Coronavirus Disease 2019 (COVID-19) Treatment Guidelines. 6/1/2023; Available at https://www.covid19treatment guidelines.nih.gov/.
49. Organization, W.H. Corticosteroids for COVID-19. 2020 6/1/2023; Available at: https://www.who.int/publications/i/item/WHO-2019-nCoV-Corticosteroids-2020.1.
50. McElvaney OJ, Curley GF, Rose-John S, et al. Interleukin-6: obstacles to targeting a complex cytokine in critical illness. Lancet Respir Med 2021;9(6):643–54.
51. Rosas IO, Diaz G, Gottlieb RL, et al. Tocilizumab and remdesivir in hospitalized patients with severe COVID-19 pneumonia: a randomized clinical trial. Intensive Care Med 2021;47(11):1258–70.
52. Gordon AC, Mouncey PR, Al-Beidh F, et al. Interleukin-6 Receptor Antagonists in Critically Ill Patients with Covid-19. N Engl J Med 2021;384(16):1491–502.
53. RECOVERY Collaborative Group. Tocilizumab in patients admitted to hospital with COVID-19 (RECOVERY): a randomised, controlled, open-label, platform trial. Lancet 2021;397(10285):1637–45.
54. Shankar-Hari M, Vale CL, Godolphin PJ, et al. Association Between Administration of IL-6 Antagonists and Mortality Among Patients Hospitalized for COVID-19: A Meta-analysis. JAMA 2021;326(6):499–518.
55. Kalil AC, Patterson TF, Mehta AK, et al. Baricitinib plus remdesivir for hospitalized adults with covid-19. N Engl J Med 2021;384(9):795–807.
56. Marconi VC, Ramanan AV, de Bono S, et al. Efficacy and safety of baricitinib for the treatment of hospitalised adults with COVID-19 (COV-BARRIER): a randomised, double-blind, parallel-group, placebo-controlled phase 3 trial. Lancet Respir Med 2021;9(12):1407–18.
57. Rubin R. Baricitinib is first approved COVID-19 immunomodulatory Treatment. JAMA 2022;327(23):2281.
58. Maslove DM, Tang B, Shankar-Hari M, et al. Redefining critical illness. Nat Med 2022;28(6):1141–8.
59. Reilly JP, Calfee CS, Christie JD. Acute respiratory distress syndrome phenotypes. Semin Respir Crit Care Med 2019;40(1):19–30.
60. Calfee CS, Delucchi K, Parsons PE, et al. Subphenotypes in acute respiratory distress syndrome: latent class analysis of data from two randomised controlled trials. Lancet Respir Med 2014;2(8):611–20.
61. Famous KR, Delucchi K, Ware LB, et al. Acute respiratory distress syndrome subphenotypes respond differently to randomized fluid management strategy. Am J Respir Crit Care Med 2017;195(3):331–8.
62. Sinha P, Delucchi KL, Thompson BT, et al. Latent class analysis of ARDS subphenotypes: a secondary analysis of the statins for acutely injured lungs from sepsis (SAILS) study. Intensive Care Med 2018;44(11):1859–69.
63. Sinha P, Delucchi KL, Chen Y, et al. Latent class analysis-derived subphenotypes are generalisable to observational cohorts of acute respiratory distress syndrome: a prospective study. Thorax 2022;77(1):13–21.
64. Calfee CS, Delucchi KL, Sinha P, et al. Acute respiratory distress syndrome subphenotypes and differential response to simvastatin: secondary analysis of a randomised controlled trial. Lancet Respir Med 2018;6(9):691–8.
65. Sinha P, Meyer NJ, Calfee CS. Biological phenotyping in sepsis and acute respiratory distress syndrome. Annu Rev Med 2023;74:457–71.

66. McAuley DF, Laffey JG, O'Kane CM, et al. Simvastatin in the acute respiratory distress syndrome. N Engl J Med 2014;371(18):1695–703.

67. Brower RG, Lanken PN, MacIntyre N, et al. Higher versus lower positive end-expiratory pressures in patients with the acute respiratory distress syndrome. N Engl J Med 2004;351(4):327–36.

68. Meyer NJ, Reilly JP, Anderson BJ, et al. Mortality benefit of recombinant human interleukin-1 receptor antagonist for sepsis varies by initial interleukin-1 receptor antagonist plasma concentration. Crit Care Med 2018;46(1):21–8.

69. Giavridis T, van der Stegen SJC, Eyquem J, et al. CAR T cell-induced cytokine release syndrome is mediated by macrophages and abated by IL-1 blockade. Nat Med 2018;24(6):731–8.

70. Strati P, Ahmed S, Kebriaei P, et al. Clinical efficacy of anakinra to mitigate CAR T-cell therapy-associated toxicity in large B-cell lymphoma. Blood Adv 2020; 4(13):3123–7.

71. Shakoory B, Carcillo JA, Chatham WW, et al. Interleukin-1 receptor blockade is associated with reduced mortality in sepsis patients with features of macrophage activation syndrome: reanalysis of a prior phase III trial. Crit Care Med 2016; 44(2):275–81.

72. Kyriazopoulou E, Huet T, Cavalli G, et al. Effect of anakinra on mortality in patients with COVID-19: a systematic review and patient-level meta-analysis. Lancet Rheumatol 2021;3(10):e690–7.

73. Sinha P, Calfee CS, Cherian S, et al. Prevalence of phenotypes of acute respiratory distress syndrome in critically ill patients with COVID-19: a prospective observational study. Lancet Respir Med 2020;8(12):1209–18.

74. Beitler JR, Thompson BT, Baron RM, et al. Advancing precision medicine for acute respiratory distress syndrome. Lancet Respir Med 2022;10(1):107–20.

75. Truwit JD, Truwit JD, Bernard GR, et al. Rosuvastatin for sepsis-associated acute respiratory distress syndrome. N Engl J Med 2014;370(23):2191–200.

76. Toner P, Boyle AJ, McNamee JJ, et al. Aspirin as a treatment for ARDS: a randomized, placebo-controlled clinical trial. Chest 2022;161(5):1275–84.

77. Richardson P, Griffin I, Tucker C, et al. Baricitinib as potential treatment for 2019-nCoV acute respiratory disease. Lancet 2020;395(10223):e30–1.

78. Gao Smith F, Perkins GD, Gates S, et al. Effect of intravenous beta-2 agonist treatment on clinical outcomes in acute respiratory distress syndrome (Balti-2): a multicentre, randomised controlled trial. Lancet 2012;379(9812):229–35.

79. Matthay MA, Brower RG, Carson S, et al. Randomized, placebo-controlled clinical trial of an aerosolized beta(2)-agonist for treatment of acute lung injury. Am J Respir Crit Care Med 2011;184(5):561–8.

80. Aman J, Duijvelaar E, Botros L, et al. Imatinib in patients with severe COVID-19: a randomised, double-blind, placebo-controlled, clinical trial. Lancet Respir Med 2021;9(9):957–68.

81. Ranieri VM, Pettilä V, Karvonen MK, et al. Effect of intravenous interferon beta-1a on death and days free from mechanical ventilation among patients with moderate to severe acute respiratory distress syndrome: a randomized clinical trial. JAMA 2020;323(8):725–33.

82. Brower RG, Matthay MA, Morris A, et al. Ventilation with lower tidal volumes as compared with traditional tidal volumes for acute lung injury and the acute respiratory distress syndrome. N Engl J Med 2000;342(18):1301–8.

83. Dellinger RP, Zimmerman JL, Taylor RW, et al. Effects of inhaled nitric oxide in patients with acute respiratory distress syndrome: results of a randomized phase II trial. Inhaled Nitric Oxide in ARDS Study Group. Crit Care Med 1998;26(1):15–23.

84. Guerin C, Reignier J, Richard JC, et al. Prone positioning in severe acute respiratory distress syndrome. N Engl J Med 2013;368(23):2159–68.
85. Shanholtz CB, Terrin ML, Harrington T, et al. Design and rationale of the CHILL phase II trial of hypothermia and neuromuscular blockade for acute respiratory distress syndrome. Contemp Clin Trials Commun 2023;33:101155.
86. Liu D, Ahmet A, Ward L, et al. A practical guide to the monitoring and management of the complications of systemic corticosteroid therapy. Allergy Asthma Clin Immunol 2013;9(1):30.

Fluid Management in Acute Respiratory Failure

Shewit P. Giovanni, MD, MSc[a],*, Kevin P. Seitz, MD, MSc[b],
Catherine L. Hough, MD, MSc[a]

KEYWORDS

- fluid management • Respiratory failure • ARDS

KEY POINTS

- Optimal fluid management in patients with acute respiratory failure is challenging to standardize, given the heterogeneity of timing and the associated acute and chronic conditions.
- Liberal and conservative fluid strategies are likely complementary and ongoing assessment in the same patient is recommended to optimize tissue perfusion and avoid volume overload.
- A conservative fluid strategy following initial resuscitation may be beneficial with minimal harm in patients with acute respiratory distress syndrome and patients with concomitant respiratory failure and sepsis.
- The ideal type of fluid, volume, and timing of diuresis during shock and after resolution of shock in acute respiratory failure remains unclear.
- Studies identifying sub-phenotypes of patients who will benefit from conservative or liberal fluid management are urgently needed.

INTRODUCTION

Acute respiratory failure (ARF) is a challenging condition with significant variability in definition,[1] which encompasses patients with progressive and acute hypoxemia, hypercapnia, or respiratory distress related to a variety of cardiorespiratory or systemic diseases such as sepsis. Acute respiratory distress syndrome (ARDS) is a serious form of ARF defined by non-cardiogenic pulmonary edema and acute hypoxemia, triggered by various pulmonary and non-pulmonary insults.[2]

The ideal fluid management in ARF would avoid impairing respiratory mechanics and gas exchange while still ensuring adequate tissue perfusion. Critically ill patients

[a] Division of Pulmonary, Allergy and Critical Care Medicine, Oregon Health & Science University, 3181 Southwest Sam Jackson Park Road, Mailing Code UHN67, Portland, OR 97239, USA;
[b] Department of Allergy, Pulmonary, and Critical Care Medicine, Vanderbilt University Medical Center, T-1215 Medical Center North, 1161 21st Avenue South, Nashville, TN 37232, USA
* Corresponding author.
E-mail address: giovanni@ohsu.edu

Crit Care Clin 40 (2024) 291–307
https://doi.org/10.1016/j.ccc.2024.01.004
0749-0704/24/© 2024 Elsevier Inc. All rights reserved.

(with hemodynamic instability) often require early intravenous fluid administration to support cardiac output, and inadequate initial fluid resuscitation may worsen mortality.[3] While there are no standardized society guideline recommendations for optimal fluid management in ARF, the majority of our understanding of fluid management comes from research in patients with ARDS and sepsis.

This review will describe the pathophysiology of ARDS and how it relates to fluid management, considerations in patients with or at risk for ARDS, ARF,and sepsis, fluid choice, post-hospital outcomes related to fluid management, metrics to guide fluid therapy, and provide a framework for fluid management depending on the clinical setting. A conservative or restrictive fluid strategy focuses on minimizing fluids during and after the resuscitative phase, and potentially adding active diuresis to reduce total fluid balance during non-resuscitative phase. A liberal fluid strategy has no restriction of intravenous fluids in the resuscitative phase and lacks protocolized active fluid removal during the recovery phase.

CONSIDERING THE PATHOPHYSIOLOGY IN ACUTE RESPIRATORY DISTRESS SYNDROME IN FLUID MANAGEMENT

In ARDS, healthy pulmonary endothelium is compromised with excessive inflammation leading to increased pulmonary endothelial and epithelial permeability, leakage of protein-rich fluid into the alveolar space, impaired fluid removal, and disrupted alveolar barrier function.[4] This can increase pulmonary hydrostatic pressures, decrease oncotic pressures, and disrupt the pressure gradient leading to significant interstitial and alveolar flooding (ie, pulmonary edema).[4] Hypothesized benefits of a conservative strategy include decreasing hydrostatic pressures and right ventricular pressures, increasing oncotic pressures, and decreasing plasma levels of angiopoietin-2 which could have a protective effect on the vascular endothelium.[5]

Excessive fluid administration could exacerbate the underlying pathophysiology in ARDS and worsen pulmonary edema. However, hypotension and subsequent decreased cardiac output and pulmonary blood flow in patients with ARDS can worsen alveolar and physiologic dead space.[6] Since the majority of patient with ARDS die from multiorgan system failure,[7] resuscitation can be imperative. Unfortunately, the right strategy to maintain tissue perfusion while limiting pulmonary edema is uncertain.

A HISTORICAL SHIFT IN FLUID MANAGEMENT

Researchers have compared liberal versus conservative strategies in patients with ARDS for more than 30 years.[8–10] Arguments for a liberal strategy, the historically conventional practice, were based on the benefit of end-organ perfusion and oxygen delivery, hypothesizing that focusing on lowering the pulmonary capillary wedge pressures (PCWP) during pulmonary edema would not be beneficial and could be harmful in patients with multiorgan system involvement particularly in shock and acute kidney injury.[11] Additionally, there was significant provider practice variation in the dose of fluids given in early liberal strategies ranging from a fluid balance of 4 L at day 4 in ARMA (the low tidal volume ventilation study in ARDS) and ALVEOLI (higher vs. lower PEEP study in ARDS)[12,13] and up to 20L at day 14 in a randomized controlled trial (RCT) of 113 ARDS patients.[14]

Early studies suggested that a conservative strategy (guided by extravascular lung water assessments)[15] in patients with ARDS and acute lung injury (ALI) may decrease pulmonary artery pressures[15] and increase intensive care unit (ICU) and ventilator-free days and that a negative cumulative fluid balance and reduced PCWP could improve overall survival.[14,16–18] Although findings were limited by the observational nature of some studies and significant confounding by severity of illness and small cohort size, it signified a paradigm shift.

This debate persisted until the landmark large multicenter RCT, the Fluid and the Catheter Treatment Trial (FACTT), was published in 2006. Using a factorial design, FACTT included 1001 patients within 48 hours of diagnosis of ALI or ARDS randomized to either a conservative or liberal fluid strategy, guided by either pulmonary artery catheters (PAC) or central venous catheters (CVC).[19] FACTT used strict protocols to guide active diuresis, vasoactive medications, and fluid boluses and targeted a higher central venous pressure (CVP) or PCWP in the liberal group and a lower goal in the conservative group. The protocol deferred to clinician-driven management in the presence of shock and held diuresis for 12 hours. While there was no difference in the primary outcome of 60-day mortality (25% vs 28%, $P = .30$), the conservative group had significantly more ventilator and ICU-free days and a significant difference in cumulative fluid balance (-136 mL in the conservative group vs nearly 7L in the liberal group). Notably, a conservative approach did not increase the incidence or duration of shock or acute kidney injury. Also importantly, there was no benefit of randomization to pulmonary artery catheter-based guidance. These studies suggest that there are potential clinical benefits and notably minimal harm with a conservative approach to fluid management in patients in ARDS who have no evidence of ongoing shock. Further studies are needed to understand the effect of fluid management strategies on mortality, management in patients with ARDS and concomitant shock, and the optimal approach to fluid and diuretic administration.

FLUID MANAGEMENT IN PATIENTS AT RISK OF ACUTE RESPIRATORY DISTRESS SNDROME

Research on strategies to prevent development and progression of ARDS is lacking and findings in published observational studies are limited by potential indication bias. However, a positive fluid balance in a patient at risk of ARDS has been associated with a higher incidence of ARDS and increased mortality.[20] An analysis of 455 patients with sepsis identified that 92% of the patients who developed ARDS had hypoproteinemia at study entry and the severity of hypoproteinemia was identified as the strongest predictor for development of ARDS,[21] a finding confirmed in patients with septic shock.[22] The low oncotic pressure associated with hypoproteinemia can facilitate hydrostatic pulmonary edema.

It is unclear how to mitigate the risk of hypoproteinemia. Colloids (such as albumin) may increase oncotic pressure and minimize volume overload. Although use of colloids has been evaluated in ARDS and ALI,[23–25] no studies exist in patients at risk of ARDS. Use of other fluid types (ie, hypertonic saline compared to normal saline) is also mixed.[26,27] A recent large multicenter RCT, Crystalloid Liberal or Vasopressors Early Resuscitation in Sepsis (CLOVERS) trial, compared a restrictive strategy focusing on early vasopressor use to a liberal strategy during the first 24 hours of treatment in 1563 patients with sepsis-induced hypotension and did not demonstrate a difference between the groups in the development of ARDS within the first 7 days of randomization.[28] More research is required on the impact of fluid management in this population.

FLUID MANAGEMENT IN ACUTE RESPIRATORY FAILURE AND SEPTIC SHOCK

ARF rarely occurs in isolation, and is common in patients with sepsis.[3] Sepsis is a syndrome of dysregulated immune response to severe infection causing organ dysfunction with hypotension and hypoperfusion, associated with a short-term mortality of up to 15%.[29] Treatment of patients with sepsis includes prompt delivery of antibiotics for the infection and administration of intravenous fluids and vasopressors to address hypoperfusion and shock.[30,31] ARF and sepsis are linked by multiple causal pathways. A pulmonary infection can cause respiratory failure and sepsis, non-pulmonary infections with sepsis are a risk factor for ARDS,[32] and treatment for sepsis with intravenous fluids can lead to iatrogenic respiratory failure by pulmonary edema.[33] As a result, fluid management in patients with sepsis and ARF can present opposing priorities for the clinician; fluid resuscitation to support perfusion and fluid removal for respiratory failure. This dilemma creates 2 research questions: first, whether the fluid strategy affects outcomes for patients with sepsis and ARF, and second, whether fluid strategy for sepsis affects the risk of subsequent respiratory failure.

In resuscitation for sepsis, guidelines have recommended initial treatment with at least 30 mL/kg (mL/kg) of intravenous fluids based largely on an RCT in 2001 that administered this large, weight-based volume of fluid as a component of multiple interventions given early in the care of patients with sepsis, termed "early goal-directed therapy (EGDT)."[31] Similarly, an observational study of patients with ARDS from sepsis suggested that inadequate initial resuscitation during usual care was associated with worse survival.[3] Three subsequent multi-center trials (ProCESS,[34] ARISE,[35] ProMISe[36]) compared EGDT to usual care for sepsis. A patient-level meta-analysis of these trials found that the EGDT strategy did not affect mortality overall or in the subgroup of patients with ARF on invasive mechanical ventilation (Adjusted Odds Ratio (AOR) 0.87 (0.55–1.37), $P = .55$).[37] For respiratory failure as an outcome of fluid strategy, EGDT was associated with a small increase in the odds of receiving mechanical ventilation (AOR 1.05 (0.89–1.24), $P = .04$). These studies demonstrated that EGDT protocols did not provide a benefit over usual care, but the degree to which additional fluid in the EGDT group affected respiratory failure is complicated by the comparison of the multiple EGDT therapies to variable usual care, which still included substantial fluid use.

In resource-limited settings, multiple trials have shown more direct evidence of harm from fluid administration in sepsis, particularly related to respiratory failure. In Zambia, the Simplified Severe Sepsis Protocol (SSSP-1) tested a sepsis protocol of early fluid use among 109 patients with severe sepsis and the trial was stopped early due to higher mortality in patients with hypoxemia randomized to the protocol.[38] The subsequent Simplified Severe Sepsis Protocol −2 (SSSP-2) trial excluded patients with respiratory failure and stopped giving fluids if patients were developing respiratory failure.[39] The group receiving the sepsis protocol received more fluids and had a higher rate of in-hospital mortality (48.1% vs 33.0%, $P = .03$). More patients in the sepsis protocol group experienced worsening hypoxemia or tachypnea as well (36% vs 22% ($P = .03$)).

In high-resource settings, 2 prospective trials inform fluid administration for patients with sepsis and ARF. The Fluid Responsiveness Evaluation in Sepsis-Associated Hypotension (FRESH) was a multicenter trial that randomized 150 patients with septic shock to an intervention arm with protocolized testing of fluid responsiveness to guide fluid therapy for the first 72 hours versus usual care. The protocolized group received a lower total volume of fluid compared to usual care with an average of 1.4 L less cumulative fluid balance, the study's primary outcome. Fewer patients randomized to the intervention arm subsequently received mechanical ventilation (17.7% vs 34.1%, $P = .04$), a provocative finding suggesting need for further evaluation.[40]

The CLOVERS trial more specifically addressed the effect of fluid volume during resuscitation for sepsis on patient outcomes, including respiratory sequelae.[16] Overall, 9.4% of the patients had respiratory failure requiring assisted ventilation. In the first 24 hours after enrollment, patients in the restrictive strategy group received a median 1.3 L of fluid (IQR 0.6–2.3) and those in the liberal group received 3.4 L (IQR 2.5–4.5 L).

Both groups experienced a similar primary outcome of 90-day mortality, and all respiratory outcomes were also similar. While CLOVERS demonstrated the safety of a restrictive approach to initial fluid resuscitation in sepsis, it did not suggest a unique benefit for respiratory failure. Two ongoing additional trials of initial fluid-volume strategy in sepsis (NCT04569942, NCT05179499) will further inform this question.

After an initial bolus of fluid for patients with sepsis, additional fluids to maintain hemodynamic goals may be beneficial, ineffective, or harmful. Several observational studies have found a more positive fluid balance is associated with increased morbidity and mortality.[33,41] The recent Conservative versus Liberal Approach to Fluid Therapy of Septic Shock in Intensive Care (CLASSIC) trial compared fluid management strategies after initial resuscitation among 1554 critically ill patients with sepsis and within 12 hours of the onset of shock.[42] The restrictive group was permitted fluid only under strict physiologic criteria to treat severe hypoperfusion with small volume boluses, while the standard-fluid group was not limited. At 5 days after enrollment, the median difference in fluid administered was 1.9 L and in cumulative fluid balance between groups was 0.7 L. The primary outcomes of death at 90 days showed no difference between the groups. Assessing the sub-group of patients with respiratory failure on ventilatory support at enrollment, however, demonstrated heterogeneity of treatment effect ($P = .03$) with an absolute difference in mortality of -5.1% (95%CI: -11.3%-1.6%) favoring the restrictive strategy. Among all patients in the trial, both groups had a similar respiratory failure outcome in ventilator-free days. Despite the relatively small separation between groups achieved by the restrictive fluid strategy, these data provide provocative evidence supporting a restrictive strategy for fluid administration in patients with sepsis and respiratory failure after the initial fluid bolus.

After resolution of shock from sepsis, very few trials have prospectively studied strategies for fluid removal by diuresis. In the FACTT trial, 70% of the patients had sepsis or pneumonia, suggesting that conclusions about the benefit of fluid limitation and diuresis in ARF can also be applied for patients with sepsis and ARF. A feasibility trial comparing a conservative fluid management strategy including diuretics to usual care enrolled 30 patients recovering from sepsis and was unable to achieve a meaningful difference in mean daily fluid balance to continue with a larger clinical trial, highlighting the difficulties in achieving substantial fluid removal in critically ill adults.[43]

Until recently, few trials had addressed fluid management strategies for patients who had both ARDS and sepsis.[44] While patients with sepsis are felt to need some intravenous fluids for resuscitation to meet physiologic targets, the optimal amount is not known. But recent data, particularly from CLOVERS and CLASSIC trials, suggest that a more conservative fluid management strategy in patients with respiratory failure and sepsis is safe and that it may even be beneficial in patients in the days following resuscitation. Across many trials, patients with sepsis are at risk of respiratory failure and protocols that increase fluid administration increase this risk. Each trial protocol provides different measures by which to individualize the treatment of sepsis with fluids to achieve physiologic parameters (eg, monitoring strategies, measures of fluid responsiveness). Minimizing variation in protocols is an important area for future trials to elucidate treatment effects and identify the best fluid management strategy for most patients.

LONG-TERM OUTCOMES OF FLUID MANAGEMENT IN ACUTE RESPIRATORY DISTRESS SYNDROME

There is a lack of studies informing the impact of fluid management strategy on long-term outcomes after ARF. Jolley and colleagues conducted a secondary analysis of the FACTT cohort to determine whether race modified the effect of fluid administration strategy on 1-year morality after ARDS.[45] The study included 655 non-Hispanic White and Black patients and demonstrated that conservative fluid management was associated with improved 1 year survival after ARDS only for Black patients (38% vs 54%, $P = .03$) and overall, there was a significant interaction between identified race and fluid treatment group ($P = .012$). While more studies are needed in this area, this suggests that the effect of fluid management strategy on longer term outcomes may not be homogenous across patient subgroups.

Mikkelsen and colleagues conducted neuropsychological testing of survivors enrolled in the FACTT trial by phone at 2 and 12 months after hospital discharge, and 75 patients (7.5% of the patients in FACTT) completed all testing.[46,47] Randomization to the conservative fluid management arm was independently associated with cognitive impairment at follow-up. This surprising finding has no obvious mechanistic cause, as physiologic parameters like cardiac index or systolic blood pressure were similar between the study groups and thus do not suggest reduced cerebral perfusion occurred in the conservative fluid group. The sample of patients in this secondary analysis was highly vulnerable to selection bias due to patients lost to follow-up or the competing risk of death, which limits the interpretation of this study.

Among patients with septic shock who were enrolled in the CLASSIC trial, a follow-up study obtained 1-year accounted for cognitive outcomes of 86.3% of enrolled patients' Mini MoCA tool[48] in 568 survivors. However, there was no difference in cognitive testing among survivors (adjusted odds ratio 1.01 (95%CI: 0.95–1.07)) or all patients accounting for those who were known to have died. The authors also found no difference in mortality or health-related quality of life by the fluid strategy assigned in the trial. Overall, the potential impact of fluid management strategies on post-hospital patient-centered outcomes in survivors of ARF remains largely unknown.

FLUID CHOICE IN ACUTE RESPIRATORY FAILURE AND ACUTE RESPIRATOR DISTRESS SYNDROME

Ideally, intravenous fluids would provide hemodynamic benefit by expanding intravascular volume to increase cardiac output without worsening interstitial edema like that seen in ARDS. No fluid type is without physiologic complications, but those available for use can be divided into 2 categories: colloids and crystalloids. Colloids such as human serum albumin are fluids that contain large molecules such which cannot readily pass through healthy capillary membranes into interstitial spaces, while crystalloids are solutions of electrolytes in water that can easily do so.

Colloids are of particular interest in patients with respiratory failure given hypoproteinemia is associated with ARDS as a risk factor. The Saline versus Albumin Fluid Evaluation (SAFE) trial randomized 6997 critically ill adult patients to a 4% albumin solution or normal saline for resuscitation. There was no difference in mortality among the groups and among the prespecified subgroup of patients with ARDS.[25] A follow-up trial, the Albumin Italian Outcome Sepsis (ALBIOS) trial, enrolled only patients with sepsis and used 20% albumin to achieve a target serum album level.[49] The ALBIOS trial found no difference between groups in the primary outcome, and the secondary and tertiary respiratory outcomes were also not different.

In addition to its role as a resuscitation fluid, colloids have also been used to facilitate fluid removal. Martin and colleagues randomized 37 patients with hypoproteinemia and ARDS to receive furosemide and albumin compared to furosemide with placebo.[24] The combination of albumin and furosemide improved outcomes, demonstrating the albumin was beneficial for diuresis but showed no difference in patient-centered outcomes.[24] A systematic review and meta-analysis of the 206 patients randomized to colloid therapy versus crystalloid in ARDS reinforced the limitations of these available data and the importance of larger trials to inform this question.[50]

Crystalloid fluids are one of the most commonly administered therapies to hospitalized adults, and they are typically categorized into unbalanced (eg, saline (0.9% sodium chloride)) or balanced (eg, Lactated Ringer's, Normosol-R) solutions. While saline includes supra-physiologic concentrations of chloride, balanced solutions contain an organic anion which allows for a reduced concentration of chloride and a more neutral pH compared to the more acidemic saline. Several large, randomized trials have been completed in the last 10 years to compare balanced solutions versus saline[51–54] and a Bayesian meta-analysis using data from 34,450 trial participants concluded with an 89.5% probability that balanced crystalloid solutions were associated with lower mortality compared to saline.[55] No analysis examined the subgroup with respiratory failure, but these patients were well represented as many of the thousands of critically-ill patients were receiving invasive mechanical ventilation in the SMART[51] (34%), BASICS[53] (44%), and PLUS[54](79%) trials. These trials found no effect from crystalloid fluid types on the number of days alive and free of mechanical ventilation outcome, suggesting that patients with respiratory failure are unlikely to derive unique benefit from balanced solutions.

REVIEW OF PROPOSED METRICS TO GUIDE FLUID RESUSCITATION IN ACUTE RESPIRATORY FAILURE

Diagnostic metrics ideally should be used to assess hemodynamics and guide fluid responsiveness in ARF particularly in patients with persistent circulatory failure (shock) where the goal is to resuscitate and optimize tissue perfusion. An ideal metric would be easy and safe to measure, consistent, reliable in predicting fluid responsiveness, and proven to lead to improved patient outcomes. No such metric has been identified solely for this purpose.

Extravascular Lung Water

Extravascular lung water (EVLW) is the volume of water in the lungs (normal index is < 7 mL/kg of ideal body weight) and a prognostic predictor of mortality in critically ill patients and ARDS.[56–58] EVLW can correlate with the severity of pulmonary edema with an increase up to 40 to 50 mL/kg body weight and it has been recommended as a potential quantitative parameter to guide fluid management in ARDS. An RCT of 101 critically ill patients compared a protocol of fluid management targeting a lower EVLW to a protocol based on PCWP with a primary outcome of development or resolution of pulmonary edema[15] Fluid restriction based on EVLW was associated with fewer ventilator, ICU days and a nearly neutral cumulative fluid balance over 3 days compared to a 2 L fluid excess in the PCWP group. Another small study comparing EVLW to PCWP for fluid management in 29 patients with ARDS found that utilizing EVLW reduced ventilator and ICU days.[59] However, while EVLW may be a useful tool to indicate fluid accumulation in lungs, the diagnostic framework for bedside measurement (transpulmonary thermodilution) and interpretation can be complex and it is not widely utilized in clinical practice yet. Further larger studies are needed and recently completed (HEAL Study, NCT00624650) to confirm its use for lung-targeted fluid strategies compared to metrics such as CVP and urine output in management of ARF.

Central Venous Pressure and Pulmonary Artery Wedge Pressure

CVP, commonly measured in critically ill patients via an indwelling CVC, may be used to measure intravascular volume as a surrogate for volume overload or right ventricular

(RV) failure. Studies have demonstrated poor correlation with other measures of fluid status. However, the FACTT study demonstrated that a CVP-guided strategy decreased duration of mechanical ventilation.[19] Notably, in the last 20 years since, fewer patients are managed with CVCs, further challenging implementation of the FACTT approach. Reducing pulmonary artery wedge pressure (PAWP) in ARDS with fluid restriction had been suggested to reduce mortality and increase ventilator-free days although studies have been limited by exclusion criteria and difficulty generalizing results to all ARDS patients[15] and sample size.[58] Overall, the routine use of the PACs to measure PAWP and guide fluid management is not recommended due to increased complications compared to CVCs with no improvement in mortality or organ function.[60]

Pulse Pressure Variation (PPV)

The respiratory variation of continuous PPV—difference between systolic and diastolic pressure—may be utilized as a reflection of ventricular stroke volume and and position on the Frank–Starling curve in patients with sinus rhythm. However, this method has not been validated and underperforms in patients with ARDS particularly due to the use of low tidal volumes in this population, and it may lead to increased false-positive rates in patients with RV dysfunction (a marker of potential fluid overload).[61,62]

Echocardiography/Ultrasound

The use of lung ultrasound to measure EVLW and detect aeration changes related to fluid administration may be used to detect pulmonary edema in patients with ARDS.[63,64] However, studies were small and the role of this tool in guiding fluid management in ARF needs further clarification. Critical care echocardiography is another important tool to assess hemodynamics in ventilated patients. Dynamic parameters such as the respiratory variations of the inferior vena cava diameter and Doppler velocity in the left ventricular outflow tract may be used to predict fluid responsiveness in ventilated patients. The ratio of right ventricle to left ventricule end-diastolic area could also provide evidence of RV dilatation and RV failure, with some limitations such as inter-operator variability.[65,66] End-expiratory and end-inspiratory occlusion changes on aortic doppler velocity can accurately predict fluid responsiveness in critical ill mechanically ventilated patients with ARF.[67] Other parameters such as measuring respiratory variation of the superior vena cava[65] may be useful in ARDS patients due to high sensitivity to predict fluid responsiveness. However, this is not a readily accessible metric as measurement requires the use of transesophageal echocardiography.

SPECIFIC CONSIDERATIONS IN ACUTE RESPIRATORY FAILURE AND RELATED FLUID STRATEGY

Surgical Patients

Patients with ARDS due to trauma may benefit from a strategy of diuresis and albumin to improve fluid balance and oxygenation.[23] Furthermore, a post-hoc analysis of surgical patients with ALI and ARDS in the FACTT cohort identified increased ventilator-free and ICU-free days with a conservative strategy.[68] Studies in the literature evaluating intra-operative and post-operative fluid administration in surgical patients have demonstrated an association between excessive fluid administration and incidence of postoperative pulmonary complications (ALI and ARDS) and a reduction in these complications in patients managed with a restrictive fluid strategy intra-operatively.[69] Based on current evidence, a restrictive strategy may be beneficial in

Table 1
Summary of select key studies assessing fluid management strategies in adult patients with or at risk of acute respiratory failure

Topic	Study Name, Author, Year	Study Design and Aim	Population	N	Key Findings
Patients with ARDS or ALI	FACTT,[19] NHLBI ARDS Clinical Trials Network, 2006	RCT comparing a conservative and liberal strategy within 48 h of ARDS/ALI diagnosis using strict protocols of fluid boluses, vasoactive medications, or diuresis guided by specific CVP or PCWP goals	ALI or ARDS	1001	No difference in 60-d mortality (primary outcome), incidence, or prevalence of shock or use of dialysis; improved oxygenation index and increased vent-free and ICU-free d with conservative strategy; significant difference in cumulative fluid balance (−136 mL in the conservative group compared to nearly 7L in liberal group)
	Sakr et al,[20] 2005	Multicenter observational study to evaluate variables and ventilator strategy associated with mortality	ALI and ARDS	3147	Positive fluid balance was associated with increased mortality
Patients at risk of ARDS	Mangiarlardi et al,[21] 2000	Multicenter observational study to evaluate outcomes in pts with hypoproteinemia compared to patients with normal serum total protein levels	Severe sepsis	455	92% of patients who developed ARDS had borderline or overt hypoproteinemia; associated with fluid retention, weight gain, prolonged mechanical ventilation, and mortality
	Chang et al,[22] 2014	Retrospective cohort study to examine associations between volume of IV fluids administered in resuscitative phase of sepsis and septic shock and development of ARDS	Severe sepsis and septic shock	296	No significant association between volume of IV fluids administered in the first 24 h of hospitalization and development of ARDS; serum albumin and APACHE II score on admission were most informative for development of ARDS

(continued on next page)

Table 1
(continued)

Topic	Study Name, Author, Year	Study Design and Aim	Population	N	Key Findings
Patients with severe sepsis or septic shock	CLOVERS,[28] PETAL network, 2023	Multicenter RCT compared a restrictive fluid strategy (with early vasopressor usage) to a liberal fluid strategy in sepsis-induced hypotension	Severe sepsis and septic shock	1503	No difference in 90-d mortality (primary outcome), vent-free d, ICU-free d, intubation from mechanical ventilation by d 27 or ARDS onset between d 1 and d 7
	FRESH,[40] Douglas et al, 2020	Multicenter RCT evaluating whether resuscitation (fluid bolus or increase in vasoactive medications) guided by dynamic assessment of FR (PLR) compared to usual care improved patient outcomes	Septic shock	150	Fluid balance at 72 h or ICU discharge (primary outcome) was significantly lower in intervention arm compared to usual care (1.3 L vs 2.02 L, $P = .021$); fewer patients in intervention arm required RRT (5.1% vs 17.5%, $P = .04$) or mechanical ventilation (17.7% vs 34.1%, $P = .04$)
	CLASSIC,[44] Meyhoff et al, 2016	Multicenter RCT comparing a restrictive strategy guided by strict physiologic criteria to standard care	Septic shock	1554	No difference in 90-d mortality (primary outcome); similar respiratory failure outcomes in vent-free d; in sub-group of patients with respiratory failure on ventilatory support (invasive or NIPPV) at enrollment, P-value for heterogeneity was 0.03 with an absolute difference in mortality of −5.1% favoring the restrictive fluid strategy

Fluid choice in ARF or ARDS				
SAFE,[50] Finfer et al, 2004	Multicenter RCT comparing FR with 4% albumin or normal saline	Critically ill patients	6997	No difference in 28-d mortality among groups (primary outcome) and no difference in mortality among pre-specified subgroup of patients with ARDS; no difference in vent-free d
ALBIOS,[51] Caironi et al, 2004	Multicenter RCT comparing 20% albumin and crystalloid or crystalloid alone	Severe sepsis	1818	No difference in 28-d or 90-d mortality among groups (primary outcome) or vent-free d
Martin et al,[23] 2002	Multicenter RCT comparing 5 d of 25 g of albumin q8 hours and continuous diuresis (furosemide) or dual placebo targeted to diuresis, weight loss, and serum total protein	Mechanically ventilated pts with ALI and hypoproteinemia	37	Improvements in the PaO_2/FiO_2 ratio in the treatment group within 24 h (from 171 to 236, $P = .02$); no difference in mortality or respiratory mechanics
Martin et al,[24] 2005	Multicenter RCT comparing furosemide with albumin or furosemide with placebo for 72 h, titrated to fluid loss and normalization of serum total protein concentration	Mechanically ventilated patients with ALI/ARDS and hypoproteinemia	40	Albumin-treated patients had greater increases in oxygenation (primary outcome) from baseline (mean change in PaO_2/FiO_2: +43 vs −24 mm Hg at 24 h and +49 vs −13 mm Hg at d 3), serum total protein (1.5 vs 0.5 g/dL at d 3), and net fluid loss (−5480 vs −1490 mL at d 3) throughout the study period (all $P<.05$)

Abbreviations: ALI, acute lung injury; APACHE II, acute physiology and chronic health evaluation; ARDS, acute respiratory distress syndrome; ARF, acute respiratory failure; CVP, central venous pressure; Fio₂, fraction of inspired oxygen; FR, fluid resuscitation; ICU, intensive care unit; IV, intravenous; NHLBI, national heart, Lung, and Blood Institute; NIPPV, non-invasive positive pressure ventilation; PaO₂, partial pressure of oxygen; PCWP, pulmonary capillary wedge pressure; PLR, passive leg raise; RCT, randomized controlled trial; RRT, renal replacement therapy.

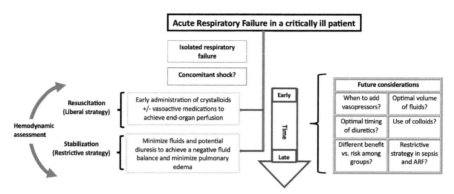

Fig. 1. Acute respiratory failure in a critically ill paitient. (Image created using Miro.)

surgical patients to minimize risk of ARF; however, the ideal fixed volume of fluids and type of fluid therapy are not well defined.[70]

Individualized approach

Given the multiple different etiologies of ARF with varying responses to treatment, this may lead to difficulty identifying a unifying strategy for fluid management. One proposal to address heterogeneity is identifying sub-phenotypes to distinguish who will respond to a specific therapy. Through latent class analysis of ARDS cohorts, 2 sub-phenotypes (hyperinflammatory and less inflammatory) were recently identified and have shown differing responses to ventilator strategies and inflammatory markers.[71] Famous and colleagues completed a secondary analysis of the FACTT study and demonstrated that a conservative fluid management strategy led to worse survival in the hyper-inflammatory phenotype of ARDS compared to the less inflammatory phenotype which had improved mortality with conservative fluid management.[72]

DISCUSSION

The accumulation of studies suggests fluid management in ARF is not as simple as an isolated liberal or conservative strategy for all patients (**Table 1**). These strategies are complementary and clinicians should personalize fluid management based on hemo-dynamic assessment, the clinical context, and response to ongoing therapy (**Fig. 1**). Ideally, this would mean consistently prioritizing a conservative fluid strategy in the absence of shock to facilitate weaning from mechanical ventilation and minimizing pulmonary edema.

GAPS IN LITERATURE

Future studies should address how to balance fluid strategy in patients with concom-itant shock and ARF, long-term outcomes, the optimal choice and quantity of fluid, timing of initiation of diuretics, and the proper hemodynamic metrics to guide fluid management.

SUMMARY

Research assessing fluid management in ARF has largely focused on patients with ARDS where hypoxemia can be exacerbated by leaky membrane permeability and non-cardiogenic pulmonary edema. While the optimal approach is unclear, studies suggest a conservative fluid management in patients with ARF who are not in shock is a safe strategy. More work is needed to understand the ideal approach for individual patients.

CLINICS CARE POINTS

> - There is evidence that a conservative fluid strategy in patients with ARDS who are no longer in shock is minimally harmful and should be the standard approach in this population. While studies suggest this may also be beneficial in patients with ARF and sepsis, more research is needed in patients at risk of ARDS.
>
> - While fluids are commonly used in critically ill patients, this can be harmful if administered inappropriately and it is imperative to consider the indication, dose, timing, and safety profile as analogous to the prescription of any other drug in critical care.
>
> - Fluid management may influence long-term outcomes and research on developing a personalized approach to fluid management and the appropriate volume and type of fluid to administer is urgently needed.

DISCLOSURE

The authors have nothing to disclose.

FUNDING

KS received support from NIH/NHLBI grant T32HL087738, CH received support from NIH grant K24141526. The authors have no conflicts of interest to disclose.

REFERENCES

1. Hakim R, Watanabe-Tejada L, Sukhal S, et al. Acute respiratory failure in randomized trials of noninvasive respiratory support: A systematic review of definitions, patient characteristics, and criteria for intubation. J Crit Care 2020;57:141–7.
2. ARDS Definition Task Force, Ranieri VM, Rubenfeld GD, et al. Acute respiratory distress syndrome: the Berlin Definition. JAMA 2012;307(23):2526–33.
3. Murphy CV, Schramm GE, Doherty JA, et al. The importance of fluid management in acute lung injury secondary to septic shock. Chest 2009;136(1):102–9.
4. Meyer NJ, Gattinoni L, Calfee CS. Acute respiratory distress syndrome. Lancet 2021;398(10300):622–37.
5. Huppert LA, Matthay MA, Ware LB. Pathogenesis of acute respiratory distress syndrome. Semin Respir Crit Care Med 2019;40(1):31–9.
6. Leigh JM. Pulmonary circulation and ventilation. Postgrad Med J 1974;50(587): 562–5.
7. Wang CY, Calfee CS, Paul DW, et al. One-year mortality and predictors of death among hospital survivors of acute respiratory distress syndrome. Intensive Care Med 2014;40(3):388–96.
8. Hyers TM. ARDS: the therapeutic dilemma. Chest 1990;97(5):1025.
9. Schuller D, Mitchell JP, Calandrino FS, et al. Fluid balance during pulmonary edema. Is fluid gain a marker or a cause of poor outcome? Chest 1991;100(4): 1068–75.
10. Hudson LD. Fluid management strategy in acute lung injury. Am Rev Respir Dis 1992;145(5):988–9.
11. Schuster DP. The case for and against fluid restriction and occlusion pressure reduction in adult respiratory distress syndrome. New Horiz 1993;1(4):478–88.

12. Acute Respiratory Distress Syndrome Network, Brower RG, Matthay MA, et al. Ventilation with lower tidal volumes as compared with traditional tidal volumes for acute lung injury and the acute respiratory distress syndrome. N Engl J Med 2000;342(18):1301–8.

13. Brower RG, Lanken PN, MacIntyre N, et al. Higher versus lower positive end-expiratory pressures in patients with the acute respiratory distress syndrome. N Engl J Med 2004;351(4):327–36.

14. Simmons RS, Berdine GG, Seidenfeld JJ, et al. Fluid balance and the adult respiratory distress syndrome. Am Rev Respir Dis 1987;135(4):924–9.

15. Mitchell JP, Schuller D, Calandrino FS, et al. Improved outcome based on fluid management in critically ill patients requiring pulmonary artery catheterization. Am Rev Respir Dis 1992;145(5):990–8.

16. Humphrey H, Hall J, Sznajder I, et al. Improved survival in ARDS patients associated with a reduction in pulmonary capillary wedge pressure. Chest 1990;97(5): 1176–80.

17. Rosenberg AL, Dechert RE, Park PK, et al, NIH NHLBI ARDS Network. Review of a large clinical series: association of cumulative fluid balance on outcome in acute lung injury: a retrospective review of the ARDSnet tidal volume study cohort. J Intensive Care Med 2009;24(1):35–46.

18. Cooke CR, Shah CV, Gallop R, et al. A simple clinical predictive index for objective estimates of mortality in acute lung injury. Crit Care Med 2009;37(6):1913–20.

19. National Heart, Lung, and Blood Institute Acute Respiratory Distress Syndrome (ARDS) Clinical Trials Network, Wiedemann HP, Wheeler AP, et al. Comparison of two fluid-management strategies in acute lung injury. N Engl J Med 2006; 354(24):2564–75.

20. Sakr Y, Vincent JL, Reinhart K, et al. High tidal volume and positive fluid balance are associated with worse outcome in acute lung injury. Chest 2005;128(5): 3098–108.

21. Mangialardi RJ, Martin GS, Bernard GR, et al. Hypoproteinemia predicts acute respiratory distress syndrome development, weight gain, and death in patients with sepsis. Ibuprofen in Sepsis Study Group. Crit Care Med 2000;28(9): 3137–45.

22. Chang DW, Huynh R, Sandoval E, et al. Volume of fluids administered during resuscitation for severe sepsis and septic shock and the development of the acute respiratory distress syndrome. J Crit Care 2014;29(6):1011–5.

23. Martin GS, Mangialardi RJ, Wheeler AP, et al. Albumin and furosemide therapy in hypoproteinemic patients with acute lung injury. Crit Care Med 2002;30(10): 2175–82.

24. Martin GS, Moss M, Wheeler AP, et al. A randomized, controlled trial of furosemide with or without albumin in hypoproteinemic patients with acute lung injury. Crit Care Med 2005;33(8):1681–7.

25. Finfer S, Bellomo R, Boyce N, et al. A comparison of albumin and saline for fluid resuscitation in the intensive care unit. N Engl J Med 2004;350(22):2247–56.

26. Mattox KL, Maningas PA, Moore EE, et al. Prehospital hypertonic saline/dextran infusion for post-traumatic hypotension. The U.S.A. Multicenter Trial. Ann Surg 1991;213(5):482–91.

27. Bulger EM, May S, Kerby JD, et al. Out-of-hospital hypertonic resuscitation after traumatic hypovolemic shock: a randomized, placebo controlled trial. Ann Surg 2011;253(3):431–41.

28. National Heart, Lung, and Blood Institute Prevention and Early Treatment of Acute Lung Injury Clinical Trials Network, Shapiro NI, Douglas IS, et al. Early Restrictive

or Liberal Fluid Management for Sepsis-Induced Hypotension. N Engl J Med 2023;388(6):499–510.

29. Rhee C, Dantes R, Epstein L, et al. Incidence and Trends of Sepsis in US Hospitals Using Clinical vs Claims Data, 2009-2014. JAMA 2017;318(13):1241–9.

30. Evans L, Rhodes A, Alhazzani W, et al. Surviving sepsis campaign: international guidelines for management of sepsis and septic shock 2021. Intensive Care Med 2021;47(11):1181–247.

31. Rivers E, Nguyen B, Havstad S, et al. Early goal-directed therapy in the treatment of severe sepsis and septic shock. N Engl J Med 2001;345(19):1368–77.

32. Bellani G, Laffey JG, Pham T, et al. Epidemiology, Patterns of Care, and Mortality for Patients With Acute Respiratory Distress Syndrome in Intensive Care Units in 50 Countries. JAMA 2016;315(8):788–800.

33. Mitchell KH, Carlbom D, Caldwell E, et al. Volume Overload: Prevalence, Risk Factors, and Functional Outcome in Survivors of Septic Shock. Ann Am Thorac Soc 2015;12(12):1837–44.

34. ProCESS Investigators, Yealy DM, Kellum JA, et al. A randomized trial of protocol-based care for early septic shock. N Engl J Med 2014;370(18):1683–93.

35. ARISE Investigators, ANZICS Clinical Trials Group, Peake SL, et al. Goal-directed resuscitation for patients with early septic shock. N Engl J Med 2014;371(16): 1496–506.

36. Mouncey PR, Osborn TM, Power GS, et al. Trial of early, goal-directed resuscitation for septic shock. N Engl J Med 2015;372(14):1301–11.

37. Investigators PRISM, Rowan KM, Angus DC, et al. Early, Goal-Directed Therapy for Septic Shock - A Patient-Level Meta-Analysis. N Engl J Med 2017;376(23): 2223–34.

38. Andrews B, Muchemwa L, Kelly P, et al. Simplified severe sepsis protocol: a randomized controlled trial of modified early goal-directed therapy in Zambia. Crit Care Med 2014;42(11):2315–24.

39. Andrews B, Semler MW, Muchemwa L, et al. Effect of an Early Resuscitation Protocol on In-hospital Mortality Among Adults With Sepsis and Hypotension: A Randomized Clinical Trial. JAMA 2017;318(13):1233–40.

40. Douglas IS, Alapat PM, Corl KA, et al. Fluid Response Evaluation in Sepsis Hypotension and Shock: A Randomized Clinical Trial. Chest 2020;158(4):1431–45.

41. Neyra JA, Li X, Canepa-Escaro F, et al. Cumulative Fluid Balance and Mortality in Septic Patients With or Without Acute Kidney Injury and Chronic Kidney Disease. Crit Care Med 2016;44(10):1891–900.

42. Meyhoff TS, Hjortrup PB, Wetterslev J, et al. Restriction of Intravenous Fluid in ICU Patients with Septic Shock. N Engl J Med 2022;386(26):2459–70.

43. Semler MW, Janz DR, Casey JD, et al. Conservative Fluid Management After Sepsis Resuscitation: A Pilot Randomized Trial. J Intensive Care Med 2020; 35(12):1374–82.

44. Silversides JA, Major E, Ferguson AJ, et al. Conservative fluid management or deresuscitation for patients with sepsis or acute respiratory distress syndrome following the resuscitation phase of critical illness: a systematic review and meta-analysis. Intensive Care Med 2017;43(2):155–70.

45. Jolley SE, Hough CL, Clermont G, et al. Relationship between Race and the Effect of Fluids on Long-term Mortality after Acute Respiratory Distress Syndrome. Secondary Analysis of the National Heart, Lung, and Blood Institute Fluid and Catheter Treatment Trial. Ann Am Thorac Soc 2017;14(9):1443–9.

46. Mikkelsen ME, Christie JD, Lanken PN, et al. The Adult Respiratory Distress Syndrome Cognitive Outcomes Study. Am J Respir Crit Care Med 2012;185(12): 1307–15.
47. Kjær MBN, Meyhoff TS, Sivapalan P, et al. Long-term effects of restriction of intravenous fluid in adult ICU patients with septic shock. Intensive Care Med 2023; 49(7):820–30.
48. Wong A, Nyenhuis D, Black SE, et al. Montreal Cognitive Assessment 5-minute protocol is a brief, valid, reliable, and feasible cognitive screen for telephone administration. Stroke 2015;46(4):1059–64.
49. Caironi P, Tognoni G, Masson S, et al. Albumin replacement in patients with severe sepsis or septic shock. N Engl J Med 2014;370(15):1412–21.
50. Uhlig C, Silva PL, Deckert S, et al. Albumin versus crystalloid solutions in patients with the acute respiratory distress syndrome: a systematic review and meta-analysis. Crit Care 2014;18(1):R10.
51. Semler MW, Self WH, Wanderer JP, et al. Balanced Crystalloids versus Saline in Critically Ill Adults. N Engl J Med 2018;378(9):829–39.
52. Self WH, Semler MW, Wanderer JP, et al. Balanced Crystalloids versus Saline in Noncritically Ill Adults. N Engl J Med 2018;378(9):819–28.
53. Zampieri FG, Machado FR, Biondi RS, et al. Effect of Intravenos Fluid Treatment With a Balanced Solution vs 0.9% Saline Solution on Mortality in Critically Ill Patients: The BaSICS Randomized Clinical Trial. JAMA 2021;326(9):1–12.
54. Finfer S, Micallef S, Hammond N, et al. Balanced Multielectrolyte Solution versus Saline in Critically Ill Adults. N Engl J Med 2022;386(9):815–26.
55. Hammond NE, Zampieri FG, Di Tanna GL, et al. Balanced Crystalloids versus Saline in Critically Ill Adults — A Systematic Review with Meta-Analysis. NEJM Evidence 2022;1(2):EVIDoa2100010.
56. Sakka SG, Klein M, Reinhart K, et al. Prognostic value of extravascular lung water in critically ill patients. Chest 2002;122(6):2080–6.
57. Jozwiak M, Silva S, Persichini R, et al. Extravascular lung water is an independent prognostic factor in patients with acute respiratory distress syndrome. Crit Care Med 2013;41(2):472–80.
58. Phillips CR, Chesnutt MS, Smith SM. Extravascular lung water in sepsis-associated acute respiratory distress syndrome: indexing with predicted body weight improves correlation with severity of illness and survival. Crit Care Med 2008;36(1):69–73.
59. Hu W, Lin CW, Liu BW, et al. Extravascular lung water and pulmonary arterial wedge pressure for fluid management in patients with acute respiratory distress syndrome. Multidiscip Respir Med 2014;9(1):3.
60. National Heart, Lung, and Blood Institute Acute Respiratory Distress Syndrome (ARDS) Clinical Trials Network, Wheeler AP, Bernard GR, et al. Pulmonary-artery versus central venous catheter to guide treatment of acute lung injury. N Engl J Med 2006;354(21):2213–24.
61. Lakhal K, Ehrmann S, Benzekri-Lefèvre D, et al. Respiratory pulse pressure variation fails to predict fluid responsiveness in acute respiratory distress syndrome. Crit Care 2011;15(2):R85.
62. Mahjoub Y, Pila C, Friggeri A, et al. Assessing fluid responsiveness in critically ill patients: False-positive pulse pressure variation is detected by Doppler echocardiographic evaluation of the right ventricle. Crit Care Med 2009;37(9):2570–5.
63. Zhao Z, Jiang L, Xi X, et al. Prognostic value of extravascular lung water assessed with lung ultrasound score by chest sonography in patients with acute respiratory distress syndrome. BMC Pulm Med 2015;15:98.

64. Caltabeloti F, Monsel A, Arbelot C, et al. Early fluid loading in acute respiratory distress syndrome with septic shock deteriorates lung aeration without impairing arterial oxygenation: a lung ultrasound observational study. Crit Care 2014; 18(3):R91.
65. Vignon P, Repessé X, Bégot E, et al. Comparison of Echocardiographic Indices Used to Predict Fluid Responsiveness in Ventilated Patients. Am J Respir Crit Care Med 2017;195(8):1022–32.
66. Vieillard-Baron A, Prigent A, Repessé X, et al. Right ventricular failure in septic shock: characterization, incidence and impact on fluid responsiveness. Crit Care 2020;24(1):630.
67. Jozwiak M, Depret F, Teboul JL, et al. Predicting Fluid Responsiveness in Critically Ill Patients by Using Combined End-Expiratory and End-Inspiratory Occlusions With Echocardiography. Crit Care Med 2017;45(11):e1131–8.
68. Stewart RM, Park PK, Hunt JP, et al. Less is more: improved outcomes in surgical patients with conservative fluid administration and central venous catheter monitoring. J Am Coll Surg 2009;208(5):725–35 [discussion 735-737].
69. Arslantas MK, Kara HV, Tuncer BB, et al. Effect of the amount of intraoperative fluid administration on postoperative pulmonary complications following anatomic lung resections. J Thorac Cardiovasc Surg 2015;149(1):314–20, 321.e1.
70. Bundgaard-Nielsen M, Secher NH, Kehlet H. "Liberal" vs. "restrictive" perioperative fluid therapy–a critical assessment of the evidence. Acta Anaesthesiol Scand 2009;53(7):843–51.
71. Calfee CS, Delucchi K, Parsons PE, et al. Subphenotypes in acute respiratory distress syndrome: latent class analysis of data from two randomised controlled trials. Lancet Respir Med 2014;2(8):611–20.
72. Famous KR, Delucchi K, Ware LB, et al. Acute Respiratory Distress Syndrome Subphenotypes Respond Differently to Randomized Fluid Management Strategy. Am J Respir Crit Care Med 2017;195(3):331–8.

Acute Respiratory Distress Syndrome

Definition, Diagnosis, and Routine Management

Philip Yang, MD, MSc[a],*, Michael W. Sjoding, MD, MSc[b]

KEYWORDS

- Acute respiratory distress syndrome • Heterogeneity • Phenotypes
- Lung-protective ventilation

KEY POINTS

- Acute respiratory distress syndrome (ARDS) is an acute inflammatory lung injury characterized by severe hypoxemic respiratory failure, bilateral opacities on chest imaging, and low lung compliance.
- ARDS is a heterogeneous syndrome that is the common end point of a wide variety of predisposing conditions, with complex pathophysiology and underlying mechanisms.
- Routine management of ARDS is centered on lung-protective ventilation strategies such as low tidal volume ventilation and targeting low airway pressures to avoid exacerbation of lung injury, as well as a conservative fluid management strategy.
- Advancements in molecular diagnostics and informatics tools may lead to a refined ARDS definition, improved understanding of ARDS heterogeneity and ARDS subphenotypes, and facilitate the development of novel therapeutic approaches.

INTRODUCTION

Acute respiratory distress syndrome (ARDS) is a rapidly progressive form of acute inflammatory lung injury associated with non-hydrostatic pulmonary edema and severe acute hypoxemic respiratory failure (AHRF).[1] It represents approximately 10% of all intensive care unit (ICU) admissions and 23% of all patients requiring mechanical ventilation.[2] However, clinicians frequently fail to recognize patients with ARDS in clinical practice and implement appropriate treatment strategies.[2] Furthermore, ARDS is a clinically heterogeneous syndrome with complex pathophysiology and underlying

[a] Division of Pulmonary, Allergy, Critical Care, and Sleep Medicine, Emory University, 6335 Hospital Parkway, Physicians Plaza Suite 310, Johns Creek, GA 30097, USA; [b] Division of Pulmonary and Critical Care Medicine, University of Michigan, 2800 Plymouth Road, NCRC, Building 16, G027W, Ann Arbor, MI 48109, USA
* Corresponding author. 6335 Hospital Parkway, Physicians Plaza Suite 310, Johns Creek, GA 30097.
E-mail address: philip.yang@emory.edu

Crit Care Clin 40 (2024) 309–327
https://doi.org/10.1016/j.ccc.2023.12.003
0749-0704/24/© 2023 Elsevier Inc. All rights reserved.

mechanisms, which has significantly limited the development of simple diagnostic tests or targeted pharmacologic therapies for ARDS that improve patient outcomes.[3] As such, ARDS continues to be associated with high mortality of up to 46% in severe cases.[1,2] The current management strategies for ARDS are largely limited to a few supportive measures that are centered around mechanical ventilation strategies aimed at avoiding further lung injury ("lung-protective ventilation" [LPV]). This article first reviews the current conceptual and clinical definitions of ARDS, current limitations in ARDS definition and diagnosis, and strategies to address those limitations. Then, it reviews the routine management strategies for ARDS, including noninvasive forms of respiratory support, invasive mechanical ventilation (IMV) with LPV strategies, and conservative fluid management.

CURRENT ACUTE RESPIRATORY DISTRESS SYNDROME DEFINITION, LIMITATIONS, AND PROPOSED CHANGES
Acute Respiratory Distress Syndrome Definition

ARDS is conceptually understood as an acute, diffuse, inflammatory lung injury leading to increased pulmonary vascular permeability and non-hydrostatic pulmonary edema, causing loss of aerated lung tissue, increased physiologic dead space, increased lung weight, and decreased lung compliance.[1] ARDS can arise from one of the many risk factors and predisposing conditions, which have historically been divided into "direct" and "indirect" causes of lung injury (**Table 1**).[4,5] Among the potential causes, pneumonia, aspiration of gastric contents, and sepsis are the most common causes of ARDS.[4] These conditions are heterogeneous in nature but eventually lead to the common pathway of acute inflammatory lung injury, resulting in the clinical findings of severe hypoxemic respiratory failure and bilateral pulmonary opacities on chest imaging.[1]

The formal clinical definition of ARDS has been updated several times because the initial description of the syndrome in a case series by Ashbaugh and colleagues.[6] This article focuses on the Berlin definition of ARDS published in 2012 (**Table 2**),[1] whose criteria are retained in the recently published Global Definition of ARDS[7] that builds on the Berlin definition. The Berlin definition was developed to address several limitations of its immediate predecessor, the American-European Consensus Conference (AECC) definition[5] for acute lung injury (ALI), and ARDS. Specifically, the Berlin definition explicitly defined "acute" as a 7-day period following a known clinical insult, required a positive end-expiratory pressure (PEEP) ≥ 5 cmH$_2$O (or continuous positive airway pressure [CPAP] ≥ 5 cmH$_2$O for patients with mild ARDS on noninvasive ventilation [NIV]) when evaluating oxygenation, and provided clarifications regarding

Table 1
Risk factors and predisposing conditions for acute respiratory distress syndrome

Direct Lung Injury	Indirect Lung Injury
• Pneumonia (bacterial, viral, or fungal)	• Sepsis from non-pulmonary source
• Aspiration of gastric contents	• Trauma or burn injury
• Toxic inhalational injury	• Pancreatitis
• Near drowning	• Drug overdose
• Pulmonary contusion	• Transfusion of blood products (transfusion-related acute lung injury [TRALI])
	• Cardiopulmonary bypass
	• Reperfusion edema after lung transplantation or embolectomy

Table 2
The Berlin definition of acute respiratory distress syndrome and mortality rates for different severity categories

Criteria	Definition		
Timing	Within 1 week of a known clinical insult or new or worsening respiratory symptoms		
Chest imaging	Bilateral opacities that are not fully explained by effusions, lobar/lung collapse, or nodules		
Origin of edema	Respiratory failure not fully explained by cardiac failure or fluid overload		
Hypoxemia		Mortality (Ranieri et al,[1] 2012)	Mortality (Bellani et al,[2] 2016)
Mild	200 mm Hg < $Pao_2/Fio_2 \leq 300$ mm Hg with PEEP or CPAP ≥ 5 cmH$_2$O	27%	34.9%
Moderate	100 mm Hg < $Pao_2/Fio_2 \leq 200$ mm Hg with PEEP ≥ 5 cmH$_2$O	32%	40.3%
Severe	$Pao_2/Fio_2 \leq 100$ mm Hg with PEEP ≥ 5 cmH$_2$O	45%	46.1%

Abbreviations: CPAP, continuous positive airway pressure; Pao_2/Fio_2, partial pressure arterial oxygen to fraction of inspired oxygen ratio; PEEP, positive end-expiratory pressure.

exclusion of hydrostatic edema without the use of pulmonary artery catheters (PACs).[1] It also defined three mutually exclusive severity categories of hypoxemia based on partial pressure of arterial oxygen to fraction of inspired oxygen (Pao_2/Fio_2) ratio, with more severe categories of hypoxemia correlating with increased mortality and decreased ventilator-free days (see **Table 2**).[1,2]

Limitations of the Berlin Acute Respiratory Distress Syndrome Definition

Although the Berlin definition of ARDS was developed to address some of the limitations of its predecessors, it is also not without its own shortcomings. First, the Berlin definition requires a patient to receive positive pressure ventilation, undergo arterial blood gas (ABG) sampling, and have either a chest radiograph or computed tomography (CT) performed to satisfy all of its diagnostic criteria. However, such diagnostic and therapeutic modalities may be difficult to obtain for all patients who are at risk of developing ARDS, especially in those who are being treated outside of ICU or in settings with limited resources.[8,9]

Second, a stated goal of the Berlin definition task force was to improve the reliability of the ARDS definition, particularly the interpretation of chest radiographs for bilateral opacities that has low interobserver reliability even among ARDS experts.[10] However, recent studies continue to demonstrate low interobserver reliability of chest radiograph interpretation for bilateral airspace opacities, which is the main driver of disagreements between physicians when identifying ARDS.[11] Efforts to improve reliability by training physicians and clinical research coordinators with a set of standard chest radiographs developed by the ARDS definition task force were ineffective,[12,13] highlighting the problematic nature of this essential criterion of the ARDS definition.

A third limitation of the Berlin definition is that it encompasses a heterogeneous syndrome with complex pathophysiology and underlying mechanisms and is inherently broad, nonspecific, and imprecise.[3] As a result, there is no standardized, gold-standard diagnostic test for ARDS.[3] The clinical manifestations of ARDS have been correlated with the histopathologic finding of diffuse alveolar damage (DAD) characterized by capillary congestion, pulmonary edema, injury to alveolar lining and endothelial cells, and hyaline membrane formation.[6,14] However, DAD is not the sole pathologic correlate of ARDS and was present in only 45% of patients with ARDS in an autopsy series.[15] Although DAD was more common in patients who met criteria for severe ARDS for more than 72 hours (69%),[15] it was still not a uniform finding, highlighting the clinical and pathologic heterogeneity of ARDS.

Underrecognition of Acute Respiratory Distress Syndrome in Clinical Practice

A related concern about the Berlin definition is that it may be difficult to operationalize at the bedside, resulting in poor recognition of ARDS in clinical practice and failure to administer evidence-based therapies for ARDS.[16] This was most clearly demonstrated in a large international prospective cohort study reporting that only 60% of ARDS cases were recognized by clinicians, with an increase in clinician recognition rates with increasing severity.[2] Moreover, clinician recognition of ARDS at the time of fulfilling ARDS criteria was even lower at 34%, suggesting that ARDS diagnosis was delayed in a substantial proportion of patients.[2] Additional studies have also reported poor clinician recognition rates of ARDS, ranging between 31% and 70%.[17–19]

Missed or delayed diagnoses of ARDS negatively impact the implementation of treatment measures that improve outcomes in ARDS. Several studies have reported overall low adherence to low tidal volume ventilation (LTVV) and substantial delays between ARDS onset and initiation of LTVV, thought to be at least partially due to poor recognition of ARDS.[2,19,20] Clinician recognition of ARDS has been associated with the use of LTVV and higher PEEP, as well as greater use of adjunctive measures such as prone positioning and neuromuscular blockade.[2,19] Therefore, improved methods to facilitate ARDS recognition may be important for timely implementation of appropriate therapies.

Modifications to the Berlin Acute Respiratory Distress Syndrome Definition

To address the concerns regarding the Berlin definition of ARDS, several proposals for modifications have been made. These proposals generally attempt to increase the applicability of the ARDS definition to capture patients who demonstrate clinical features of ARDS but do not strictly satisfy the current Berlin definition or are receiving care in settings where certain diagnostic tests are unavailable. For example, high-flow nasal oxygen (HFNO) has become increasingly popular for treatment of hypoxemic respiratory failure and ARDS since 2012, especially during the recent COVID-

19 pandemic.[21] However, the low-level positive pressure generated by HFNO is highly variable and cannot reliably satisfy the PEEP requirement of the Berlin definition.[22] In addition, some of the diagnostic testing modalities specified in the Berlin definition, such as ABG and radiographic testing, may not be readily available in settings with limited health care resources.[8,9]

One of the earlier proposals for modifying the Berlin definition, called the Kigali modification,[8] tried to address some of these issues. It proposed.

1. Removal of a PEEP requirement, to allow patients to be diagnosed without positive pressure ventilation
2. An oxygenation cutoff based on oxygen saturation by pulse oximetry (SpO_2) to Fio_2 ratio $\leq$315, in lieu of the Pao_2/Fio_2 ratio that requires ABG testing
3. The use of lung ultrasound as an acceptable imaging modality to assess for bilateral opacities, in addition to plain radiograph and CT.

In the original cohort study conducted in Kigali, Rwanda, these modifications allowed for identification of ARDS in patients who otherwise would not have fully satisfied the Berlin definition yet had severe hypoxemia with a high mortality of 50%.[8] Even in resource-rich settings, the Kigali modification could prove beneficial by facilitating earlier ARDS diagnosis in patients outside of the ICU who are not receiving positive pressure ventilation and avoiding the need for ABG testing and imaging modalities that use ionizing radiation.[9]

More recently, the Global Definition of ARDS[7] was published, which sought to build on the Berlin definition and address similar concerns discussed above. It includes components that are very similar to the Kigali modification, including.

1. Allowing HFNO with a minimum flow rate of 30 L/min, or NIV or CPAP with at least 5 cmH2O of end-expiratory pressure
2. Allowing either Pao_2/Fio_2 $\leq$300 or SpO_2/Fio_2 $\leq$315 with SpO_2 $\leq$97% to identify hypoxemia
3. Adding ultrasound as a modality of imaging to identify bilateral opacities
4. Not requiring PEEP, oxygen flow, or specific respiratory support devices to diagnose ARDS in resource variable settings.

In both proposed modifications, lung ultrasound can be used to identify bilateral opacities. However, the specific lung ultrasound findings of bilateral opacities have varied across studies. In the Kigali modification, bilateral opacities were identified by ultrasound findings of "B-lines" (an imaging artifact consistent with alveolar-interstitial edema) and/or consolidation without associated effusion in at least one area on each side of the chest.[8] However, a recent study proposed a more detailed, quantitative evaluation method called the lung ultrasound ARDS score that was validated against chest x-ray or CT images when available.[23] This score is calculated based on weighting the presence and type of abnormal ultrasound findings in 12 regions of the chest (six areas in each hemithorax), including the presence of abnormal pleural lines, B-lines, or consolidations.[23] Validation studies of these approaches in prospective studies across diverse populations will be necessary to demonstrate generalizability and standardize the ultrasound examination to support ARDS diagnosis.[24] Additional concerns regarding the use of ultrasound for ARDS diagnosis include inter-operator variability depending on the sonographer's training and external factors that make it difficult to obtain ultrasound images, such as obesity, catheters, and lines.[23,24] Owing to these limitations, the Global Definition of ARDS does not formally include specific ultrasound findings or scoring systems as a part of the definition.[7] Nonetheless, there is growing evidence to support the use of ultrasound for identifying bilateral opacities and to promote training in the use of lung ultrasound in evaluating patients with ARDS.[7]

EMERGING APPROACHES FOR IMPROVING THE ACUTE RESPIRATORY DISTRESS SYNDROME DEFINITION AND DIAGNOSIS

The above modifications to the ARDS definition will make it more inclusive and easier to be applied in wider clinical contexts, which may allow for increased inclusion into future epidemiologic studies, clinical research, and clinical trials for ARDS. However, these modifications may also make the ARDS definition more nonspecific and will not address the issues related to poor reliability and heterogeneity of the Berlin definition. Therefore, additional methods spanning molecular diagnostics and informatics domains are being studied to improve the reliability of the Berlin definition and to advance the pathophysiologic understanding of ARDS. Although all of these techniques require additional research before incorporation into a new ARDS definition, they all share a common goal of improving ARDS identification and phenotyping to facilitate earlier delivery of tailored interventions (**Fig. 1**).

Biomarkers for Improving Acute Respiratory Distress Syndrome Identification and Phenotyping

Several candidate biomarkers measured in serum or plasma have been studied for use in improving identification and risk stratification of patients with ARDS (**Table 3**). Measuring several of these biomarkers together may offer better diagnostic and prognostic accuracy than individual biomarkers by themselves, though studies differ with regard to which biomarkers are measured together.[25–27] Although most studies have focused on blood biomarkers, some studies have examined biomarkers from other body compartments, such as protein biomarkers from bronchoalveolar lavage fluid[28–30] and volatile organic compounds in exhaled breath condensates.[31,32] Advanced molecular techniques such as metabolomics[29,33–36] and proteomics[37–39] have also been explored to help identify ARDS and understand the details of its pathophysiology.

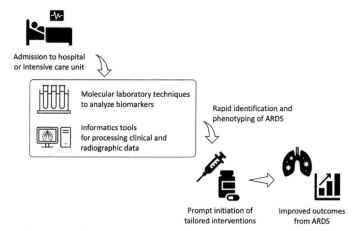

Fig. 1. Clinical and scientific tools being researched to improve identification and phenotyping of acute respiratory distress syndrome (ARDS).

Biomarkers have also played an important role in understanding the pathophysiologic heterogeneity of ARDS. Earlier studies in this area focused on correlating the biomarker profiles with the clinical risk factors or etiologies of ARDS. For example, surfactant protein-A (SP-A) and surfactant protein-D (SP-D) levels were shown to be higher in patients with ARDS from pneumonia than in patients with ARDS from trauma.[40] Another study demonstrated that von Willebrand factor (vWF) levels were lower in patients with trauma-associated ARDS compared with those with other causes of ARDS and lower in patients with indirect ARDS compared with those with direct ARDS.[41] Angiopoietin-2 (Ang-2) and SP-D were shown to correlate with ARDS from indirect versus direct lung injury, respectively, suggesting distinct mechanisms of lung injury caused by different etiologies of ARDS.[42]

More recently, sophisticated statistical methods analyzing both biomarker and clinical data have been used to divide patients into ARDS subphenotypes, thereby reducing the heterogeneity of patients within the groups. In secondary analyses of several ARDS clinical trials, latent class analysis (LCA) has consistently identified two distinct subphenotypes of ARDS based on clinical and laboratory data.[43–46]

Table 3
Select candidate biomarkers for acute respiratory distress syndrome identification and risk stratification

Biomarker	Mechanistic Involvement in Acute Respiratory Distress Syndrome (ARDS)
Soluble receptor for advanced glycation end products (sRAGE)[25,26,90–92]	Marker of lung epithelial injury. Extracellular domain of multiligand receptor expressed on alveolar type 1 cells and may be a causal intermediate in sepsis-induced ARDS.
Surfactant protein-D (SP-D)[26,40,93,94]	Marker of lung epithelial injury. Synthesized in alveolar type 2 cells and non-ciliated bronchiolar epithelium, involved in lung inflammation.
Angiopoietin-2 (Ang-2)[25,95,96]	Marker of lung endothelial injury. Binds Tie2 receptors on lung endothelial cells and impairs endothelial barrier function.
Von Willebrand factor (vWF)[41,95]	Marker of lung endothelial injury. Glycoprotein involved with hemostasis, released by endothelial cells in endothelial injury.
Soluble intercellular adhesion molecule-1 (sICAM-1)[30,97]	Marker of both lung epithelial and endothelial injury. Expressed on both alveolar epithelial and vascular endothelial cells, involved in neutrophil recruitment into the lung.
Interleukin-6 and interleukin-8[25,98]	Nonspecific pro-inflammatory cytokine.
Tumor necrosis factor-α (TNF-α)[25,98]	Nonspecific pro-inflammatory cytokine.
Soluble tumor necrosis factor receptor (sTNFR)-1 and −2[99]	Binds circulating TNF-α and regulates inflammatory response.
Plasminogen activator inhibitor-1 (PAI-1)[100,101]	Inhibitor of fibrinolysis contributes to fibrin deposition in alveolar spaces.

One of the two subphenotypes was characterized by elevated levels of inflammatory biomarkers, such as interleukin (IL)-6, IL-8, soluble tumor necrosis factor receptor (sTNFR)-1, and plasminogen activator inhibitor (PAI)-1.[43–46] This subphenotype, labeled the "hyper-inflammatory" phenotype, was consistently associated with higher mortality and worse clinical outcomes compared with the "hypo-inflammatory" phenotype. More strikingly, the hyper-inflammatory subphenotype seemed to benefit significantly from higher PEEP strategy,[43] simvastatin therapy,[44] and liberal fluid strategy,[45] whereas the hypo-inflammatory subphenotype had no benefit or even harm from such therapies. The subphenotypes were subsequently validated in two prospective observational cohorts of ARDS patients, further supporting their generalizability.[47] These results indicate that biomarkers can be informative for identifying ARDS subphenotypes with unique biological characteristics and treatment responses and have the potential to inform future clinical trials.

However, significant challenges still remain in the application of biomarkers in clinical settings. Many biomarker studies show significant variations in patient populations and methodology, making it difficult to establish the optimal timing and method of biomarker measurement. There is also no consensus regarding which biomarker, or panel of biomarkers, most reliably identify ARDS or its subphenotypes. In the studies of LCA-derived ARDS subphenotypes, attempts to develop parsimonious models using just three to five biomarkers and clinical variables (instead of > 30 variables included in the full models) found slightly different sets of biomarkers to be useful for identifying the ARDS subphenotypes.[43,45,46] Moreover, many of the promising biomarkers are not yet available for rapid measurement in clinical laboratories, and the capability to measure the biomarkers in real time still needs to be developed.[44,46] Further research is necessary to standardize the methods and timing of biomarker measurement, validate the reproducibility of biomarker-based ARDS identification and phenotyping across diverse populations, and determine whether personalized treatment strategies based on subphenotypes can indeed improve outcomes.[48]

Informatics Approaches for Improving Reliability of Acute Respiratory Distress Syndrome Recognition

The wealth of clinical data available in electronic medical record (EMR) systems has led to the development of several promising informatics techniques to improve ARDS detection. If deployed, these tools could help to improve the poor recognition of ARDS in clinical practice. Although clinical scores for early identification of ARDS such as the Lung Injury Prediction Score[49] were developed previously, many of its components required manual chart review by clinicians, making it difficult to automate within EMR. Other earlier studies examined automated, rule-based "sniffer" tools that analyzed EMR data to screen patients who may have ARDS, relying primarily on qualifying Pao_2/Fio_2 ratios and keywords contained in chest imaging reports (such as "bilateral," "infiltrates," and "edema").[50,51] Recent advances in machine learning (ML) and artificial intelligence techniques have led to the further development of sophisticated models that can process a large amount of clinical information to identify ARDS earlier in its course.[52–55] Given the poor reliability of chest imaging interpretation, methods incorporating chest radiographs — such as natural language processing applied to radiology reports[56] and deep convolutional neural network to detect ARDS findings on chest radiograph images[57] — have also been studied with promising results.

Although most informatics tools focus on improving the reliability and timeliness of ARDS identification, they have been used to corroborate the aforementioned hyper- and hypo-inflammatory subphenotypes of ARDS[58,59] as well as to explore a novel previously undefined phenotypes of ARDS.[60] These phenotypes demonstrate different treatment responses and distinct clinical characteristics and may have implications for designing and selecting patients for future clinical trials in ARDS.

There are still numerous barriers that need to be overcome before the novel informatics tools for ARDS can be implemented in clinical settings. Most existing studies use retrospective data or secondary analyses of clinical trials, and more prospective studies are needed to validate the model performance and generalizability, especially across different institutions with different patient populations, data recording practices, and/or data processing capabilities.[61] It is also unclear whether the ML model predictions can facilitate meaningful clinical interventions or prevention of ARDS that would not have been possible otherwise,[61] given the rapid onset of ARDS and narrow therapeutic window.[2,62] In addition, the inner workings of the so-called "black-box" algorithms need to be evaluated for their physiologic validity and credibility.[61]

ROUTINE MANAGEMENT STRATEGIES FOR ACUTE RESPIRATORY DISTRESS SYNDROME

Current management strategies for ARDS mainly consist of supportive care, including various modalities of oxygen support and mechanical ventilation strategies designed to reduce further lung injury LPV). Numerous clinical trials of potential ARDS therapies have failed to demonstrate benefit, and no specific pharmacologic therapy currently exists,[3] which is likely explained by the significant clinical and pathophysiologic heterogeneity of patients meeting the current ARDS definition.

Noninvasive Modalities of Oxygen Support

The Berlin definition of ARDS specifies that a patient should be receiving positive pressure ventilation with at least 5 cmH$_2$O of PEEP to satisfy the definition of ARDS based on the fact that PEEP can markedly affect oxygenation and the Pao$_2$/Fio$_2$ ratio.[1] The PEEP requirement could be met during administration of noninvasive positive pressure ventilation (NIPPV) for patients with mild ARDS. HFNO, a newer modality of noninvasive respiratory support that also provides variable levels of PEEP, emerged after the Berlin definition was established. The recent increase in the use of HFNO for treatment of AHRF and ARDS has resulted in the inclusion of HFNO in the new Global Definition of ARDS described above.[7]

However, it is important to note that the benefit of HFNO or NIPPV for improving outcomes from ARDS has not been clearly demonstrated in clinical trials. The results of individual clinical trials of HFNO conducted in various clinical contexts (both before and during the COVID-19 pandemic) have not individually demonstrated a convincing benefit of HFNO therapy, with mixed signals for mortality benefit or intubation rates when compared with standard oxygen therapy or NIPPV.[63–66] A subsequent pooled analyses of these clinical trials and additional studies found potential benefit of HFNO for preventing intubation, but not for reducing mortality.[48] Clinical trials comparing HFNO and NIPPV also have not demonstrated a clear mortality benefit of either treatment modality and have produced somewhat conflicting results for reducing intubation rates.[63,64,67,68] In addition, when the results of several clinical trials comparing conventional oxygen therapy to NIPPV were analyzed for the development of the European Society of Intensive Care Medicine (ESICM) guidelines, there was no significant benefit of NIPPV over conventional therapy for reducing intubation or mortality, leading the guideline committee to not recommend one therapy over the other.[48] Although NIPPV may have a strong physiologic rationale, these potential benefits may be countered by its potential harms including poor patient tolerance, impaired ability to clear secretions, increased risk of patient self-induced lung injury, and delayed intubation.[48] NIPPV via helmet interface was also explored as an alternative to the traditional face mask in a small single-center trial,[69] but additional data to support its utility are lacking.

As a consequence, the only affirmative recommendation regarding noninvasive respiratory support in the recent ESICM ARDS guidelines is for using HFNO over conventional oxygen therapy to reduce the risk of intubation (but not to reduce mortality).[48] Otherwise, the ESICM guidelines do not make a recommendation for or against the use of HFNO versus NIPPV or NIPPV versus conventional oxygen therapy.[48] For patients with AHRF or ARDS who are initiated on HFNO therapy, clinical scores such as the respiratory rate-oxygenation index (defined as SpO_2/FiO_2 ratio divided by the respiratory rate) can be helpful for evaluating the risk of HFNO failure and determining whether or not HFNO therapy can be continued.[70,71] However, many patients with ARDS will develop worsening respiratory failure and will ultimately require endotracheal intubation and IMV.

Lung-Protective Ventilation

Once a patient with ARDS is placed on IMV, supportive management is centered on "lung-protective" mechanical ventilation strategies to mitigate several potential mechanisms of ventilator-induced lung injury in ARDS. First, atelectasis and pulmonary edema reduce aerated lung volumes in patients with ARDS. In such cases, even "normal" tidal volumes that may be physiologic for uninjured lungs may nonetheless result in regional overdistention of aerated lung in ARDS and cause "volutrauma."[72] A related mechanism of injury is "barotrauma," which also results from regional lung overdistension (with or without increased airway pressures) and can lead to alveolar rupture, air leaks, and other complications such as pneumothorax and pneumomediastinum.[73] In addition, repetitive opening and closing of alveoli with tidal breaths and the corresponding shearing injury to the lungs may amplify regional lung strain, resulting in "atelectrauma."[73,74] Together, these mechanisms exacerbate and perpetuate lung epithelial and endothelial injury associated with ARDS, which then leads to release of pro-inflammatory mediators and worsening systemic inflammation ("biotrauma").[4,73] As such, mechanical ventilation strategies in ARDS should be optimized to minimize further lung injury.

This is first achieved by ensuring that patients receive low tidal volumes to reduce volutrauma and overdistension injury. In a landmark randomized controlled trial (RCT) from the ARDS network, patients receiving low tidal volume ventilation strategy (initial tidal volume of 6 mL per kg of ideal body weight [IBW] and targeting plateau pressure ≤ 30 cmH$_2$O) had significantly lower mortality and higher 28-day ventilator-free days compared with those receiving "traditional" tidal volume ventilation strategy (initial tidal volume of 12 mL per kg of IBW and targeting plateau pressure ≤ 50 cmH$_2$O), causing the trial to be stopped early.[72] Of note, the low tidal volume ventilation group had higher PEEP and FiO_2 requirements as well as more respiratory acidosis than the traditional ventilation group, but nonetheless had greater reductions in plasma IL-6 concentrations, indicating reduced inflammatory response with lower tidal volumes.[72] Based on the results of this trial and analysis of other studies, multiple society guidelines for ARDS all recommend strategies that limit tidal volumes (4–8 mL/ kg of IBW) and plateau pressures (<30 cmH$_2$O).[48,75]

Another important consideration in minimizing further lung injury is using higher PEEP, though the benefits of this strategy are less clearly defined than those of low tidal volume ventilation. Although it was believed that higher PEEP may improve alveolar recruitment and minimize lung injury associated with cyclical alveolar collapse, there were also concerns regarding the potential harms of higher PEEP such as lung overdistension and circulatory depression.[74] Three large RCTs did not demonstrate a significant mortality benefit for the higher PEEP strategy, though there were some improvements in oxygenation and other secondary end points with the higher PEEP strategy.[76–78] When the individual patient data from these three trials were pooled in a meta-analysis, there was potential benefit of higher PEEP strategy in patients with moderate or severe ARDS (Pao_2/Fio_2 $\leq$200 mm Hg), but not in patients with mild ARDS.[74] Secondary analysis of additional clinical trials also did not demonstrate a significant difference in mortality or other clinical outcomes with higher PEEP strategy[75] and using esophageal pressure monitoring (as an estimate of pleural pressure) to guide PEEP titration also did not demonstrate improved outcomes from ARDS compared with empirical high-PEEP strategy.[79] As such, the ideal method for titrating or setting PEEP is not clearly established, and the guidelines do not make clear recommendations for higher PEEP strategy (one guideline with conditional recommendation for higher PEEP strategy and another with no recommendation).[48,75]

Additional studies have suggested that it is not necessarily the PEEP itself, but rather the combined effect of tidal volume and PEEP on airway pressures and lung mechanics that may have a stronger impact on lung injury and clinical outcomes. In a secondary analysis of individual patient data from nine ARDS clinical trials, the driving pressure (defined as the plateau pressure minus PEEP, which is equal to the ratio of tidal volume to respiratory system compliance and is a surrogate for cyclic lung strain with each tidal breath) was examined as an independent variable associated with survival.[80] The study showed that lower driving pressure (indicating lower tidal volume in relation to a given respiratory system compliance) was most strongly associated with survival and that changes in the plateau pressure or PEEP were not individually associated with survival unless they led to a concurrent reduction in the driving pressure. This study provided insight that higher PEEP strategy may be beneficial only if the increased PEEP improves alveolar recruitment and lung mechanics such that the same tidal volume can be delivered with a lower lung strain.[80]

Although the optimal strategy for adjusting ventilator settings in ARDS remains unclear based on available evidence, dynamic adjustment of tidal volume and PEEP to achieve low plateau pressure and perhaps low driving pressure is a reasonable approach. Based on the currently available guidelines,[48,75] a possible starting point would be to set a tidal volume of around 6 mL/kg of IBW (acceptable range 4–8 mL/kg of IBW) and following the protocol for higher PEEP strategy that was used in one of three RCTs mentioned above (ALVEOLI [Assessment of Low Tidal Volume and Elevated End-Expiratory Volume to Obviate Lung Injury],[76] LOV [Lung Open Ventilation] Study,[77] EXPRESS [Expiratory Pressure][78]), then monitoring the resulting changes in airway pressures. Subsequently, the ventilator settings should be adjusted incrementally to achieve plateau pressure $\leq$30 cmH_2O and driving pressure $\leq$15 cmH_2O while carefully monitoring for potential complications such as excessive impairments in oxygenation, acid–base balance, or hemodynamics.

Conservative Fluid Strategy

Although it is not explicitly discussed in either of the recent ARDS guidelines, another important supportive measure in ARDS is conservative fluid strategy. Although restricting fluid intake and increasing urinary output are thought to be beneficial for decreasing lung edema and improving clinical outcomes, such strategy may cause decreased cardiac output and worsening of non-pulmonary organ function.[81] This risk–benefit balance was assessed in the FACTT trial,[81] in which patients with ARDS were assigned to either conservative versus liberal fluid strategies and either PAC versus central venous catheter in a two-by-two factorial design. The participants' central venous pressure or pulmonary artery occlusion pressure, systemic mean arterial pressure, urine output, and cardiac index were measured to determine their fluid status and prescribe appropriate interventions, consisting of various combinations of fluid, vasopressors, inotropes, and/or diuretics depending on their randomization assignment. Although there was no difference in 60-day mortality between the conservative versus liberal fluid groups, the conservative fluid group had higher 28-day ventilator-free days and ICU-free days, as well as better lung injury scores and oxygenation indexes, without an increase in non-pulmonary organ failures.[81] A subsequent secondary analysis of this trial demonstrated potential differences in treatment responses to fluid strategies between ARDS subphenotypes,[45] but a separate RCT dedicated to evaluating this matter has not been conducted. The exact protocol used in the FACTT trial is difficult to follow, but conservative fluid strategy aimed at reducing fluid intake and increasing urinary output is considered beneficial for improving lung function and is generally preferred in patients with ARDS.

DISCUSSION

This article has focused on the current definition of ARDS and routine management strategies for ARDS that should be applied to nearly all patients with ARDS with only rare exceptions. However, such strategies entail general supportive ventilator management and fluid strategies, rather than targeting a specific ARDS pathophysiologic process. Even adjunctive and rescue therapies for ARDS—such as prone positioning, neuromuscular blockade, corticosteroids, and extracorporeal membrane oxygenation—merely seek to improve oxygenation/ventilation and reduce further lung injury, rather than address the underlying pathologic process. This may explain, at least partially, why mortality from ARDS has not improved significantly in recent years[82] despite some decline noted during the first decade of the 2000s.[83] This stagnation of improvements in ARDS mortality bears some resemblance to the failure of recent RCTs in sepsis[84–86] to replicate the benefits of early goal-directed therapy,[87] highlighting the need for improved recognition of ARDS as well as specific targeted therapies to further improve outcomes.

At the heart of this problem lies the clinical and pathophysiologic heterogeneity of patients meeting the current definition of ARDS. The AECC and Berlin definitions proved useful for establishing a uniform definition of ALI/ARDS and creating a framework for performing many of the practice-informing clinical trials. However, "lumping" different disease processes into a single syndromic definition and then attempting study treatments that target specific pathologic processes has proven exceedingly difficult. This problem has even led to criticisms about the utility and validity of ARDS as a clinical entity, along with suggestions to avoid the term "ARDS" in favor of more specific nomenclature based on concrete pathologic processes (eg, "pneumococcal respiratory distress," or "hypo- vs hyper-inflammatory lung failure").[88,89] In some ways, this is broadly consistent with the recent trends favoring precision medicine approaches in ARDS research, with an increasing focus on "splitting" ARDS into subphenotypes and endotypes that may respond differently to treatments. With the continued advancements in molecular techniques and informatics tools, this approach may lead to a more granular and refined understanding of the heterogeneous syndrome of ARDS. Such efforts could enable opportunities for innovative clinical trial design using prognostic and predictive enrichment to discovery of novel targeted therapies that may move us beyond the routine supportive therapies for ARDS.

SUMMARY

In summary, ARDS is a severe form of acute inflammatory lung injury that develops secondary to an inciting clinical event, which then leads to non-cardiogenic pulmonary edema, severe hypoxemic respiratory failure, bilateral opacities on chest imaging, and low lung compliance. Despite decades of research, mortality from ARDS remains high, with further improvements in outcomes being hindered by the clinical and pathologic heterogeneity inherent in its syndromic definition, underrecognition in clinical practice, and lack of therapies targeting specific pathologic processes in ARDS. The main treatment strategies for ARDS are supportive measures consisting of noninvasive oxygen support and IMV, LPV strategies, and conservative fluid strategy. The proposed changes to the clinical definition of ARDS, in combination with the advancements in clinical, laboratory, and informatics methods for diagnosing and phenotyping ARDS, may enable innovative approaches to ARDS clinical trials, discovery of novel ARDS therapies, and improvements in clinical outcomes from ARDS.

CLINICS CARE POINTS

- Acute respiratory distress syndrome (ARDS) is currently defined by the Berlin definition, but this definition may soon be updated to allow ARDS to be diagnosed with the use of (1) high-flow nasal oxygen (HFNO), without a requirement for positive end-expiratory pressure (PEEP); (2) SpO_2/Fio_2 criteria to identify hypoxia, without the need for arterial blood gas testing; and (3) ultrasound as an additional modality of imaging to identify bilateral opacities.

- HFNO and noninvasive ventilation are reasonable modalities of oxygen support in patients who are developing ARDS or have mild ARDS, but many patients with ARDS will subsequently require invasive mechanical ventilation.

- Lung-protective ventilation strategy in ARDS consists of delivering low tidal volumes (4–8 mL per kg of ideal body weight) to avoid lung overdistension and optimizing PEEP to promote alveolar recruitment such that plateau and driving pressures, which are surrogate measures of mechanical stress on the lungs, are minimized.

- Conservative fluid strategy should also be applied to ARDS patients to reduce lung edema, by reducing fluid intake and increasing urinary output within safe limits.

DISCLOSURE

The authors have no disclosures.

FUNDING

Dr Sjoding is supported by the National Heart, Lung, and Blood Institute (NHLBI) of the National Institutes of Health (NIH) under award number R01HL158626. The content is solely the responsibility of the authors and does not necessarily represent the official views of the National Institutes of Health.

REFERENCES

1. Ranieri V, Rubenfeld G, Thompson B, et al. Acute respiratory distress syndrome: the berlin definition. JAMA 2012;307(23):2526–33.
2. Bellani G, Laffey J, Pham T, et al, LUNG SAFE Investigators, ESICM Trials Group. Epidemiology, patterns of care, and mortality for patients with acute

respiratory distress syndrome in intensive care units in 50 countries. JAMA 2016;315(8):788–800.

3. Reilly JP, Calfee CS, Christie JD. Acute respiratory distress syndrome phenotypes. Semin Respir Crit Care Med 2019;40(1):19–30.

4. Thompson BT, Chambers RC, Liu KD. Acute respiratory distress syndrome. N Engl J Med 2017;377(6):562–72.

5. Bernard G, Artigas A, Brigham K, et al. The American-European consensus conference on ARDS. definitions, mechanisms, relevant outcomes, and clinical trial coordination. Am J Respir Crit Care Med 1994;149(3 Pt 1):818–24.

6. Ashbaugh DG, Bigelow DB, Petty TL, et al. Acute respiratory distress in adults. Lancet 1967;2(7511):319–23.

7. Matthay MA, Arabi Y, Arroliga AC, et al. A new global definition of acute respiratory distress syndrome. Am J Respir Crit Care Med 2023. https://doi.org/10.1164/rccm.202303-0558WS.

8. Riviello ED, Kiviri W, Twagirumugabe T, et al. Hospital incidence and outcomes of the acute respiratory distress syndrome using the Kigali modification of the berlin definition. Am J Respir Crit Care Med 2016;193(1):52–9.

9. Riviello ED, Buregeya E, Twagirumugabe T. Diagnosing acute respiratory distress syndrome in resource limited settings: the kigali modification of the berlin definition. Curr Opin Crit Care 2017;23(1):18–23.

10. Rubenfeld GD, Caldwell E, Granton J, et al. Interobserver variability in applying a radiographic definition for ARDS. Chest 1999;116(5):1347–53.

11. Sjoding MW, Hofer TP, Co IC, et al. Interobserver reliability of the berlin ARDS definition and strategies to improve the reliability of ARDS diagnosis. Chest 2018;153(2):361–7.

12. Peng JM, Qian CY, Yu XY, et al, China Critical Care Clinical Trial Group CCCCTG. Does training improve diagnostic accuracy and inter-rater agreement in applying the Berlin radiographic definition of acute respiratory distress syndrome? A multicenter prospective study. Crit Care 2017;21(1):12.

13. Goddard SL, Rubenfeld GD, Manoharan V, et al. The randomized educational acute respiratory distress syndrome diagnosis study: a trial to improve the radiographic diagnosis of acute respiratory distress syndrome. Crit Care Med 2018;46(5):743–8.

14. Katzenstein AL, Bloor CM, Leibow AA. Diffuse alveolar damage–the role of oxygen, shock, and related factors. A review. Am J Pathol 1976;85(1):209–28.

15. Thille AW, Esteban A, Fernandez-Segoviano P, et al. Comparison of the Berlin definition for acute respiratory distress syndrome with autopsy. Am J Respir Crit Care Med 2013;187(7):761–7.

16. Bellani G, Pham T, Laffey JG. Missed or delayed diagnosis of ARDS: a common and serious problem. Intensive Care Med 2020;46(6):1180–3.

17. Ferguson ND, Frutos-Vivar F, Esteban A, et al. Acute respiratory distress syndrome: underrecognition by clinicians and diagnostic accuracy of three clinical definitions. Crit Care Med 2005;33(10):2228–34.

18. Frohlich S, Murphy N, Doolan A, et al. Acute respiratory distress syndrome: underrecognition by clinicians. J Crit Care 2013;28(5):663–8.

19. Schwede M, Lee RY, Zhuo H, et al. Clinician recognition of the acute respiratory distress syndrome: risk factors for under-recognition and trends over time. Crit Care Med 2020;48(6):830–7.

20. Weiss CH, Baker DW, Weiner S, et al. Low tidal volume ventilation use in acute respiratory distress syndrome. Crit Care Med 2016;44(8):1515–22.

21. Crimi C, Pierucci P, Renda T, et al. High-flow nasal cannula and COVID-19: a clinical review. Respir Care 2022;67(2):227–40.

22. Parke R, McGuinness S, Eccleston M. Nasal high-flow therapy delivers low level positive airway pressure. Br J Anaesth 2009;103(6):886–90.

23. Smit MR, Hagens LA, Heijnen NFL, et al, DARTS Consortium members. Lung ultrasound prediction model for acute respiratory distress syndrome: a multicenter prospective observational study. Am J Respir Crit Care Med 2023; 207(12):1591–601.

24. Ware LB. Improving acute respiratory distress syndrome diagnosis: is lung ultrasound the answer? Am J Respir Crit Care Med 2023;207(12):1548–9.

25. Fremont RD, Koyama T, Calfee CS, et al. Acute lung injury in patients with traumatic injuries: utility of a panel of biomarkers for diagnosis and pathogenesis. J Trauma 2010;68(5):1121–7.

26. Ware LB, Koyama T, Zhao Z, et al. Biomarkers of lung epithelial injury and inflammation distinguish severe sepsis patients with acute respiratory distress syndrome. Crit Care 2013;17(5):R253.

27. Ware LB, Koyama T, Billheimer DD, et al, NHLBI ARDS Clinical Trials Network. Prognostic and pathogenetic value of combining clinical and biochemical indices in patients with acute lung injury. Chest 2010;137(2):288–96.

28. Albertine KH, Soulier MF, Wang Z, et al. Fas and fas ligand are up-regulated in pulmonary edema fluid and lung tissue of patients with acute lung injury and the acute respiratory distress syndrome. Am J Pathol 2002;161(5):1783–96.

29. Evans CR, Karnovsky A, Kovach MA, et al. Untargeted LC-MS metabolomics of bronchoalveolar lavage fluid differentiates acute respiratory distress syndrome from health. J Proteome Res 2014;13(2):640–9.

30. Agouridakis P, Kyriakou D, Alexandrakis MG, et al. The predictive role of serum and bronchoalveolar lavage cytokines and adhesion molecules for acute respiratory distress syndrome development and outcome. Respir Res 2002;3:25.

31. Bos LDJ, Schultz MJ, Sterk PJ. Exhaled breath profiling for diagnosing acute respiratory distress syndrome. BMC Pulm Med 2014;14:1–9.

32. Bos LDJ, Weda H, Wang Y, et al. Exhaled breath metabolomics as a noninvasive diagnostic tool for acute respiratory distress syndrome. Eur Respir J 2014;44(1): 188–97.

33. Stringer KA, Serkova NJ, Karnovsky A, et al. Metabolic consequences of sepsis-induced acute lung injury revealed by plasma 1H-nuclear magnetic resonance quantitative metabolomics and computational analysis. Am J Physiol Lung Cell Mol Physiol 2011;300(1):L4–11.

34. Stringer KA, Jones AE, Puskarich MA, et al. 1H-nuclear magnetic resonance (NMR)-detected lipids associated with apoptosis differentiate early acute respiratory distress syndrome (ARDS) from sepsis. Am J Respir Crit Care Med 2014;189:A5000.

35. Esper AM, Park Y, Martin GS, et al. Metabolomic analysis in sepsis and ARDS. Am J Respir Crit Care Med 2013;187:A2223.

36. Yang P, Hu X, Iffrig E, et al. Serial metabolomic analyses in sepsis-induced acute respiratory distress syndrome. Am J Respir Crit Care Med 2022;205:A5139.

37. Bowler RP, Dudag B, Chan ED, et al. Proteomic analysis of pulmonary edema fluid and plasma in patients with acute lung injury. Am J Physiol Lung Cell Mol Physiol 2004;286(6):L1095–104.

38. de Torre C, Ying SX, Munson PJ, et al. Proteomic analysis of inflammatory biomarkers in bronchoalveolar lavage. Proteomics 2006;6(13):3949–57.

39. Chen X, Shan Q, Jiang L, et al. Quantitative proteomic analysis by iTRAQ for identification of candidate biomarkers in plasma from acute respiratory distress syndrome patients. Biochem Biophys Res Commun 2013;441(1):1–6.
40. Eisner M, Parsons P, Matthay M, et al. Plasma surfactant protein levels and clinical outcomes in patients with acute lung injury. Thorax 2003;58(11):983–8.
41. Ware LB, Eisner MD, Thompson BT, et al. Significance of Von Willebrand factor in septic and nonseptic patients with acute lung injury. Am J Respir Crit Care Med 2004;170(7):766–72.
42. Calfee CS, Janz DR, Bernard GR, et al. Distinct molecular phenotypes of direct vs indirect ARDS in single-center and multicenter studies. Chest 2015;147(6): 1539–48.
43. Calfee CS, Delucchi K, Parsons PE, et al, NHLBI ARDS Network. Subphenotypes in acute respiratory distress syndrome: latent class analysis of data from two randomised controlled trials. Lancet Respir Med 2014;2(8):611–20.
44. Calfee CS, Delucchi KL, Sinha P, et al, Irish Critical Care Trials Group. Acute respiratory distress syndrome subphenotypes and differential response to simvastatin: secondary analysis of a randomised controlled trial. Lancet Respir Med 2018;6(9):691–8.
45. Famous KR, Delucchi K, Ware LB, et al, ARDS Network. Acute respiratory distress syndrome subphenotypes respond differently to randomized fluid management strategy. Am J Respir Crit Care Med 2017;195(3):331–8.
46. Sinha P, Delucchi KL, Thompson BT, et al, NHLBI ARDS Network. Latent class analysis of ARDS subphenotypes: a secondary analysis of the statins for acutely injured lungs from sepsis (SAILS) study. Intensive Care Med 2018;44(11): 1859–69.
47. Sinha P, Delucchi KL, Chen Y, et al. Latent class analysis-derived subphenotypes are generalisable to observational cohorts of acute respiratory distress syndrome: a prospective study. Thorax 2022;77(1):13–21.
48. Grasselli G, Calfee CS, Camporota L, et al, European Society of Intensive Care Medicine Taskforce on ARDS. ESICM guidelines on acute respiratory distress syndrome: definition, phenotyping and respiratory support strategies. Intensive Care Med 2023;49(7):727–59.
49. Gajic O, Dabbagh O, Park P, et al, U.S. Critical Illness and Injury Trials Group: Lung Injury Prevention Study Investigators USCIITG-LIPS. Early identification of patients at risk of acute lung injury: evaluation of lung injury prediction score in a multicenter cohort study. Am J Respir Crit Care Med 2011;183(4):462–70.
50. Herasevich V, Yilmaz M, Khan H, et al. Validation of an electronic surveillance system for acute lung injury. Intensive Care Med 2009;35(6):1018–23.
51. Koenig HC, Finkel BB, Khalsa SS, et al. Performance of an automated electronic acute lung injury screening system in intensive care unit patients. Crit Care Med 2011;39(1):98–104.
52. Le S, Pellegrini E, Green-Saxena A, et al. Supervised machine learning for the early prediction of acute respiratory distress syndrome (ARDS). J Crit Care 2020;60:96–102.
53. Zeiberg D, Prahlad T, Nallamothu BK, et al. Machine learning for patient risk stratification for acute respiratory distress syndrome. PLoS One 2019;14(3): e0214465.
54. Singhal L, Garg Y, Yang P, et al. eARDS: a multi-center validation of an interpretable machine learning algorithm of early onset Acute Respiratory Distress Syndrome (ARDS) among critically ill adults with COVID-19. PLoS One 2021;16(9): e0257056.

55. Wu W, Wang Y, Tang J, et al. Developing and evaluating a machine-learning-based algorithm to predict the incidence and severity of ARDS with continuous non-invasive parameters from ordinary monitors and ventilators. Comput Methods Programs Biomed 2023;230:107328.

56. Afshar M, Joyce C, Oakey A, et al. A computable phenotype for acute respiratory distress syndrome using natural language processing and machine learning. AMIA Annu Symp Proc 2018;2018:157–65.

57. Sjoding MW, Taylor D, Motyka J, et al. Deep learning to detect acute respiratory distress syndrome on chest radiographs: a retrospective study with external validation. Lancet Digit Health 2021;3(6):e340–8.

58. Maddali MV, Churpek M, Pham T, et al, LUNG SAFE Investigators and the ESICM Trials Group. Validation and utility of ARDS subphenotypes identified by machine-learning models using clinical data: an observational, multicohort, retrospective analysis. Lancet Respir Med 2022;10(4):367–77.

59. Sinha P, Churpek MM, Calfee CS. Machine learning classifier models can identify acute respiratory distress syndrome phenotypes using readily available clinical data. Am J Respir Crit Care Med 2020;202(7):996–1004.

60. Bai Y, Xia J, Huang X, et al. Using machine learning for the early prediction of sepsis-associated ARDS in the ICU and identification of clinical phenotypes with differential responses to treatment. Front Physiol 2022;13:1050849.

61. Wong AI, Cheung PC, Kamaleswaran R, et al. Machine learning methods to predict acute respiratory failure and acute respiratory distress syndrome. Front Big Data 2020;3:579774.

62. Shari G, Kojicic M, Li G, et al. Timing of the onset of acute respiratory distress syndrome: a population-based study. Respir Care 2011;56(5):576–82.

63. Frat JP, Thille AW, Mercat A, et al, FLORALI Study Group, REVA Network. High-flow oxygen through nasal cannula in acute hypoxemic respiratory failure. N Engl J Med 2015;372(23):2185–96.

64. Azoulay E, Lemiale V, Mokart D, et al. Effect of high-flow nasal oxygen vs standard oxygen on 28-day mortality in immunocompromised patients with acute respiratory failure: the high randomized clinical trial. JAMA 2018;320(20):2099–107.

65. Frat JP, Quenot JP, Badie J, et al, SOHO-COVID Study Group and the REVA Network. Effect of high-flow nasal cannula oxygen vs standard oxygen therapy on mortality in patients with respiratory failure due to COVID-19: the SOHO-COVID randomized clinical trial. JAMA 2022;328(12):1212–22.

66. Perkins GD, Ji C, Connolly BA, et al, RECOVERY-RS Collaborators. Effect of noninvasive respiratory strategies on intubation or mortality among patients with acute hypoxemic respiratory failure and COVID-19: the RECOVERY-RS randomized clinical trial. JAMA 2022;327(6):546–58.

67. Grieco DL, Menga LS, Cesarano M, et al, COVID-ICU Gemelli Study Group. Effect of helmet noninvasive ventilation vs high-flow nasal oxygen on days free of respiratory support in patients with COVID-19 and moderate to severe hypoxemic respiratory failure: the HENIVOT randomized clinical trial. JAMA 2021;325(17):1731–43.

68. Nair PR, Haritha D, Behera S, et al. Comparison of High-flow nasal cannula and noninvasive ventilation in acute hypoxemic respiratory failure due to severe COVID-19 pneumonia. Respir Care 2021;66(12):1824–30.

69. Patel BK, Wolfe KS, Pohlman AS, et al. Effect of noninvasive ventilation delivered by helmet vs face mask on the rate of endotracheal intubation in patients with

acute respiratory distress syndrome: a randomized clinical trial. JAMA 2016; 315(22):2435–41.

70. Roca O, Messika J, Caralt B, et al. Predicting success of high-flow nasal cannula in pneumonia patients with hypoxemic respiratory failure: the utility of the ROX index. J Crit Care 2016;35:200–5.

71. Roca O, Caralt B, Messika J, et al. An index combining respiratory rate and oxygenation to predict outcome of nasal high-flow therapy. Am J Respir Crit Care Med 2019;199(11):1368–76.

72. Brower R, Matthay M, Morris A, et al. Ventilation with lower tidal volumes as compared with traditional tidal volumes for acute lung injury and the acute respiratory distress syndrome. N Engl J Med 2000;342(18):1301–8.

73. Slutsky AS, Ranieri VM. Ventilator-induced lung injury. N Engl J Med 2013; 369(22):2126–36.

74. Briel M, Meade M, Mercat A, et al. Higher vs lower positive end-expiratory pressure in patients with acute lung injury and acute respiratory distress syndrome: systematic review and meta-analysis. JAMA 2010;303(9):865–73.

75. Fan E, Del Sorbo L, Goligher EC, et al, American Thoracic Society, European Society of Intensive Care Medicine, and Society of Critical Care Medicine. An official American thoracic society/European society of intensive care medicine/society of critical care medicine clinical practice guideline: mechanical ventilation in adult patients with acute respiratory distress syndrome. Am J Respir Crit Care Med 2017;195(9):1253–63.

76. Brower RG, Lanken PN, MacIntyre N, et al, National Heart, Lung, and Blood Institute ARDS Clinical Trials Network. Higher versus lower positive end-expiratory pressures in patients with the acute respiratory distress syndrome. N Engl J Med 2004;351(4):327–36.

77. Meade MO, Cook DJ, Guyatt GH, et al, Lung Open Ventilation Study Investigators. Ventilation strategy using low tidal volumes, recruitment maneuvers, and high positive end-expiratory pressure for acute lung injury and acute respiratory distress syndrome: a randomized controlled trial. JAMA 2008;299(6):637–45.

78. Mercat A, Richard JCM, Vielle B, et al, Expiratory Pressure Express Study Group. Positive end-expiratory pressure setting in adults with acute lung injury and acute respiratory distress syndrome: a randomized controlled trial. JAMA 2008;299(6):646–55.

79. Beitler JR, Sarge T, Banner-Goodspeed VM, et al, EPVent-2 Study Group. Effect of titrating positive end-expiratory pressure (peep) with an esophageal pressure-guided strategy vs an empirical high peep-fio2 strategy on death and days free from mechanical ventilation among patients with acute respiratory distress syndrome: a randomized clinical trial. JAMA 2019;321(9):846–57.

80. Amato MB, Meade MO, Slutsky AS, et al. Driving pressure and survival in the acute respiratory distress syndrome. N Engl J Med 2015;372(8):747–55.

81. Wiedemann HP, Wheeler AP, Bernard GR, et al. Comparison of two fluid-management strategies in acute lung injury. N Engl J Med 2006;354(24):2564–75.

82. Parcha V, Kalra R, Bhatt SP, et al. Trends and geographic variation in acute respiratory failure and ARDS mortality in the United States. Chest 2021;159(4): 1460–72.

83. Cochi SE, Kempker JA, Annangi S, et al. Mortality trends of acute respiratory distress syndrome in the United States from 1999 to 2013. Ann Am Thorac Soc 2016;13(10):1742–51.

84. Investigators A, Group ACT, Peake SL, et al. Goal-directed resuscitation for patients with early septic shock. N Engl J Med 2014;371(16):1496–506.

85. Pro Cl, Yealy DM, Kellum JA, et al. A randomized trial of protocol-based care for early septic shock. N Engl J Med 2014;370(18):1683–93.
86. Mouncey PR, Osborn TM, Power GS, et al, ProMISe Trial Investigators. Trial of early, goal-directed resuscitation for septic shock. N Engl J Med 2015; 372(14):1301–11.
87. Rivers E, Nguyen B, Havstad S, et al, Early Goal-Directed Therapy Collaborative Group. Early goal-directed therapy in the treatment of severe sepsis and septic shock. N Engl J Med 2001;345(19):1368–77.
88. Vincent JL, Slutsky AS. We've never seen a patient with ARDS. Intensive Care Med 2020;46(12):2133–5.
89. Gattinoni L, Marini JJ. Isn't it time to abandon ARDS? The COVID-19 lesson. Crit Care 2021;25(1):326.
90. Jones TK, Feng R, Kerchberger VE, et al. Plasma sRAGE Acts as a genetically regulated causal intermediate in sepsis-associated acute respiratory distress syndrome. Am J Respir Crit Care Med 2020;201(1):47–56.
91. Calfee CS, Ware LB, Eisner MD, et al, NHLBI ARDS Network. Plasma receptor for advanced glycation end products and clinical outcomes in acute lung injury. Thorax 2008;63(12):1083–9.
92. Jabaudon M, Futier E, Roszyk L, et al. Soluble form of the receptor for advanced glycation end products is a marker of acute lung injury but not of severe sepsis in critically ill patients. Crit Care Med 2011;39(3):480–8.
93. Park J, Pabon M, Choi AMK, et al. Plasma surfactant protein-D as a diagnostic biomarker for acute respiratory distress syndrome: validation in US and Korean cohorts. BMC Pulm Med 2017;17(1):204.
94. Determann R, Royakkers A, Haitsma J, et al. Plasma levels of surfactant protein D and KL-6 for evaluation of lung injury in critically ill mechanically ventilated patients. BMC Pulm Med 2010;10(6).
95. Van Der Heijden M, Van Nieuw Amerongen GP, Koolwijk P, et al. Angiopoietin-2, permeability oedema, occurrence and severity of ALI/ARDS in septic and non-septic critically ill patients. Thorax 2008;63(10):903–9.
96. Agrawal A, Matthay MA, Kangelaris KN, et al. Plasma angiopoietin-2 predicts the onset of acute lung injury in critically ill patients. Am J Respir Crit Care Med 2013;187(7):736–42.
97. Calfee CS, Eisner MD, Parsons PE, et al, NHLBI Acute Respiratory Distress Syndrome Clinical Trials Network. Soluble intercellular adhesion molecule-1 and clinical outcomes in patients with acute lung injury. Intensive Care Med 2009; 35(2):248–57.
98. Terpstra ML, Aman J, Van Nieuw Amerongen GP, et al. Plasma biomarkers for acute respiratory distress syndrome: a systematic review and Meta-Analysis. Crit Care Med 2014;42(3):691–700.
99. Parsons PE, Matthay MA, Ware LB, et al, National Heart LBIARDSCTN. Elevated plasma levels of soluble TNF receptors are associated with morbidity and mortality in patients with acute lung injury. Am J Physiol Lung Cell Mol Physiol 2005; 288(3):L426–31.
100. Ware LB, Matthay MA, Parsons PE, et al, National Heart, Lung, and Blood Institute Acute Respiratory Distress Syndrome Clinical Trials Network. Pathogenetic and prognostic significance of altered coagulation and fibrinolysis in acute lung injury/acute respiratory distress syndrome. Crit Care Med 2007;35(8):1821–8.
101. Prabhakaran P, Ware LB, White KE, et al. Elevated levels of plasminogen activator inhibitor-1 in pulmonary edema fluid are associated with mortality in acute lung injury. Am J Physiol Lung Cell Mol Physiol 2003;285(1):L20–8.

Adjunctive Therapies in Acute Respiratory Distress Syndrome

Megan Trieu, MD[a], Nida Qadir, MD[b],*

KEYWORDS

- Acute respiratory distress syndrome • Prone positioning • Recruitment maneuvers
- Neuromuscular blockade • Corticosteroids • Pulmonary vasodilators
- Extracorporeal membrane oxygenation

KEY POINTS

- The evidence basis for most adjunctive therapies is limited to patients with early moderate to severe acute respiratory distress syndrome (ARDS).
- Despite being underused in clinical practice, prone positioning has the strongest supporting evidence of all adjunctive therapies in ARDS and is recommended for patients with $Pao_2/Fio_2 < 150$ mm Hg.
- Corticosteroids may improve outcomes in early ARDS but should be avoided as late salvage therapy (>14 days after ARDS onset).
- Extracorporeal membrane oxygenation should be considered in select patients with early severe ARDS, particularly those with $Pao_2/Fio_2 < 80$ mm Hg or pH < 7.25 with $PaCO_2 \geq 60$ mm Hg despite optimal medical management.
- Although the routine use of neuromuscular blocking agents, pulmonary vasodilators, and brief recruitment maneuvers is not recommended, these therapies may have specific roles in select patients.

INTRODUCTION

Since the acute respiratory distress syndrome (ARDS) was first described in 1967, significant advances have been made in understanding its epidemiology, pathogenesis, and management.[1] Supportive care with lung-protective mechanical ventilation (LPV) remains a fundamental part of clinical care, demonstrating benefit in ARDS of all

a Division of Pulmonary Critical Care Sleep Medicine and Physiology, Department of Medicine, University of California San Diego, 9300 Campus Point Drive, #7381, La Jolla, CA 92037-1300, USA; b Division of Pulmonary Critical Care and Sleep Medicine, Department of Medicine, David Geffen School of Medicine, University of California Los Angeles, 10833 Le Conte Avenue, Room 43-229 CHS, Los Angeles, CA 90095, USA
* Corresponding author. 10833 Le Conte Avenue, Room 43-229 CHS, Los Angeles, CA 90095.
E-mail address: nqadir@mednet.ucla.edu

Crit Care Clin 40 (2024) 329–351
https://doi.org/10.1016/j.ccc.2023.12.004
criticalcare.theclinics.com

severities. Despite the advent of LPV, mortality remains high,[2–5] particularly for patients with moderate to severe ARDS, whose reported mortality rates exceed 40%. Over the years, numerous adjunctive therapies have also been investigated and subsequently become important tools for clinical care.[6] However, although lung-protective ventilation has been shown to be beneficial in all patients with ARDS, adjunctive therapies come with both risks and benefits and their evidence basis is largely limited to those with moderate to severe ARDS. As such, patient and illness characteristics must be taken into consideration before their implementation. In this review, the authors provide a framework for adjunctive therapies for patients with ARDS (**Fig. 1**), focusing on summarizing supporting evidence and discussing considerations for their use.

PRONE POSITIONING

Prone positioning has been evaluated as a strategy for improving oxygenation and respiratory mechanics in patients with severe ARDS (**Fig. 2**). In the supine position, there is atelectasis and alveolar flooding of dependent dorsal lung tissue, where blood flow is the greatest, leading to the loss of functional lung volume and ventilation–perfusion (V/Q) mismatch.[7] When a patient is positioned prone, gravitational forces shift from the dorsal to ventral lung regions, allowing for alveolar recruitment of dorsal lung and drainage of secretions from previously dependent airways.[8] Although this also results in ventral lung compression, conformational shape-matching, the tendency of lung to maintain the same volume within its surrounding chest cavity favors ventral expansion,

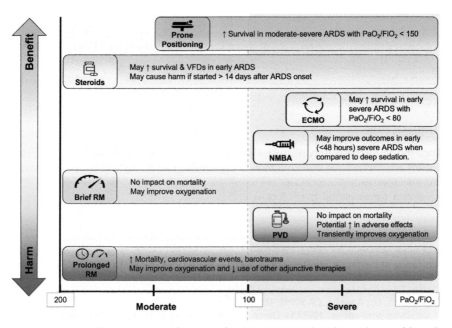

Adjunctive Therapies in Moderate and Severe ARDS

Fig. 1. Adjunctive therapies in moderate and severe ARDS ranked by evidence of benefit versus harm. ECMO, extracorporeal membrane oxygenation; NMBA, neuromuscular blocking agents; P/F, Pao_2:Fio_2 ratio; PVD, pulmonary vasodilators; RM, recruitment maneuvers; VFD, ventilator-free day.

SUPINE

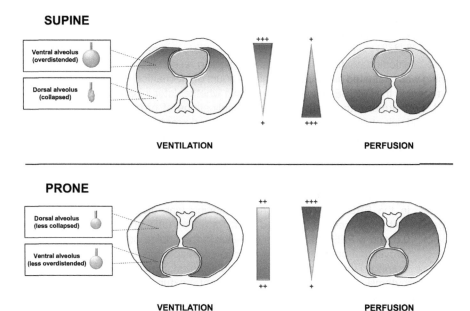

Fig. 2. Physiologic effects of prone positioning compared with supine positioning in ARDS, depicted in an axial view of the thorax. Perfusion remains relatively constant in both supine and prone positions, with the majority of blood flow supplying dorsal lung, independently of the gravitational gradient. In the supine position, ventral alveoli are overdistended and dorsal alveoli are collapsed, resulting in loss of functional lung volume and V/Q mismatch. In the prone position, gravitational forces shift from dorsal to ventral lung regions, allowing for alveolar recruitment of dorsal lung. Ventral lung compression is offset by conformational shape-matching, which favors ventral expansion in the prone position, thereby reducing ventral alveoli overdistension. These effects of prone positioning allow for a more homogenous distribution of ventilation and lung stress and enhance V/Q matching.

which partially offsets the impact of gravitational forces on the ventral lung. As a result, the ventral alveoli are less overdistended, and ventilation is more homogenous.[9] Meanwhile, perfusion remains relatively constant in both supine and prone positions, independent of gravitational forces. Altogether, these effects of prone positioning improve oxygenation by enhancing V/Q matching and minimize ventilator-induced lung injury (VILI) by distributing the stress and strain more uniformly within the lungs.

Early studies demonstrated that prone positioning improved oxygenation but did not provide significant survival benefit in a broad population of patients with ARDS.[10–12] However, subsequent meta-analyses suggested that prone positioning may have additional benefit in patients with severe hypoxemia.[13,14] In 2013, the landmark Prone Positioning in Severe Acute Respiratory Distress Syndrome (PROSEVA) trial investigated the effects of early and prolonged prone positioning in moderate–severe ARDS. In this trial, 466 patients with ARDS and a PaO_2/FiO_2 ratio of less than 150 mm Hg on an FiO_2 of ≥ 0.6 and a PEEP of ≥ 5 cm H_2O after 12 to 24 hours of mechanical ventilation were randomized to prone positioning for ≥ 16 hours per day or supine positioning. Patients assigned to the prone group had decreased 28-day mortality (16.0% vs 32.8%, $P < .001$) without increased incidence of complications.[15] Since PROSEVA, additional meta-analyses have illustrated similar mortality benefit with prone positioning, particularly if applied for at least 12 hours per day.[16,17]

The use of prone positioning for the management of ARDS is currently strongly recommended by consensus society guidelines for patients with a PaO_2/FiO_2 ratio < 150 mm Hg.[18,19,20] However, the optimal timing, duration, and patient selection criteria for prone positioning continue to be areas of ongoing research and debate. Prone positioning was evaluated as an early (within 24 hours of mechanical ventilation) adjunctive treatment in the PROSEVA trial; it is unknown whether later initiation is similarly beneficial. Furthermore, there are potential complications of prone positioning, with an increased risk of endotracheal tube obstruction and pressure sores noted in a pooled analysis.[19] Potential excess sedation and decreased mobility due to proning are also factors that have not yet been systematically evaluated; additional contraindications and possible complications of prone positioning are listed in **Table 1**.

With regard to duration, individual proning sessions of at least 12 hours per day are recommended, but overall duration of therapy and criteria for discontinuation remains unclear. In the PROSEVA trial, prone positioning was discontinued if there was improvement in oxygenation (defined as a Pao_2/Fio_2 ratio of $\geq$150 mm Hg on an Fio_2 of $\leq$0.6 and a PEEP of $\leq$10 cm of water in the supine position for > 4 hours); lack of improvement or worsening oxygenation or respiratory mechanics; or adverse events occurring in the prone position (ie, cardiac arrest, hemodynamic instability, unstable arrhythmia, massive hemoptysis, accidental extubation, mainstem bronchus intubation, or endotracheal tube obstruction).[15] However, the use of lack of improvement in gas exchange as a criteria for discontinuing prone positioning is debatable, as other studies suggest that the survival benefit seen with prone positioning may not depend on improvement in gas exchange and may instead be related to reduction in VILI.[21] The ideal duration is, therefore, based on a balance between the benefits of prone positioning and the risks of likely increased sedation requirements and decreased mobility.

Despite evidence of mortality benefit, prone positioning remains underused. In pre-COVID-19 cohorts, it was used in just 6% to 11% of patients with moderate to severe ARDS, less frequently than any other adjunct except extracorporeal membrane

Table 1 Contraindications and possible complications of prone positioning	
Contraindications	**Possible Complications**
Absolute Contraindications	
Spinal instability	Tube or line dislodgment
Increased intracranial pressure	Endotracheal tube obstruction
Massive hemoptysis	Brachial plexus injury
Abdominal compartment syndrome	Pressure ulcers
	Vomiting
Relative Contraindications	Elevated intra-abdominal pressure
Severe hemodynamic instability	Facial or ocular edema
Unstable arrhythmia	Excess sedation
Unstable facial, pelvic, or femur fracture	Prolonged immobility
Open abdominal wound	
Anterior chest tube	
Recent tracheal surgery	
Recent sternotomy	
Pregnancy (late-term)	

oxygenation (ECMO), a significantly more invasive and expensive therapy.[6,22,23] Although prone positioning was used more frequently during the COVID-19 pandemic (up to 39%–70% of patients with ARDS), its usage remains highly variable among institutions and it is unclear whether this increased use will persist.[24,25] Several barriers may contribute to the low rates of prone positioning. Clinician-level factors may include underrecognition of ARDS, a lack of familiarity and comfort with prone positioning, or a lack of belief in its utility. Variability in clinician understanding of indications for proning may also be a factor, as it is frequently viewed as a rescue maneuver for refractory severe hypoxemia as opposed to a management strategy to mitigate VILI.[26] Moreover, although prone positioning does not necessarily require specialized beds or equipment, it is a resource-intensive technique that involves a coordinated effort from a multidisciplinary team, including nurses, respiratory therapists, and physicians.[27] The logistics of safely proning a patient may pose challenges in some health care settings, particularly in resource-limited situations. Continued efforts must be made to overcome these barriers through education and institutional protocols.

RECRUITMENT MANEUVERS

Recruitment maneuvers, used as part of an "open lung approach" (OLA), are intended to improve oxygenation and compliance by reopening atelectatic alveoli and preventing cyclical collapse.[28] The rationale behind this strategy is to counteract alveolar derecruitment, which may occur due to low tidal volume ventilation, inadequate positive end-expiratory pressure (PEEP), or absorption atelectasis due to administration of high Fio_2. Various recruitment maneuver techniques have been described (**Fig. 3**), including sustained insufflation (increasing airway pressure to 35–40 cm H_2O for 30–40 seconds),[29–32] sighs (transient, cyclical increases in airway pressure to 30–45 cm H_2O),[33,34] and staircase recruitment (fixed inspiratory pressure or tidal volume

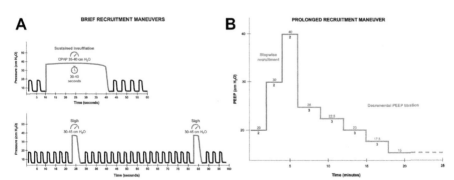

Fig. 3. Recruitment maneuver techniques. (*A*) Pressure versus time curve during brief recruitment maneuvers. Sustained insufflation (increase in airway pressure for 30–40 seconds) is depicted in the top graph, whereas sighs (transient cyclic increases in airway pressure) are depicted in the lower graph. (*B*) An example of a prolonged recruitment maneuver. This schematic depicts the recruitment maneuvers used in the PHARLAP trial.[41] Subjects were given boluses of neuromuscular blocking agents and placed on pressure control ventilation with an inspiratory pressure of 15 cm H_2O. PEEP was then increased stepwise to 20 cm H_2O, 30 cm H_2O, and 40 cm H_2O for 2 minutes each, followed by decremental titration first to 25 cm H_2O, and then by 2.5-cm H_2O for 3 minutes each until desaturation, or a minimum PEEP of 15 cm H_2O was achieved. CPAP, continuous positive pressure ventilation; PEEP, positive end expiratory pressure.

with stepwise increases in PEEP to 35–45 cm H_2O followed by decremental PEEP titration).[35–38]

While promising from a pathophysiologic perspective, application of recruitment maneuvers in clinical practice remains controversial. Although the American Thoracic Society recently issued a strong recommendation against the use of prolonged recruitment maneuvers (PEEP $\geq$ 35 cm H_2O for > 60 seconds), there is uncertainty about the potential benefit of brief recruitment maneuvers.[20] While both prolonged and brief recruitment maneuvers improve hypoxemia, their effects on gas exchange may be variable and transient.[39] Conducting recruitment maneuvers also frequently requires the use of neuromuscular blockade and comes with risk of hemodynamic instability and barotrauma. These risks are especially pronounced with prolonged recruitment maneuvers. The Alveolar Recruitment for Acute Respiratory Distress Syndrome (ART) trial randomized 1010 patients with moderate to severe ARDS to a conventional low PEEP strategy versus an OLA consisting of staircase recruitment maneuvers with pressure control ventilation at 15 cm H_2O and PEEP increased stepwise to 25 cm H_2O, 30 cm H_2O, and 35 cm H_2O for 1 minute each, followed by decremental PEEP titration to best respiratory compliance. The experimental strategy resulted in increased mortality, decreased ventilator-free days, and higher rates of barotrauma.[40] Similarly, the Maximal Recruitment Open Lung Ventilation in Acute Respiratory Distress Syndrome investigators also examined the impact of OLA in patients with moderate to severe ARDS compared with a conventional low PEEP strategy. The intervention included staircase recruitment maneuvers with pressure control ventilation at 15 $\pm$ 3 cm H_2O and PEEP increased stepwise to 20 cm H_2O, 30 cm H_2O, and 40 cm H_2O for 2 minutes each, followed by decremental PEEP titration first to 25 cm H_2O, and then by 2.5-cm H_2O steps for 3 minutes each until oxygen saturation decreased by $\geq$ 2% or a minimum PEEP of 15 cm H_2O was reached. This trial was stopped early due to the findings of the ART trial and concern for potential harm in the OLA, but found that the open lung intervention was associated with increased incidence of cardiovascular events, decreased use of additional adjunctive therapies (ie, prone positioning, inhaled nitric oxide [iNO], and ECMO), and no difference in mortality or ventilator-free days.[41]

Although brief recruitment maneuvers may be safer than prolonged maneuvers,[29,30,34] hemodynamic instability can still occur[31] and benefit in patient-centered outcomes has not yet been demonstrated.[42] Nevertheless, there may be specific clinical scenarios in which recruitment maneuvers have utility, such as de-recruitment after disconnection from positive pressure or refractory hypoxemia. In situations where recruitment maneuvers are considered, brief maneuvers should be utilized, neuromuscular blockade should be administered beforehand, and the clinical team should both monitor for and be prepared to respond to hemodynamic instability and barotrauma.

NEUROMUSCULAR BLOCKING AGENTS

The role of neuromuscular blocking agents (NMBAs) in the management of ARDS has been debated for decades. Their proposed mechanism of benefit is by minimizing many forms of patient–ventilator asynchrony, thus reducing ventilator-associated lung injury (VALI) and its associated sequelae. NMBAs also decrease metabolic activity, thereby reducing oxygen consumption and carbon dioxide production. However, although NMBAs are widely available and logistically easy to administer, there are many caveats to their use, one of which is that using NMBAs requires deep sedation, whereas current clinical practice guidelines recommend the use of lighter sedation.[43] In addition, there is potentially an increased risk of intensive care unit (ICU)-acquired weakness, particularly when used in conjunction with systemic corticosteroids,[44] although this association has primarily been seen in older case series, with more recent data suggesting against a causal relationship.[45] Of note, although several NMBAs have been used for the management of ARDS, cisatracurium, a newer nondepolarizing agent, has no known association with ICU-acquired weakness. It is also associated with a decrease in inflammatory cytokines independently of its impact on VALI and was used in the largest randomized controlled trials (RCTs) assessing NMBA use in ARDS, suggesting that it may be a preferable NMBA.[46]

The use of cisatracurium in ARDS has been assessed in two large RCTs, the first of which was the ARDS et Curarisation Systematique (ACURASYS) trial.[47] In this double-blinded RCT, 340 patients with early (within <48 hours of onset) moderate–severe ARDS ($Pao_2/Fio_2 < 150$ mm Hg) were randomized to 48 hours of continuous cisatracurium versus placebo. Patients in the control arm received deep sedation to maintain blinding. The results suggested that cisatracurium reduced 90-day mortality (31.6% vs 40.7%, $P = .08$, hazard ratio 0.68 [95% CI, 0.48–0.98], $P = .04$). However, there were several limitations to this study; among the most notable was that deep sedation in the control arm is not comparable to current ICU practices of light sedation and/or daily awakenings.

In light of these limitations, the use of neuromuscular blockade was subsequently reevaluated in the larger Reevaluation of Systemic Early Neuromuscular Blockade (ROSE) trial, an unblinded RCT of 1006 patients with early (within <48 hours of onset) moderate–severe ARDS ($Pao_2/Fio_2 < 150$ mm Hg on PEEP $\geq$ 8 cm H_2O) comparing 48 hours of continuous cisatracurium to usual care with light sedation.[48] There was no difference between the two groups with regard to hospital mortality, ventilator-free days, ICU-free days, or hospital-free days. The cisatracurium group was less mobile while in the hospital and had more adverse cardiovascular events. Importantly, they did not have an increased risk of ICU-acquired weakness, but it is crucial to note that this was in the setting of short-term cisatracurium administration, and the risks of longer term infusion remain unknown. There were some key differences in the design of these trials that may have contributed to the discrepancy in their findings. The more contemporary ROSE trial used lighter sedation targets in the control group in accordance with current standard of care, whereas deep sedation was used in the ACURASYS trial. In addition, the ROSE trial also used a higher PEEP strategy than the ACURASYS trial. Finally, the use of prone positioning was lower in the ROSE trial than in the ACURASYS trial.

Based on the results of these trials, the routine use of NMBAs is not currently recommended for the management of ARDS. Nevertheless, they may have utility in select patients and are one of the most frequently used adjunctive therapies.[6,22] Although the use of NMBAs does not confer a mortality benefit when compared to light sedation, pooled analyses demonstrate a possible reduction in mortality in comparison to deep sedation, particularly in early (< 48 hours since onset) severe ARDS.[20] Additionally, NMBAs may improve oxygenation and reduce risk of barotrauma.[49] Accordingly, they may be useful for patients with refractory hypoxemia despite ventilator optimization, particularly in individuals already receiving deep sedation, and could also be considered before pursuing more invasive therapies, such as ECMO. In addition, severe patient–ventilator asynchrony can result in VALI, increased mortality, prolonged duration of mechanical ventilation, longer ICU and hospital lengths of stay, and worsened comfort and quality of sleep.[50] When severe asynchrony persists despite ventilator optimization, NMBAs can mitigate these risks by facilitating passive ventilation. These benefits must be balanced with the potential short-term risk of increased cardiovascular events, presumably from exposure to deeper sedation, and the theoretic long-term risks associated with immobility. Importantly, NMBAs were used for up to 48 hours in a majority of study patients; the risks associated with longer duration of use are unknown and may be increased.

CORTICOSTEROIDS

Corticosteroids are potent anti-inflammatory agents routinely used in the treatment of various ARDS-related conditions, including septic shock, hypoxemic respiratory failure due to COVID-19, and severe community-acquired pneumonia.[51-55] They have been theorized to similarly benefit patients with ARDS by suppressing the synthesis of pro-inflammatory cytokines. Corticosteroids are the most commonly used adjunctive therapy, applied in more than 40% of patients with moderate to severe ARDS.[22] The high frequency of use, compared with other adjunctive strategies, likely reflects its widespread availability, low cost, and ease of administration.

Studies evaluating the effect of systemic corticosteroids in ARDS have yielded variable results, suggesting that the impact of corticosteroid use may be influenced by timing or duration of therapy, ARDS etiology, or other patient factors. In an early trial comparing the administration of high-dose methylprednisolone (30 mg/kg every 6 hours for 24 hours) with placebo in 99 patients with ARDS, no difference was found in 45-day mortality.[56] In contrast, a larger multicenter RCT comparing more modest doses of methylprednisolone (1 mg/kg daily for 14 days, followed by taper for up to 28 days) to placebo for early (within 72 hours of onset) ARDS, demonstrated decreased ICU mortality (20.6% vs 42.9%; $P = .03$), days of mechanical ventilation, and ICU length of stay in patients receiving corticosteroids.[57] More recently, the dexamethasone in ARDS (DEXA-ARDS) trial, an unblinded RCT of 277 patients comparing a 10-day regimen of dexamethasone with placebo in early (within 30 hours of onset) ARDS, found that dexamethasone increased ventilator-free days (12.3 ± 9.9 vs 7.5 ± 9.0 days; $P < .0001$) and decreased 60-day mortality (21% vs 36%; $P < .0047$),[58] although there were some limitations of this trial, including the exclusion of a large number of patients and slow enrollment occurring over 5 years. During the COVID-19 pandemic, several RCTs also found that corticosteroids improved outcomes in COVID-19-related ARDS, and two separate meta-analyses have demonstrated a reduction in mortality and duration of mechanical ventilation, with higher rates of survival in patients receiving longer courses (> 7 days).[59,60]

Although the overall body of evidence on corticosteroids in ARDS points toward benefit, it is important to note that most trials demonstrating positive outcomes have used corticosteroids as an early intervention in ARDS, and these results have not been replicated in later ARDS. The Late Steroids Rescue Study, a multicenter RCT assessed the use of corticosteroids in patients with ARDS for ≥ 7 days, found that although corticosteroids increased in the number of ventilator-free days and shock-free days, they did not decrease overall 60- or 180-day mortality, and there was a concerning increase in mortality in the subset of patients given corticosteroids more than 14 days after onset of ARDS.[61]

There are several important caveats to take into account when considering the use of corticosteroids. It is crucial to recognize that ARDS is a heterogeneous syndrome with varying underlying causes, some of which may derive greater benefit from this intervention than others. As such, corticosteroids may be most useful in patients with concurrent conditions that are typically steroid-responsive, such as shock or community-acquired pneumonia. Corticosteroids are also not without risk, and there are limited data about possible adverse effects in patients with ARDS, such as secondary infections, neuromuscular weakness, gastrointestinal bleeding, and severe hyperglycemia.

Studies assessing the short-term use of corticosteroids in other patient populations have demonstrated the potential for harm.[62,63] They should be used with caution in patients at greater risk for these complications, such as the immunocompromised, individuals with metabolic syndrome, or patients with concern for active mycobacterial, fungal, or parasitic infections. In addition, benefits conferred by corticosteroids are likely limited to early ARDS, and they should be avoided as a late salvage therapy (after 14 days since ARDS onset) as they may be associated with increased mortality in this context.

Finally, there is currently no consensus regarding specific agent, dosing, timing, and duration of corticosteroid administration in ARDS. Most trials have used different regimens (**Table 2**); although any of these could reasonably be used in a clinical context, the Society of Critical Care Medicine and European Society of Critical Care Medicine guidelines currently recommend methylprednisolone 1 mg/kg/day tapered slowly over 14 days—methylprednisolone due to its greater penetration into lung tissue and a longer course with taper to minimize the chance of deterioration from potential development of a reconstituted inflammatory response.[64] Of note, these guidelines were published in 2017 before the DEXA-ARDS trial and RCTs on COVID-related ARDS. Further research is necessary to determine the optimal regimen to establish a standard protocol for implementation.

PULMONARY VASODILATORS

Selective pulmonary vasodilators, such as iNO and inhaled prostacyclin, are sometimes used as a rescue therapy in patients with refractory hypoxemia. Because they are administered via inhalation, these agents can localize to well-aerated alveoli, causing selective vasodilation of ventilated capillary vessels, thereby improving V/Q matching and oxygenation.[65,66] The reduction in pulmonary vascular resistance also

Table 2	
Corticosteroid regimens used in acute respiratory distress syndrome clinical trials	
Corticosteroid	**Dosing**
Dexamethasone	
Villar 2020[58]	20 mg/day × 5 d, then 10 mg/day × 5 d
Horby 2020[53]	6 mg/day × 10 d
Tomazini 2020[88]	20 mg/day × 5 d, then 10 mg/day × 5 d
Methylprednisolone	
Meduri 1998[89]	2 mg/kg/day × 14 d, then 1 mg/kg × 7 d, then 0.25 mg/kg × 3 d, then 0.125 mg/kg × 2 d
Steinberg 2006[61]	2 mg/kg PBW × 1, then 0.5 mg/kg PBW Q6H × 14 d, then 0.5 mg/kg PBW Q12H × 7 d
Meduri 2007[57]	1 mg/kg/day × 1 loading dose, then 1 mg/kg × 14 d, then 0.5 mg/kg × 7 d, then 0.25 mg/kg × 3 d, then 0.125 mg/kg × 3 d
Jeronimo 2020[90]	0.5 mg/kg × 5 d
Hydrocortisone	
Annane 2006[91]	50 mg Q6H × 7 d (in combination with fludrocortisone 50 mcg/day)
Tongyoo 2016[92]	50 mg Q6H for 7 d
Angus 2020[93]	50–100 mg Q6H × 7 d; OR shock-dependent course: 50 mg Q6H for up to 28 d

decreases right ventricular afterload, improving right ventricular function and cardiac output.[67]

Despite these features, iNO has not been shown to significantly reduce mortality, duration of mechanical ventilation, ICU length of stay, or hospital length of stay in patients with ARDS.[68–70] Although it has the potential to improve oxygenation, the effect is typically small and transient. Over time, tachyphylaxis can also develop as can V/Q mismatch from the induction of vasodilation in poorly ventilated alveoli, potentially leading to deterioration in as little as 2 to 4 days.[71] In addition, iNO is associated with an increased risk of renal failure in patients with ARDS.[72] Inhaled prostacyclin, commonly epoprostenol and more recently iloprost, may also transiently improve oxygenation.[73] Compared with iNO, inhaled prostacyclin is available at a lower cost and with a potentially safer side effect profile. However, similar to iNO, inhaled prostacyclin has not demonstrated improvement in mortality or other patient-centered outcomes.[74]

Current evidence does not support the routine use of pulmonary vasodilators as an adjunctive strategy for ARDS. However, they are used in up to 13% of patients with severe ARDS[6,22] and may have a temporizing role for patients with severe hypoxia to facilitate transportation, necessary procedures, or as a bridge to ECMO. Pulmonary vasodilators are not recommended for prolonged use unless indicated for a concurrent condition, such as underlying pulmonary hypertension.

EXTRACORPOREAL MEMBRANE OXYGENATION

Venovenous ECMO (V-V ECMO) has been increasingly adopted as an adjunctive therapy for patients with severe ARDS. V-V ECMO works by draining blood from the central venous system and passing it through a gas exchange device for oxygenation and carbon dioxide removal before returning the blood back to the venous system, thereby allowing for gas exchange while bypassing the lungs. With gas exchange facilitated by the ECMO circuit, ventilator support can be reduced, decreasing the burden of mechanical power applied to the lungs and minimizing the risk of VALI. Although the use of ECMO has increased dramatically in recent years, particularly since the 2009 H1N1 pandemic and COVID-19 pandemic, it remains an invasive, labor-intensive therapy, available only at specialized centers equipped with requisite resources and expertise.[75,76]

Two landmark trials assessing the utility of V-V ECMO for ARDS have been conducted. The first was the Conventional Ventilatory Support versus Extracorporeal Membrane Oxygenation for Severe Adult Respiratory Failure (CESAR) trial, which randomized 180 patients with severe ARDS to conventional management or referral to ECMO centers for consideration of V-V ECMO.[77] Patients allocated to consideration for treatment with ECMO had decreased death or severe disability at 6 months (47% vs 63%, relative risk 0·69; 95% CI 0·05–0·97, $P = 0·03$). However, there were several limitations to this trial. Only 75% of patients in the intervention arm actually received ECMO. In addition, conventional management was not standardized in the control arm, and few patients received prone positioning, albeit the trial was conducted before the publication of the PROSEVA trial and guidelines recommending prone positioning were issued.

V-V ECMO was reevaluated in the ECMO to Rescue Lung Injury in Severe ARDS (EOLIA) trial, which randomized 249 patients with severe ARDS to V-V ECMO or conventional management.[78] Crossover to ECMO was permitted in the control group for refractory hypoxia. Ventilator management was protocolized, and there was a high rate of other adjunctive therapy use, including prone positioning. Patients receiving

ECMO had decreased 60-day mortality (35% vs 46%, $P = .09$), although this difference did not achieve statistical significance. However, the trial had been stopped early due to predefined futility rules, as it was unlikely to achieve the anticipated absolute risk reduction of 20%, a decision that was met with some criticism and may have resulted in an inconclusive outcome.[79] With regard to adverse events, patients randomized to ECMO received more blood transfusions and had more severe thrombocytopenia but had fewer ischemic strokes and no significant difference in other safety outcomes, including massive bleeding, hemorrhagic stroke, ventilator-associated pneumonia, or pneumothorax. Subsequent pooled analyses suggest that V-V ECMO may lower mortality in very severe ARDS compared with current best practices, although the magnitude of benefit remains uncertain.[80,81]

In light of these findings, current recommendations suggest the use of V-V ECMO for patients with severe ARDS as defined by the EOLIA trial's inclusion criteria—refractory hypoxemia ($Pao_2/Fio_2 < 80$ mm Hg) or hypercapnic acidosis (pH < 7.25 with a $Paco_2 \geq 60$ mm Hg) despite optimal medical management (**Fig. 4**).[78,82] However, given the invasive and resource-intensive nature of ECMO, careful patient selection is of utmost importance and should focus on patients most likely to benefit from extracorporeal support—those with reversible etiologies of respiratory failure and minimal risk factors for futility who are early in their ARDS course. A reduction in survival after 7 days of mechanical ventilation has been seen in large cohorts,[83,84] and there was a substantially higher mortality rate (57%) in patients in the EOLIA trial who crossed over from the control arm to ECMO and thus had late initiation of extracorporeal support.[78] There are no absolute contraindications for ECMO, but patient-specific factors that decrease likelihood for survival, such as immunosuppression, multi-organ failure, life-limiting chronic conditions, severe neurologic injury, advanced age, and bleeding diathesis, should be factored into decisions regarding an individual's suitability for ECMO (see **Fig. 4**). It is also important to note that there are limited data on long-term outcomes and whether increased survival correlates with other patient-centered outcomes, such as health-related quality of life, which may influence patient preferences and selection criteria.[85] On an institutional level, volume and expertise of

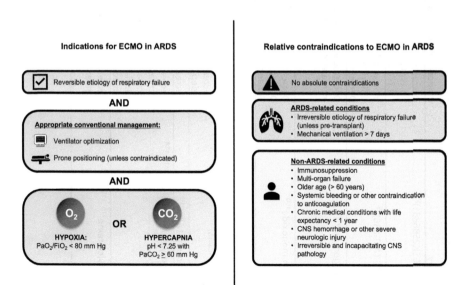

Fig. 4. Indications for and relative contraindications to ECMO in ARDS.

Table 3
Investigational therapies for acute respiratory distress syndrome

Therapy	Proposed Mechanism of Action	Results to Date	Ongoing Clinical Trials
ACE2 (GSK2586881)[94]	Decrease inflammation, vascular permeability, and fibroproliferation	No impact on oxygenation or SOFA scores	
Anti-TF (ALT-836)[95]	Inhibit thrombin formation and fibrin deposition Decrease inflammation	Safety established (phase I)	NCT00879606
Beta-agonists[96–99]	Decrease vascular permeability Increase alveolar fluid clearance	Increased mortality Possible decreased plateau pressure and improved oxygenation	NCT04193878
Carbon monoxide[100]	Decrease oxidative stress Decrease inflammation Enhance phagocytosis	Safety established (phase I) Possible improvement in LIS and SOFA scores	NCT03799874, NCT04870125
GM-CSF[101–103]	Decrease epithelial cell injury Enhance alveolar macrophage function	Possible improved oxygenation	NCT02595060
Heparin[104–107]	Decrease inflammation and fibrin deposition	Possible increased VFD	
Interferon β-1a[108,109]	Decrease vascular permeability	No impact on mortality or VFD	
Mesenchymal stromal cells[110–114]	Decrease vascular permeability Increase alveolar fluid clearance Increase secretion of anti-inflammatory and antimicrobial mediators	Safety established in phase I and IIa studies Preliminary report suggested decreased mortality and increased VFD and ICU-free days	NCT02444455 NCT03608592 NCT03042143 NCT04367077
N-acetylcysteine[115–119]	Decrease inflammation Decrease oxidative stress	No impact on mortality, oxygenation, VFD, or hospital/ICU length of stay	

Solnatide (AP 301)[120,121]	Increase alveolar fluid clearance	Possible reduction in extravascular lung water and ventilation pressures in patients with SOFA score ≥ 11	NCT03567577
Statins[122–125]	Decrease inflammation	No impact on mortality or VFD Possible benefit in hyperinflammatory subphenotype (exploratory study)	
Streptokinase[107]	Decrease intra-alveolar fibrin clot to aid alveolar re-expansion	Improved oxygenation, lung compliance, and ICU mortality	
Surfactant[126–129]	Replace deficient or dysfunctional endogenous surfactant	No impact on mortality or oxygenation	
Vitamin C[130]	Decrease inflammation Enhance alveolar epithelial barrier function Decrease microvascular thrombosis	No impact on SOFA scores Possible decreased mortality and hospital/ICU length of stay in patients with sepsis and ARDS (exploratory analyses)	NCT04291508

Abbreviations: ACE2, angiotensin-converting enzyme 2; anti-TF, anti-tissue factor antibody; LIS, lung injury score; SOFA, sequential, organ failure assessment score; VFD, ventilator-free days.

ECMO centers may also impact outcomes, as more experienced centers tend to achieve lower mortality rates although with higher resource utilization.[86,87] In addition, the staffing, equipment, and other requirements necessary for ECMO are substantial and may have implications for institutional resource allocation. Further research is needed to address these considerations and provide more comprehensive insights into the use of ECMO in ARDS.

FUTURE DIRECTIONS

In addition to the numerous adjunctive therapies discussed in this article, other emerging therapies are being explored (**Table 3**), with several clinical trials currently in progress. These investigations aim to uncover new treatment options for patients with ARDS. Although remarkable progress has been achieved in further investigating existing adjunctive therapies for ARDS, several important questions remain. First, it is important to evaluate the impact of using multiple therapies simultaneously and determine whether their combination yields synergistic or antagonistic effects. In practice, adjunctive therapies are most frequently used in combination,[22] despite minimal evidence on the impact of using them in this fashion. Understanding which therapies may be synergistic has the potential to maximize treatment efficacy and optimize patient outcomes. Second, the heterogeneity of treatment effect in specific subgroups of patients with ARDS is a topic that warrants additional investigation, as it may be a major reason why many prior clinical trials for ARDS therapies have been "negative." Identifying patient subgroups that respond more favorably, experience limited benefits, or even suffer potential harm, from certain adjunctive therapies can help tailor treatment strategies and improve patient selection. Last, the suboptimal uptake of evidence-based adjunctive therapies must be addressed. This will likely involve a multifaceted approach, including educating clinicians to enable timely recognition of ARDS, improving guidelines and protocols, and considering potential barriers in resource-limited settings. Addressing these questions and challenges can promote the implementation and proper utilization of adjunctive therapies in ARDS, ultimately leading to improved patient care and outcomes.

SUMMARY

Adjunctive therapies are an important aspect of ARDS management, particularly for patients with moderate to severe ARDS. Although the heterogeneity of ARDS poses challenges in finding universally effective treatments, various therapies, including prone positioning, recruitment maneuvers, NMBAs, corticosteroids, pulmonary vasodilators, and ECMO, have been explored. Although the risks and evidence for benefit are variable for different therapies, each may have a role in the management of individual patients and specific clinical scenarios, and appropriate implementation requires careful consideration. Continued research efforts and an individualized approach are essential for optimizing the utilization of adjunctive therapies and improving patient outcomes in ARDS.

CLINICS CARE POINTS

- Although supportive care with lung-protective ventilation remains the cornerstone of acute respiratory distress syndrome (ARDS) management, there is a growing body of evidence supporting the use of adjunctive therapies in early ARDS, particularly in patients with moderate to severe hypoxia.

- Among adjunctive therapies for ARDS, prone positioning has the most compelling evidence of mortality benefit and is recommended for patients with Pao_2/Fio_2 <150 mm Hg.
- Corticosteroids may improve outcomes in early ARDS but should be avoided as late salvage therapy (>14 days after ARDS onset). Further research is needed to identify the optimal agent, dosing, and duration.
- Extracorporeal membrane oxygenation may improve outcomes in select patients with early severe ARDS and Pao_2/Fio_2 < 80 mm Hg or pH < 7.25 with $pCO_2 \geq$ 60 mm Hg despite optimal medical management. Patient selection should involve a multidisciplinary evaluation and include careful assessment for risk factors for futility of treatment.
- Although the impact of neuromuscular blocking agents, pulmonary vasodilators, and brief recruitment maneuvers on mortality is unclear, these therapies may have utility in carefully selected patients.

DISCLOSURE

The authors have nothing to disclose.

REFERENCES

1. Ashbaugh DG, Bigelow DB, Petty TL, et al. Acute respiratory distress in adults. Lancet Lond Engl 1967;2(7511):319–23.
2. Acute Respiratory Distress Syndrome Network, Brower RG, Matthay MA, et al. Ventilation with lower tidal volumes as compared with traditional tidal volumes for acute lung injury and the acute respiratory distress syndrome. N Engl J Med 2000;342(18):1301–8.
3. Briel M, Meade M, Mercat A, et al. Higher vs lower positive end-expiratory pressure in patients with acute lung injury and acute respiratory distress syndrome: systematic review and meta-analysis. JAMA 2010;303(9):865–73.
4. Beitler JR, Sarge T, Banner-Goodspeed VM, et al. Effect of titrating positive end-expiratory pressure (PEEP) with an esophageal pressure-guided strategy vs an empirical high PEEP-fio2 strategy on death and days free from mechanical ventilation among patients with acute respiratory distress syndrome: a randomized clinical trial. JAMA 2019;321(9):846–57.
5. National Heart, Lung, and Blood Institute Acute Respiratory Distress Syndrome ARDS Clinical Trials Network, Wiedemann HP, Wheeler AP, et al. National Heart, Lung, and Blood Institute Acute Respiratory Distress Syndrome (ARDS) Clinical Trials Network, Wiedemann HP, Wheeler AP, et al. Comparison of two fluid-management strategies in acute lung injury. N Engl J Med 2006;354(24): 2564–75.
6. Bellani G, Laffey JG, Pham T, et al. Epidemiology, patterns of care, and mortality for patients with acute respiratory distress syndrome in intensive care units in 50 countries. JAMA 2016;315(8):788–800.
7. Galiatsou E, Kostanti E, Svarna E, et al. Prone position augments recruitment and prevents alveolar overinflation in acute lung injury. Am J Respir Crit Care Med 2006;174(2):187–97.
8. van der Zee P, Gommers D. Recruitment maneuvers and higher PEEP, the so-called open lung concept, in patients with ARDS. Crit Care Lond Engl 2019; 23(1):73.
9. Gattinoni L, Taccone P, Carlesso E, et al. Prone position in acute respiratory distress syndrome. Rationale, indications, and limits. Am J Respir Crit Care Med 2013;188(11):1286–93.

10. Gattinoni L, Tognoni G, Pesenti A, et al. Effect of prone positioning on the survival of patients with acute respiratory failure. N Engl J Med 2001;345(8): 568–73.

11. Sud S, Sud M, Friedrich JO, et al. Effect of mechanical ventilation in the prone position on clinical outcomes in patients with acute hypoxemic respiratory failure: a systematic review and meta-analysis. CMAJ Can Med Assoc J J Assoc Medicale Can 2008;178(9):1153–61.

12. Taccone P, Pesenti A, Latini R, et al. Prone positioning in patients with moderate and severe acute respiratory distress syndrome: a randomized controlled trial. JAMA 2009;302(18):1977–84.

13. Alsaghir AH, Martin CM. Effect of prone positioning in patients with acute respiratory distress syndrome: a meta-analysis. Crit Care Med 2008;36(2):603–9.

14. Gattinoni L, Carlesso E, Taccone P, et al. Prone positioning improves survival in severe ARDS: a pathophysiologic review and individual patient meta-analysis. Minerva Anestesiol 2010;76(6):448–54.

15. Guérin C, Reignier J, Richard JC, et al. Prone positioning in severe acute respiratory distress syndrome. N Engl J Med 2013;368(23):2159–68.

16. Munshi L, Del Sorbo L, Adhikari NKJ, et al. Prone position for acute respiratory distress syndrome. A systematic review and meta-analysis. Ann Am Thorac Soc 2017;14(Supplement_4):S280–8.

17. Moran JL, Graham PL. Multivariate meta-analysis of the mortality effect of prone positioning in the acute respiratory distress syndrome. J Intensive Care Med 2021;36(11):1323–30.

18. Grasselli G, Calfee CS, Camporota L, et al. ESICM guidelines on acute respiratory distress syndrome: definition, phenotyping and respiratory support strategies. Intensive Care Med 2023;49(7):727–59.

19. Fan E, Del Sorbo L, Goligher EC, et al. An official American thoracic society/European society of intensive care medicine/society of critical care medicine clinical practice guideline: mechanical ventilation in adult patients with acute respiratory distress syndrome. Am J Respir Crit Care Med 2017;195(9): 1253–63.

20. Qadir N, Sahetya S, Munshi L, et al. An Update on Management of Adult Patients with Acute Respiratory Distress Syndrome: An Official American Thoracic Society Clinical Practice Guideline. Am J Respir Crit Care Med 2023. https://doi. org/10.1164/rccm.202311-2011ST.

21. Albert RK, Keniston A, Baboi L, et al. Prone position-induced improvement in gas exchange does not predict improved survival in the acute respiratory distress syndrome. Am J Respir Crit Care Med 2014;189(4):494–6.

22. Qadir N, Bartz RR, Cooter ML, et al. Variation in early management practices in moderate-to-severe ARDS in the United States: the severe ARDS: generating evidence study. Chest 2021;160(4):1304–15.

23. Duggal A, Rezoagli E, Pham T, et al. Patterns of use of adjunctive therapies in patients with early moderate to severe ARDS: insights from the LUNG SAFE study. Chest 2020;157(6):1497–505.

24. COVID-ICU Group on behalf of the REVA Network and the COVID-ICU Investigators. Clinical characteristics and day-90 outcomes of 4244 critically ill adults with COVID-19: a prospective cohort study. Intensive Care Med 2021;47(1): 60–73. https://doi.org/10.1007/s00134-020-06294-x.

25. Gupta S, Hayek SS, Wang W, et al. Factors associated with death in critically ill patients with coronavirus disease 2019 in the US. JAMA Intern Med 2020; 180(11):1436–47.

26. Guérin C, Beuret P, Constantin JM, et al. A prospective international observational prevalence study on prone positioning of ARDS patients: the APRONET (ARDS Prone Position Network) study. Intensive Care Med 2018;44(1):22–37.
27. Qadir N, Chen JT. Adjunctive therapies in ARDS: the disconnect between clinical trials and clinical practice. Chest 2020;157(6):1405–6.
28. Amato MB, Barbas CS, Medeiros DM, et al. Effect of a protective-ventilation strategy on mortality in the acute respiratory distress syndrome. N Engl J Med 1998;338(6):347–54.
29. Meade MO, Cook DJ, Guyatt GH, et al. Ventilation strategy using low tidal volumes, recruitment maneuvers, and high positive end-expiratory pressure for acute lung injury and acute respiratory distress syndrome: a randomized controlled trial. JAMA 2008;299(6):637–45.
30. Xi XM, Jiang L, Zhu B, RM group. Clinical efficacy and safety of recruitment maneuver in patients with acute respiratory distress syndrome using low tidal volume ventilation: a multicenter randomized controlled clinical trial. Chin Med J (Engl) 2010;123(21):3100–5.
31. Arnal JM, Paquet J, Wysocki M, et al. Optimal duration of a sustained inflation recruitment maneuver in ARDS patients. Intensive Care Med 2011;37(10):1588–94.
32. Constantin JM, Jabaudon M, Lefrant JY, et al. Personalised mechanical ventilation tailored to lung morphology versus low positive end-expiratory pressure for patients with acute respiratory distress syndrome in France (the LIVE study): a multicentre, single-blind, randomised controlled trial. Lancet Respir Med 2019;7(10):870–80.
33. Pelosi P, Cadringher P, Bottino N, et al. Sigh in acute respiratory distress syndrome. Am J Respir Crit Care Med 1999;159(3):872–80.
34. Mauri T, Foti G, Fornari C, et al. Sigh in patients with acute hypoxemic respiratory failure and ARDS. Chest 2021;159(4):1426–36.
35. Hodgson CL, Tuxen DV, Davies AR, et al. A randomised controlled trial of an open lung strategy with staircase recruitment, titrated PEEP and targeted low airway pressures in patients with acute respiratory distress syndrome. Crit Care Lond Engl 2011;15(3):R133.
36. Hodgson CL, Tuxen DV, Bailey MJ, et al. A positive response to a recruitment maneuver with PEEP titration in patients with ARDS, regardless of transient oxygen desaturation during the maneuver. J Intensive Care Med 2011;26(1):41–9.
37. Morán I, Blanch L, Fernández R, et al. Acute physiologic effects of a stepwise recruitment maneuver in acute respiratory distress syndrome. Minerva Anestesiol 2011;77(12):1167–75.
38. Kacmarek RM, Villar J, Sulemanji D, et al. Open lung approach for the acute respiratory distress syndrome: a pilot, randomized controlled trial. Crit Care Med 2016;44(1):32–42.
39. Brower RG, Morris A, MacIntyre N, et al. Effects of recruitment maneuvers in patients with acute lung injury and acute respiratory distress syndrome ventilated with high positive end-expiratory pressure. Crit Care Med 2003;31(11):2592–7.
40. Writing Group for the Alveolar Recruitment for Acute Respiratory Distress Syndrome Trial ART Investigators, Cavalcanti AB, Suzumura ÉA, et al. Writing Group for the Alveolar Recruitment for Acute Respiratory Distress Syndrome Trial (ART) Investigators, Cavalcanti AB, Suzumura ÉA, et al. Effect of Lung Recruitment and Titrated Positive End-Expiratory Pressure (PEEP) vs Low PEEP on Mortality in Patients With Acute Respiratory Distress Syndrome: a Randomized Clinical Trial. JAMA 2017;318(14):1335–45.

41. Hodgson CL, Cooper DJ, Arabi Y, et al. Maximal recruitment open lung ventilation in acute respiratory distress syndrome (PHARLAP). A phase II, multicenter randomized controlled clinical trial. Am J Respir Crit Care Med 2019;200(11):1363–72.

42. Pensier J, De Jong A, Hajjej Z, et al. Effect of lung recruitment maneuver on oxygenation, physiological parameters and mortality in acute respiratory distress syndrome patients: a systematic review and meta-analysis. Intensive Care Med 2019;45(12):1691–702.

43. Devlin JW, Skrobik Y, Gélinas C, et al. Clinical practice guidelines for the prevention and management of pain, agitation/sedation, delirium, immobility, and sleep disruption in adult patients in the ICU. Crit Care Med 2018;46(9):e825–73.

44. Fischer JR, Baer RK. Acute myopathy associated with combined use of corticosteroids and neuromuscular blocking agents. Ann Pharmacother 1996;30(12):1437–45.

45. Wilcox SR. Corticosteroids and neuromuscular blockers in development of critical illness neuromuscular abnormalities: a historical review. J Crit Care 2017;37:149–55.

46. Qadir N, Chang SY. Pharmacologic treatments for acute respiratory distress syndrome. Crit Care Clin 2021;37(4):877–93.

47. Papazian L, Forel JM, Gacouin A, et al. Neuromuscular blockers in early acute respiratory distress syndrome. N Engl J Med 2010;363(12):1107–16.

48. National Heart Lung, Blood Institute PETAL Clinical Trials Network, Moss M, Huang DT, et al. Early neuromuscular blockade in the acute respiratory distress syndrome. N Engl J Med 2019;380(21):1997–2008.

49. Ho ATN, Patolia S, Guervilly C. Neuromuscular blockade in acute respiratory distress syndrome: a systematic review and meta-analysis of randomized controlled trials. J Intensive Care 2020;8:12.

50. Bruni A, Garofalo E, Pelaia C, et al. Patient-ventilator asynchrony in adult critically ill patients. Minerva Anestesiol 2019;85(6):676–88.

51. Annane D, Renault A, Brun-Buisson C, et al. Hydrocortisone plus fludrocortisone for adults with septic shock. N Engl J Med 2018;378(9):809–18.

52. Venkatesh B, Finfer S, Cohen J, et al. Adjunctive glucocorticoid therapy in patients with septic shock. N Engl J Med 2018;378(9):797–808.

53. The RECOVERY Collaborative Group. Dexamethasone in hospitalized patients with covid-19. N Engl J Med 2021;384(8):693–704. https://doi.org/10.1056/NEJMoa2021436.

54. Stern A, Skalsky K, Avni T, et al. Corticosteroids for pneumonia. Cochrane acute respiratory infections group. Cochrane Database Syst Rev 2017;2017(12). https://doi.org/10.1002/14651858.CD007720.pub3.

55. Dequin PF, Meziani F, Quenot JP, et al. Hydrocortisone in severe community-acquired pneumonia. N Engl J Med 2023;388(21):1931–41.

56. Bernard GR, Luce JM, Sprung CL, et al. High-dose corticosteroids in patients with the adult respiratory distress syndrome. N Engl J Med 1987;317(25):1565–70.

57. GU Meduri, Golden E, Freire AX, et al. Methylprednisolone infusion in early severe ARDS: results of a randomized controlled trial. Chest 2007;131(4):954–63.

58. Villar J, Ferrando C, Martínez D, et al. Dexamethasone treatment for the acute respiratory distress syndrome: a multicentre, randomised controlled trial. Lancet Respir Med 2020;8(3):267–76.

59. GU Meduri, Siemieniuk RAC, Ness RA, et al. Prolonged low-dose methylpred-nisolone treatment is highly effective in reducing duration of mechanical ventilation and mortality in patients with ARDS. J Intensive Care 2018;6:53.
60. Chaudhuri D, Sasaki K, Karkar A, et al. Corticosteroids in COVID-19 and non-COVID-19 ARDS: a systematic review and meta-analysis. Intensive Care Med 2021;47(5):521–37.
61. Steinberg KP, Hudson LD, Goodman RB, et al. Efficacy and safety of corticosteroids for persistent acute respiratory distress syndrome. N Engl J Med 2006; 354(16):1671–84.
62. Waljee AK, Rogers MAM, Lin P, et al. Short term use of oral corticosteroids and related harms among adults in the United States: population based cohort study. BMJ 2017;j1415. https://doi.org/10.1136/bmj.j1415. Published online April 12.
63. Ayodele OA, Cabral HJ, McManus DD, et al. Glucocorticoids and risk of venous thromboembolism in asthma patients aged 20-59 Years in the United Kingdom's CPRD 1995-2015. Clin Epidemiol 2022;14:83–93.
64. Annane D, Pastores SM, Rochwerg B, et al. Guidelines for the diagnosis and management of critical illness-related corticosteroid insufficiency (CIRCI) in critically ill patients (Part I): society of critical care medicine (SCCM) and European society of intensive care medicine (ESICM) 2017. Crit Care Med 2017;45(12): 2078–88.
65. Zwissler B, Kemming G, Habler O, et al. Inhaled prostacyclin (PGI2) versus inhaled nitric oxide in adult respiratory distress syndrome. Am J Respir Crit Care Med 1996;154(6 Pt 1):1671–7.
66. Walmrath D, Schneider T, Schermuly R, et al. Direct comparison of inhaled nitric oxide and aerosolized prostacyclin in acute respiratory distress syndrome. Am J Respir Crit Care Med 1996;153(3):991–6.
67. Putensen C, Hörmann C, Kleinsasser A, et al. Cardiopulmonary effects of aerosolized prostaglandin E1 and nitric oxide inhalation in patients with acute respiratory distress syndrome. Am J Respir Crit Care Med 1998;157(6 Pt 1):1743–7.
68. Griffiths MJD, Evans TW. Inhaled nitric oxide therapy in adults. N Engl J Med 2005;353(25):2683–95.
69. Adhikari NKJ, Burns KEA, Friedrich JO, et al. Effect of nitric oxide on oxygenation and mortality in acute lung injury: systematic review and meta-analysis. BMJ 2007;334(7597):779.
70. Gebistorf F, Karam O, Wetterslev J, et al. Inhaled nitric oxide for acute respiratory distress syndrome (ARDS) in children and adults. Cochrane Database Syst Rev 2016;2016(6):CD002787.
71. Gerlach H, Keh D, Semmerow A, et al. Dose-response characteristics during long-term inhalation of nitric oxide in patients with severe acute respiratory distress syndrome: a prospective, randomized, controlled study. Am J Respir Crit Care Med 2003;167(7):1008–15.
72. Ruan SY, Wu HY, Lin HH, et al. Inhaled nitric oxide and the risk of renal dysfunction in patients with acute respiratory distress syndrome: a propensity-matched cohort study. Crit Care Lond Engl 2016;20(1):389.
73. Sawheny E, Ellis AL, Kinasewitz GT. Iloprost improves gas exchange in patients with pulmonary hypertension and ARDS. Chest 2013;144(1):55–62.
74. Afshari A, Bastholm Bille A, Allingstrup M. Aerosolized prostacyclins for acute respiratory distress syndrome (ARDS). Cochrane Database Syst Rev 2017; 7(7):CD007733.

75. Brodie D, Slutsky AS, Combes A. Extracorporeal life support for adults with respiratory failure and related indications: a review. JAMA 2019;322(6):557–68.

76. Organization ELS. ECLS Registry Report: International Summary.; 2023. https://www.elso.org/registry/internationalsummaryandreports/reports.aspx.

77. Peek GJ, Mugford M, Tiruvoipati R, et al. Efficacy and economic assessment of conventional ventilatory support versus extracorporeal membrane oxygenation for severe adult respiratory failure (CESAR): a multicentre randomised controlled trial. Lancet Lond Engl 2009;374(9698):1351–63.

78. Combes A, Hajage D, Capellier G, et al. Extracorporeal membrane oxygenation for severe acute respiratory distress syndrome. N Engl J Med 2018;378(21):1965–75.

79. Harrington D, Drazen JM. Learning from a trial stopped by a data and safety monitoring board. N Engl J Med 2018;378(21):2031–2.

80. Goligher EC, Tomlinson G, Hajage D, et al. Extracorporeal membrane oxygenation for severe acute respiratory distress syndrome and posterior probability of mortality benefit in a post hoc Bayesian analysis of a randomized clinical trial. JAMA 2018;320(21):2251–9.

81. Munshi L, Walkey A, Goligher E, et al. Venovenous extracorporeal membrane oxygenation for acute respiratory distress syndrome: a systematic review and meta-analysis. Lancet Respir Med 2019;7(2):163–72.

82. Tonna JE, Abrams D, Brodie D, et al. Management of adult patients supported with venovenous extracorporeal membrane oxygenation (VV ECMO): guideline from the extracorporeal life support organization (ELSO). ASAIO J Am Soc Artif Intern Organs 1992 2021;67(6):601–10.

83. Schmidt M, Bailey M, Sheldrake J, et al. Predicting survival after extracorporeal membrane oxygenation for severe acute respiratory failure. The Respiratory Extracorporeal Membrane Oxygenation Survival Prediction (RESP) score. Am J Respir Crit Care Med 2014;189(11):1374–82.

84. Schmidt M, Zogheib E, Rozé H, et al. The PRESERVE mortality risk score and analysis of long-term outcomes after extracorporeal membrane oxygenation for severe acute respiratory distress syndrome. Intensive Care Med 2013;39(10):1704–13.

85. Wilcox ME, Jaramillo-Rocha V, Hodgson C, et al. Long-term quality of life after extracorporeal membrane oxygenation in ARDS survivors: systematic review and meta-analysis. J Intensive Care Med 2020;35(3):233–43.

86. Barbaro RP, Odetola FO, Kidwell KM, et al. Association of hospital-level volume of extracorporeal membrane oxygenation cases and mortality. Analysis of the extracorporeal life support organization registry. Am J Respir Crit Care Med 2015;191(8):894–901.

87. Verma A, Hadaya J, Williamson C, et al. A contemporary analysis of the volume-outcome relationship for extracorporeal membrane oxygenation in the United States. Surgery 2023;173(6):1405–10.

88. Tomazini BM, Maia IS, Cavalcanti AB, et al. Effect of dexamethasone on days alive and ventilator-free in patients with moderate or severe acute respiratory distress syndrome and COVID-19: the CoDEX randomized clinical trial. JAMA 2020;324(13):1307–16.

89. Meduri GU, Headley AS, Golden E, et al. Effect of prolonged methylprednisolone therapy in unresolving acute respiratory distress syndrome: a randomized controlled trial. JAMA 1998;280(2):159–65.

90. Jeronimo CMP, Farias MEL, Val FFA, et al. Methylprednisolone as adjunctive therapy for patients hospitalized with coronavirus disease 2019 (COVID-19;

metcovid): a randomized, double-blind, phase IIb, placebo-controlled trial. Clin Infect Dis Off Publ Infect Dis Soc Am 2021;72(9):e373–81.

91. Annane D, Sébille V, Bellissant E, et al, Study Group. Effect of low doses of corticosteroids in septic shock patients with or without early acute respiratory distress syndrome. Crit Care Med 2006;34(1):22–30.

92. Tongyoo S, Permpikul C, Mongkolpun W, et al. Hydrocortisone treatment in early sepsis-associated acute respiratory distress syndrome: results of a randomized controlled trial. Crit Care Lond Engl 2016;20(1):329.

93. Angus DC, Derde L, Al-Beidh F, et al. Effect of hydrocortisone on mortality and organ support in patients with severe COVID-19: the REMAP-CAP COVID-19 corticosteroid domain randomized clinical trial. JAMA 2020;324(13):1317–29.

94. Khan A, Benthin C, Zeno B, et al. A pilot clinical trial of recombinant human angiotensin-converting enzyme 2 in acute respiratory distress syndrome. Crit Care Lond Engl 2017;21(1):234.

95. Morris PE, Steingrub JS, Huang BY, et al. A phase I study evaluating the pharmacokinetics, safety and tolerability of an antibody-based tissue factor antagonist in subjects with acute lung injury or acute respiratory distress syndrome. BMC Pulm Med 2012;12:5.

96. Perkins GD, McAuley DF, Thickett DR, et al. The beta-agonist lung injury trial (Balti): a randomized placebo-controlled clinical trial. Am J Respir Crit Care Med 2006;173(3):281–7.

97. National Heart, Lung, and Blood Institute Acute Respiratory Distress Syndrome ARDS Clinical Trials Network, Matthay MA, Brower RG, et al. National Heart, Lung, and Blood Institute Acute Respiratory Distress Syndrome (ARDS) Clinical Trials Network, Matthay MA, Brower RG, et al. Randomized, placebo-controlled clinical trial of an aerosolized β_2-agonist for treatment of acute lung injury. Am J Respir Crit Care Med 2011;184(5):561–8.

98. Gao Smith F, Perkins GD, Gates S, et al. Effect of intravenous β-2 agonist treatment on clinical outcomes in acute respiratory distress syndrome (Balti-2): a multicentre, randomised controlled trial. Lancet Lond Engl 2012;379(9812):229–35.

99. Festic E, Carr GE, Cartin-Ceba R, et al. Randomized clinical trial of a combination of an inhaled corticosteroid and beta agonist in patients at risk of developing the acute respiratory distress syndrome. Crit Care Med 2017;45(5):798–805.

100. Fredenburgh LE, Perrella MA, Barragan-Bradford D, et al. A phase I trial of low-dose inhaled carbon monoxide in sepsis-induced ARDS. JCI Insight 2018;3(23):e124039.

101. Matute-Bello G, Liles WC, Radella F, et al. Modulation of neutrophil apoptosis by granulocyte colony-stimulating factor and granulocyte/macrophage colony-stimulating factor during the course of acute respiratory distress syndrome. Crit Care Med 2000;28(1):1–7.

102. Presneill JJ, Harris T, Stewart AG, et al. A randomized phase II trial of granulocyte-macrophage colony-stimulating factor therapy in severe sepsis with respiratory dysfunction. Am J Respir Crit Care Med 2002;166(2):138–43.

103. Paine R, Standiford TJ, Dechert RE, et al. A randomized trial of recombinant human granulocyte-macrophage colony stimulating factor for patients with acute lung injury. Crit Care Med 2012;40(1):90–7.

104. Dixon B, Santamaria JD, Campbell DJ. A phase 1 trial of nebulised heparin in acute lung injury. Crit Care Lond Engl 2008;12(3):R64.

105. Dixon B, Schultz MJ, Smith R, et al. Nebulized heparin is associated with fewer days of mechanical ventilation in critically ill patients: a randomized controlled trial. Crit Care Lond Engl 2010;14(5):R180.

106. Dixon B, Smith R, Santamaria JD, et al. A trial of nebulised heparin to limit lung injury following cardiac surgery. Anaesth Intensive Care 2016;44(1):28–33.

107. Abdelaal Ahmed Mahmoud A, Mahmoud HE, Mahran MA, et al. Streptokinase versus unfractionated heparin nebulization in patients with severe acute respiratory distress syndrome (ARDS): a randomized controlled trial with observational controls. J Cardiothorac Vasc Anesth 2020;34(2):436–43.

108. Bellingan G, Maksimow M, Howell DC, et al. The effect of intravenous interferon-beta-1a (FP-1201) on lung CD73 expression and on acute respiratory distress syndrome mortality: an open-label study. Lancet Respir Med 2014;2(2):98–107.

109. Ranieri VM, Pettilä V, Karvonen MK, et al. Effect of intravenous interferon β-1a on death and days free from mechanical ventilation among patients with moderate to severe acute respiratory distress syndrome: a randomized clinical trial. JAMA 2020;323(8):725–33.

110. Wilson JG, Liu KD, Zhuo H, et al. Mesenchymal stem (stromal) cells for treatment of ARDS: a phase 1 clinical trial. Lancet Respir Med 2015;3(1):24–32.

111. Matthay MA, Calfee CS, Zhuo H, et al. Treatment with allogeneic mesenchymal stromal cells for moderate to severe acute respiratory distress syndrome (START study): a randomised phase 2a safety trial. Lancet Respir Med 2019; 7(2):154–62.

112. Bellingan G, Jacono F, Bannard-Smith J, et al. Primary analysis of a phase 1/2 study to assess MultiStem® cell therapy, a regenerative advanced therapy medicinal product (ATMP), in acute respiratory distress syndrome (MUST-ARDS). In: B14. Late BREAKING clinical trials. American Thoracic Society; 2019. p. A7353. https://doi.org/10.1164/ajrccm-conference.2019.199.1_MeetingAbstracts. A7353.

113. Yip HK, Fang WF, Li YC, et al. Human umbilical cord-derived mesenchymal stem cells for acute respiratory distress syndrome. Crit Care Med 2020;48(5): e391–9.

114. Lanzoni G, Linetsky E, Correa D, et al. Umbilical cord mesenchymal stem cells for COVID-19 acute respiratory distress syndrome: a double-blind, phase 1/2a, randomized controlled trial. Stem Cells Transl Med 2021;10(5):660–73.

115. Jepsen S, Herlevsen P, Knudsen P, et al. Antioxidant treatment with N-acetylcysteine during adult respiratory distress syndrome: a prospective, randomized, placebo-controlled study. Crit Care Med 1992;20(7):918–23.

116. Suter PM, Domenighetti G, Schaller MD, et al. N-acetylcysteine enhances recovery from acute lung injury in man. A randomized, double-blind, placebo-controlled clinical study. Chest 1994;105(1):190–4.

117. Bernard GR, Wheeler AP, Arons MM, et al. A trial of antioxidants N-acetylcysteine and procysteine in ARDS. The Antioxidant in ARDS Study Group. Chest 1997;112(1):164–72.

118. Domenighetti G, Suter PM, Schaller MD, et al. Treatment with N-acetylcysteine during acute respiratory distress syndrome: a randomized, double-blind, placebo-controlled clinical study. J Crit Care 1997;12(4):177–82.

119. Taher A, Lashgari M, Sedighi L, et al. A pilot study on intravenous N-Acetylcysteine treatment in patients with mild-to-moderate COVID19-associated acute respiratory distress syndrome. Pharmacol Rep PR 2021;73(6):1650–9.

120. Schwameis R, Eder S, Pietschmann H, et al. A FIM study to assess safety and exposure of inhaled single doses of AP301-A specific ENaC channel activator for the treatment of acute lung injury. J Clin Pharmacol 2014;54(3):341–50.
121. Krenn K, Lucas R, Croizé A, et al. Inhaled AP301 for treatment of pulmonary edema in mechanically ventilated patients with acute respiratory distress syndrome: a phase IIa randomized placebo-controlled trial. Crit Care Lond Engl 2017;21(1):194.
122. National Heart Lung, Blood Institute ARDS Clinical Trials Network, Truwit JD, Bernard GR, et al. Rosuvastatin for sepsis-associated acute respiratory distress syndrome. N Engl J Med 2014;370(23):2191–200.
123. McAuley DF, Laffey JG, O'Kane CM, et al. Simvastatin in the acute respiratory distress syndrome. N Engl J Med 2014;371(18):1695–703.
124. Dinglas VD, Hopkins RO, Wozniak AW, et al. One-year outcomes of rosuvastatin versus placebo in sepsis-associated acute respiratory distress syndrome: prospective follow-up of SAILS randomised trial. Thorax 2016;71(5):401–10.
125. Calfee CS, Delucchi KL, Sinha P, et al. Acute respiratory distress syndrome subphenotypes and differential response to simvastatin: secondary analysis of a randomised controlled trial. Lancet Respir Med 2018;6(9):691–8.
126. Anzueto A, Baughman RP, Guntupalli KK, et al. Aerosolized surfactant in adults with sepsis-induced acute respiratory distress syndrome. Exosurf acute respiratory distress syndrome sepsis study group. N Engl J Med 1996;334(22):1417–21.
127. Spragg RG, Lewis JF, Walmrath HD, et al. Effect of recombinant surfactant protein C-based surfactant on the acute respiratory distress syndrome. N Engl J Med 2004;351(9):884–92.
128. Spragg RG, Taut FJH, Lewis JF, et al. Recombinant surfactant protein C-based surfactant for patients with severe direct lung injury. Am J Respir Crit Care Med 2011;183(8):1055–61.
129. Willson DF, Truwit JD, Conaway MR, et al. The adult calfactant in acute respiratory distress syndrome trial. Chest 2015;148(2):356–64.
130. Fowler AA, Truwit JD, Hite RD, et al. Effect of vitamin C infusion on organ failure and biomarkers of inflammation and vascular injury in patients with sepsis and severe acute respiratory failure: the CITRIS-ALI randomized clinical trial. JAMA 2019;322(13):1261–70.

Acute Respiratory Failure in Pregnancy

Stephen E. Lapinsky, MBBCh, MSc, FRCPC[a,*],
Daniela N. Vasquez, MD[b]

KEYWORDS

- Respiratory failure • Mechanical ventilation • Pregnancy complications
- Fetal hypoxia • Obstetric delivery

KEY POINTS

- Although the fetus may be affected by abnormal maternal blood gases, data are insufficient to warrant changes to usual blood gas targets.
- The pregnant patient is at increased risk of acute respiratory distress syndrome, particularly related to certain infections such as influenza and coronavirus disease 2019.
- Mechanical ventilation should be carried out using similar parameters to those used in the non-pregnant patient.
- Although delivery may be considered in an attempt to improve the maternal respiratory condition, significant improvement does often not occur.

INTRODUCTION

Respiratory failure in pregnancy is uncommon, but with a significant increase occurring during the coronavirus disease 2019 (COVID-19) pandemic. In addition to COVID-19, pregnancy increases the risk or severity of other respiratory conditions, including asthma, aspiration, thromboembolism, and influenza pneumonitis. Furthermore, several pregnancy-specific conditions such as preeclampsia, amniotic fluid embolism, and peripartum cardiomyopathy may precipitate respiratory failure.

Management of respiratory failure during pregnancy may be altered by the changes in maternal respiratory physiology, and by the high-risk intervention of endotracheal intubation. The presence of a fetus may influence investigations and drug choices in these patients. Although limited data exist regarding the approach to prolonged mechanical ventilation management in pregnancy, increasing data are now being published. Delivery of the fetus is often considered in an attempt to improve the

[a] Mount Sinai Hospital, Toronto, Interdepartmental Division of Critical Care Medicine, University of Toronto, 600 University Avenue, Toronto M5G1X5, Canada; [b] ICU Head of Department, Sanatorio Anchorena, Tomás M. de Anchorena 1872, City of Buenos Aires, Argentina
* Corresponding author.
E-mail address: Stephen.lapinsky@utoronto.ca

Crit Care Clin 40 (2024) 353–366
https://doi.org/10.1016/j.ccc.2024.01.005
0749-0704/24/© 2024 Elsevier Inc. All rights reserved.

criticalcare.theclinics.com

maternal respiratory status, but available data suggest that benefit occurs only in a minority of patients.

MATERNO-FETAL RESPIRATORY PHYSIOLOGY

The pregnant state is associated with upper airway edema and hyperemia making endotracheal intubation potentially more difficult. The chest wall shape changes as pregnancy progresses, resulting in a decrease in functional residual capacity (FRC) by 10% to 25%, with minimal change in total lung capacity.[1] Minute ventilation increases in pregnancy reaching 40% above baseline, mediated by rising progesterone levels. This occurs via an increase in tidal volume with very little change in respiratory rate.[2] As a result, an arterial blood gas during pregnancy will demonstrate a mild, compensated respiratory alkalosis, with $PaCO_2$ falling to 28 to 32 mm Hg and plasma bicarbonate falling to 18 to 21 mEq/L.[3] An arterial blood gas in pregnancy with a $PaCO_2$ of 40 mm Hg and bicarbonate 20 mEq/L may superficially resemble a mild metabolic acidosis, but with the knowledge of the reduced normal $PaCO_2$ level, this should be recognized as a respiratory acidosis. Severe alkalosis, for example due to hyperventilation or vomiting, may cause uterine artery vasoconstriction thereby reducing uterine blood flow and resulting in fetal hypoxia.[4]

Oxygen levels should not be significantly altered by the pregnant state, although a small increase occurs due to the hypocapnia, and mild hypoxemia may be found in the supine position as FRC diminishes near term. Oxygen consumption (and CO_2 production) increases by 20% to 33% due to increased metabolic demands of the fetus and uterus. The reduced oxygen reserve in the lungs (reduced FRC) combined with the increased oxygen consumption results in the rapid development of hypoxemia during hypoventilation or apnea, as may occur during intubation.[5]

Oxygen Targets in Pregnancy

Although it is often suggested that maternal arterial oxygen levels should be maintained at greater than 70 mm Hg (or saturation >95%),[6] there are no studies to support this threshold. Maternal oxygen saturation is only one of the factors affecting fetal oxygen delivery. Uterine blood flow and therefore placental perfusion impact fetal oxygen delivery and may be adversely affected by catecholamines, alkalosis, or reduced venous return produced by elevated intrathoracic pressure during mechanical ventilation.[7] A short-term clinical study during electronic fetal monitoring used inhalation of 10% oxygen to generate controlled maternal hypoxemia (saturation <85%), with no demonstrable adverse fetal effects.[8] Hyperoxia may be harmful by increasing peripheral resistance and reducing cardiac output.[9]

Carbon Dioxide (PaCO₂) Targets in Pregnancy

The question arises as to whether the normally reduced $PaCO_2$ levels in pregnancy should be the ventilation target, and whether permissive hypercapnia is harmful. Hypocapnia and alkalosis may be harmful by reducing placental perfusion.[4] Permissive hypercapnia is accepted during pressure-limited ventilation in the non-pregnant patient, but the effects of hypercapnia on the fetus have not been adequately studied. The concerns would be a reduction in the gradient for excretion of fetal CO_2, and right-shifting the fetal oxyhemoglobin dissociation curve, adversely affecting fetal oxygen transport. Fetal acidosis may occur but likely does not have the same ominous implications for the fetus as lactic acidosis secondary to hypoxia. Several small clinical studies have not demonstrated adverse effects of short-term exposure of the fetus to hypercapnia (largely during cesarean delivery).[10,11] Case series of status asthmaticus have described severe maternal hypercapnia with $PaCO_2$ levels greater than 100 mm Hg for more than 24 hours, with good maternal and neonatal outcomes.[12] Management of CO_2 levels in the ventilated pregnant patient involves a risk-benefit balance of potentially aggravating maternal lung injury by higher tidal volume ventilation, versus the unclear adverse effects of mild hypercapnia on the fetus.

CAUSES OF ACUTE RESPIRATORY FAILURE

Respiratory failure may result from several pregnancy-specific conditions, as well as pulmonary conditions which are aggravated by the pregnant state, or conditions unrelated to pregnancy (**Table 1**).

Acute Respiratory Distress Syndrome in Pregnancy

Pregnant patients appear to be at increased risk of ARDS compared to non-pregnant patients due to the increased circulating blood volume, decreased serum albumin level, and an upregulation of components of the acute inflammatory response.[13] ARDS may be caused by conditions unique to pregnancy such as amniotic fluid embolism, conditions augmented by pregnancy such as aspiration pneumonia, or conditions unrelated to pregnancy. Although ARDS is relatively rare during pregnancy (59.6 per 100,000 live births in 2012), it has become more common recently related to the coronavirus disease 2019 (COVID-19) pandemic.[14]

Aspiration pneumonitis is a significant risk during labor and delivery due to the increase in intra-abdominal pressure, the decreased tone of the lower esophageal sphincter, and the use of the supine position for delivery.[15] Pregnant women are also more susceptible to respiratory complications of viral pneumonitis especially from COVID-19 and influenza.[14]

Amniotic fluid embolism is an uncommon but devastating pregnancy-specific condition occurring in about 7.7 per 100,000 pregnancies, with a high mortality rate and accounting for 14% of all maternal deaths.[16,17] This condition usually occurs associated with uterine manipulation or labor and delivery, and is characterized by sudden hemodynamic collapse with hypoxic respiratory failure. The pathophysiology involves inflammatory mediators from amniotic fluid entering uterine vessels, precipitating acute pulmonary hypertension and biventricular dysfunction. Survivors of the initial cardiovascular collapse may develop disseminated intravascular coagulation and ARDS.

Other conditions associated with ARDS during pregnancy are preeclampsia, sepsis especially due to pyelonephritis or puerperal infections, and transfusion-related acute

Table 1 Causes of respiratory failure in pregnancy		
Unique to Pregnancy	**Exacerbated by Pregnancy**	**Unrelated to Pregnancy**
Preeclampsia	Pulmonary edema due to	Bacterial pneumonia
Amniotic fluid embolism	preexisting cardiac	Restrictive lung disease
Pulmonary edema due to	disease	Cystic fibrosis
peripartum	Acute respiratory distress	Trauma
cardiomyopathy	syndrome	
Tocolytic pulmonary edema	Aspiration pneumonitis	
	Viral pneumonia	
	(influenza, COVID-19)	
	Pulmonary embolism	

lung injury, manifesting as sudden dyspnea during, or within 6 hours of transfusion of plasma-containing blood products.[18]

Cardiogenic Pulmonary Edema

Pulmonary edema may occur during pregnancy as a result cardiac disease, or hypertensive disorders of pregnancy. Pulmonary edema occurs in about 2.9% of patients with preeclampsia.[19] Various hemodynamic profiles have been identified in preeclampsia, including a hypodynamic type with increased systemic vascular resistance (associated with early preeclampsia) and a hyperdynamic subtype (associated with late preeclampsia).[20] Impaired systolic and diastolic function may occur.[21] The pulmonary edema commonly presents immediately postpartum due to increased central circulating volume, related to fluid administration as well as the return of blood from the contracting uterus. The low colloid oncotic pressure and abnormal vascular permeability likely also contribute.

As the blood volume and cardiac output requirements increase during pregnancy, women with pre-existing heart disease are at risk of cardiac decompensation. The peripartum period is also high risk, related to shifts in intravascular volume associated with delivery. Those with cyanotic heart disease, mitral and aortic valve stenotic lesions, or systolic dysfunction are at most risk.[22] A cardiac condition specific to pregnancy is peripartum cardiomyopathy, occurring in 1 of 1000 to 4000 pregnancies,[23] presenting with congestive heart failure. This condition is also associated with a risk of pulmonary and systemic embolization.[24]

Pulmonary Infections

Pregnancy is associated with a down regulation of cell-mediated immunity, with an intact or upregulated humoral immune response,[25] to allow tolerance to paternally derived fetal antigens. These changes to the immune system increase the pregnant person's susceptibility to certain infections.

COVID-19 infection appears to be more severe during pregnancy, with an increased risk of hospitalization and intensive care unit (ICU) admission as well as the complication of preterm birth.[26] During the COVID-19 pandemic, pregnant women requiring mechanical ventilation for respiratory failure were seen in numbers far higher than for any condition previously. Women at highest risk for severe disease were those of minority ethnicity or with diabetes, hypertensive disorders, and obesity.[26] Although case-fatality rates differed widely by geographic location and study design, a high incidence of mortality did occur in pregnant women.[27]

Influenza pneumonitis causes significant morbidity in pregnancy, and during influenza epidemics the maternal mortality rate has been higher than the general population,[28] with a marked increase in the need for ICU admission.[29] Varicella pneumonia may also be associated with increased morbidity and mortality during pregnancy, although not all studies have confirmed this increased risk.[30]

Although the incidence of community-acquired pneumonia is similar to that in the general population, pneumonia is an important cause of maternofetal morbidity and mortality.[31] An increased incidence of complications of pneumonia, including respiratory failure, may occur in pregnancy, and pneumonia may precipitate preterm labor, small-for-gestational-age, and intrauterine and neonatal death.[31] Delayed diagnosis may occur, due to inappropriate concern of radiation exposure and limitation in the use of chest imaging. Treatment uses similar antibacterials to the non-pregnant patient, but some drugs such as tetracyclines and quinolones should be avoided if possible.[31]

Other Conditions

Asthma: Asthma affects up to 10% of the general population and is therefore a common disorder in pregnancy.[32] The hormonal changes of pregnancy affects asthma in a variable way, but approximately a third of asthmatics will deteriorate during their pregnancy.[33] Drugs used in labor and delivery may affect asthma control. Oxytocin carries little risk, but 15-methyl prostaglandin F_2-alpha (carboprost, Hemabate), methylergonovine, and ergonovine may cause bronchospasm. Some narcotics (other than fentanyl) release histamine, which can worsen bronchospasm. Status asthmaticus in pregnancy is managed similarly to non-pregnant patients.[34]

Pulmonary thrombo-embolic disease: The risk of thromboembolism is significantly increased in pregnancy and it is a leading cause of maternal mortality, accounting for about 10% of pregnancy-related deaths in the United States.[35,36] The peak incidence occurs in the postpartum period, particularly after cesarean section. Diagnosis can be made by duplex ultrasonography (although false-positive Doppler results may occur), and ventilation-perfusion (V/Q) scanning or computed tomography (CT) pulmonary angiography can be safely performed during pregnancy.[37] V/Q scanning usually produces good quality scans, as these patients lack pulmonary co-morbidity, while CT angiography carries the risk of maternal breast tissue exposure to a significant dose of radiation, with concerns about an increased risk of breast cancer.[38] Both tests are associated with a low fetal radiation exposure.

VENTILATION MANAGEMENT
Airway Management

The obstetric airway should be considered a difficult airway and managed by an operator with appropriate skill. Failed intubation occurs 8 times more commonly than in other anesthetic intubations.[39] The reduced FRC and increased oxygen consumption in pregnancy result in rapid oxygen desaturation during apnea,[5] and visualization may be impaired by upper airway mucosal edema. Other factors exacerbating the situation include preeclampsia (with additional edema), mucosal bleeding (due to friability and hyperemia of the mucosa), the increase risk of aspiration (the stomach should always be considered full), and large breasts (which can obstruct the handle of the laryngoscope). A smaller size endotracheal tube may be needed, and the nasal route should be avoided. Although it is important to provide optimal pre-oxygenation, over-ventilation and respiratory alkalosis must be avoided. Additional equipment should be available, including a short handle laryngoscope and smaller size endotracheal tubes.

Non-invasive Ventilation

Non-invasive ventilation (NIV) is increasingly used for short-term ventilatory support in non-pregnant patients and avoids the complications associated with endotracheal intubation and sedation. In the pregnant patient, the use of NIV increases the risk of aspiration as a complication, but it is clearly beneficial in some situations particularly in obstetric respiratory complications which reverse rapidly.[40] NIV has been also used effectively in pregnant patients with chronic respiratory failure due to neuromuscular disease,[41] and may be useful in other common indications for NIV (eg, heart failure, obstructive airways disease), but data are lacking.

NIV was used successfully in pregnant women during the H1N1 pandemic with a report of 83 patients (45% of all those ventilated) initially receiving NIV, with invasive ventilation avoided in 46% of the NIV group.[42] NIV can be administered via a variety of interfaces including face mask, but the use of the helmet interface has also been described.[43]

In general, NIV should be reserved for the patient who is alert, protecting their airway and with good spontaneous respirations, and where the requirement for mechanical ventilation is expected to be relatively brief.

Invasive Mechanical Ventilation

Although significant knowledge has been generated over the past 20 years on the appropriate provision on non-injurious mechanical ventilation, pregnant women were predominantly excluded or not reported in these major mechanical ventilation trials. Recommendations on ventilation during pregnancy are therefore based on observational studies, physiologic concepts, and expert opinions (**Table 2**).

Low tidal volume ventilation (6–8 mL/kg of ideal body weight) is the best practice approach for patients with[44] and without ARDS.[45] Lung volumes change minimally through pregnancy although tidal volume increases,[46] and using an ideal body weight based on height remains appropriate in pregnant women. In patients with severe ARDS, the benefits of low tidal volume ventilation must be weighed against the potential fetal risks of permissive hypercapnia (see above).

The decreased FRC occurring as pregnancy progresses renders the pregnant patient susceptible to atelectasis and alveolar derecruitment. Recruitment maneuvers and higher positive end-expiratory pressure (PEEP) levels may prevent alveolar derecruitment and be beneficial.[47] However, hemodynamic monitoring must be

Table 2		
Mechanical ventilation during pregnancy: comparison with the non-pregnant patient		
Parameter	**Non-pregnant Patient**	**Pregnant Patient**
Tidal volume	6 mL/kg IBW	6 mL/kg IBW
Plateau pressure limit	< 30 cmH_2O	Higher pressures often accepted but prospective data suggest no difference compared with the non-pregnant population[48]
Oxygen saturation goal	Usually > 88%–92% Avoid hyperoxia	Often suggest > 94% but unclear if this is necessary Avoid hyperoxia
Arterial carbon dioxide ($PaCO_2$) limit	Permissive hypercapnia (sometimes as high as 100 mm Hg)	Avoid hypocapnia and alkalosis Pregnancy normal = 28–32 mm Hg Limited data on hypercapnia, but moderate levels (eg, 50 mm Hg) may be safe
Patient positioning	Semi upright (45°)	Left lateral decubitus for hemodynamics Head elevation important to avoid reflux
Prone positioning	Good data of benefit in ARDS	Technically difficult but feasible, no evidence of harm

Abbreviations: Fio_2, fraction of inspired oxygen; IBW, ideal body weight (based on height); PEEP, positive end-expiratory pressure.

considered to detect decreased cardiac output and hypotension potentially deleterious to the fetus.

Due to the reduced chest wall compliance, airway pressures in pregnant women may be expected to be higher for a given tidal volume. However, a study of 47 ventilated pregnant women with COVID-19 demonstrated that lung mechanics in these patients were similar to those from the general ICU population with COVID-19.[48] Plateau (end-inspiratory occlusion) pressure is used to assess lung overdistension and is part of the management of low tidal volume ventilation in ARDS.[44] Plateau pressure is affected by the lung and chest wall compliance in addition to lung volume and total PEEP. Even if an increase in airway pressures caused by decreased chest wall compliance does occur, this does not contribute to the transpulmonary pressure applied to the alveolus and is not harmful.[49,50]

Non-conventional Support

In the presence of intractable hypoxemia, rescue modalities such as inhaled nitric oxide (iNO) are sometimes used, based on limited clinical experience and published case reports. These have not been specifically studied in pregnancy, but iNO has been used in a small case series of pregnant patients with severe COVID-19 demonstrating improvement in hypoxemia with no adverse neonatal effects.[51] Prone positioning has been shown to have a mortality benefit in ARDS patients with a PaO_2/FiO_2 ratio less than 150,[52] but pregnant women were excluded from this study. Prone positioning may be perceived as producing adverse pressure effects on the uterus and maternal blood vessels. However, prone positioning produces largely beneficial local hemodynamic effects; a prospective study showed that it relieves uterine compression of the large maternal vessels.[53] A prospective study, as well as a small number of published case reports and conference abstracts have described successful use of prone positioning in pregnancy,[48,54,55] and algorithms have been developed specifically for pregnant patients.[56] These involve padding the chest, pelvis, and lower legs anteriorly prior to turning, "cocooning" the padded patient with a bed sheet, and then careful turning following usual protocols.

Extracorporeal life-support was utilized in pregnant patients during the 2009 H1N1 influenza epidemic and the COVID-19 pandemic, due to the large number of pregnant women with severe disease[57,58] A case series of 12 pregnant and postpartum women documents a 66% maternal and 71% neonatal survival.[57]

Adjunctive Interventions and Therapy

Imaging

The pregnant patient with respiratory failure may require chest radiography and chest computed tomography (CT), raising concerns regarding risks to the fetus. Although risks to the fetus of clinical radiological studies are very low, radiation may affect the fetus by inducing teratogenicity, carcinogenesis, and effects on brain development. Teratogenicity risks are greatest during first trimester and are related to the total dose administered (usually requiring more than 50 mGy).[59] Carcinogenesis (usually childhood leukemia) arises due to DNA mutations which can occur at any radiation dose. The risk at low fetal exposure is minimal, increasing to approximately a doubling of risk of fatal childhood cancer at a fetal dose of 50 mGy.[59] Fetal radiation exposure of a single chest X-ray during pregnancy is minimal (**Table 3**) and can be decreased by using abdominal shielding and a well collimated X-ray beam. Chest CT exposes the fetus to a higher radiation, but less than 1 mGy,[60,61] and is considered safe in pregnancy with or without contrast.[38,61]

Table 3			
Estimated fetal and maternal radiation exposure to chest imaging modalities[27,60]			
	Estimated Fetal Radiation Dose (mGy)	Effective Maternal Dose to Whole Body (mSv)	Estimated Maternal Dose to Breasts (mGy)
Chest radiography	0.002	0.1	0.04
CT	0.013–0.8	1–2.5	3
V/Q scan	0.1–0.3	4–18	0.22–0.28

While radiation exposure in pregnancy commonly generates significant concern amongst health care providers as well as the general public, the risks to the fetus are extremely low. Radiological procedures that would usually be performed in the non-pregnant patient should never be avoided, though the precautions described earlier should be taken and unnecessary studies avoided. The American College of Obstetricians and Gynecologists guidelines emphasize that "with few exceptions, radiation exposure through radiography, computed tomography (CT) scan, or nuclear medicine imaging techniques is at a dose much lower than the exposure associated with fetal harm."[59]

Drug therapy

Mechanical ventilation sometimes requires analgesic, sedative, and neuromuscular blocking (NMB) medications. There are little data on the safety of continuous analgesia and sedation in pregnant patients. Opioids are often provided to patients undergoing mechanical ventilation, and no malformations have been described with short-term use of morphine or fentanyl.[62] Although some studies have suggested a link between first trimester use of benzodiazepines and major congenital malformations, controversy exists about this association.[63,64] When administered close to delivery, benzodiazepines can cause a neonatal withdrawal syndrome or the floppy infant syndrome.[65]

No human clinical data suggest teratogenicity with the use of propofol.[62] Case reports describe its use during mechanical ventilation with no significant concern other than the development of hypotension with decreased uteroplacental perfusion. A single report describes propofol infusion in 2 pregnant women, with the development of an acidosis not typical of a propofol infusion syndrome.[66]

Dexmedetomidine, a sedative alpha-2-agonist agent, has been used during cesarean delivery both intravenously and intrathecally. A single case report describes its use as an infusion in the ICU for a ventilated pregnant.[67] Dexmedetomidine crosses the placenta[68] and its impact on the newborn is unknown. The drug may also induce uterine contractions.[62]

Neuromuscular blocking (NMB) agents may be used for prevention of ventilator dyssynchrony in ARDS. The non-depolarizing NMBs cross the placenta in variable amounts, with the fetal-maternal drug concentration ratio of atracurium, vecuronium, rocuronium, and pancuronium varying between 0.07 and 0.26.[69] The altered pharmacokinetics and dynamics in pregnancy affect dosing of these drugs. As most data on NMB were obtained during cesarean or other surgical interventions during late pregnancy,[69] little is known about the effects of a prolonged NMB infusion or exposure during the first trimester. Case reports describe potential adverse effects; administration for 10 days may have resulted in neonatal arthrogryphosis.[70] Prolonged infusion of NMBs were used by many centers in pregnant patients during the COVID-19 pandemic, but should be used with caution and for the shortest time possible.

The optimal analgesic and sedative regimen for the mechanically ventilated patients during pregnancy is not known. In 2017, the Food and Drug Administration of the

United States submitted a warning that repeated or lengthy use of general anesthetic or sedative drugs in pregnant women during their third trimester may affect the development of children's brains.[71] The statement is controversial as it was based largely on animal studies and human data are inconclusive. Nevertheless, minimizing sedation is the standard of care for all ICU patients,[72] and this practice is even more relevant in the pregnant patient.

ROLE OF DELIVERY

While it may be considered that urgent delivery of the pregnant patient with respiratory failure may be beneficial for the mother's respiratory status and for the fetus,[73] this benefit to the mother has not been demonstrated in all studies.[74–76] A retrospective study evaluated the respiratory effects of delivery in 10 women ventilated with respiratory failure.[76] Only 6 patients demonstrated improvement in oxygenation or compliance.[76] A case series evaluated 71 pregnant women requiring mechanical ventilation, who underwent cesarean delivery within 48 hours of intubation.[77] Those with an obstetric cause for ARDS (eg, preeclampsia) did show an improvement in oxygenation and a shorter duration of ventilation, but this was not observed in women with non-obstetric causes for ARDS.[77] A retrospective study analyzed 27 women with COVID-19 who delivered while on mechanical ventilation.[78] Oxygenation and driving pressure, a parameter associated with lung injury, improved after delivery predominantly in obese patients, although some women deteriorated after delivery. In fact, considerable interindividual variability was acknowledged as a limitation by the authors.[78]

Prospective data collection has significant advantages in this situation, and a study of 47 pregnant women with COVID-19, who delivered while invasively ventilated, tracked respiratory parameters before and after delivery.[48] Although PaO_2/FiO_2 ratio increased somewhat after delivery (from a mean of 134 to 192 mm Hg over 24 h), no improvement was noted in static compliance, plateau pressure, or driving pressure.

Overall, these data demonstrate the lack of universal improvement in compliance and driving pressure with delivery. Although a small improvement in oxygenation occurred in some cases, this cannot be used as a surrogate for improved outcomes.[79] Usual obstetric indications should drive the decision for delivery (which may include severe fetal distress related to the hypoxic maternal environment), but routine delivery is not appropriate. The mode of delivery should be based on usual obstetric principles; while cesarean section allows more rapid delivery in the critically ill patient, the increased physiologic stress may be associated with higher mortality in these patients.[80] The ICU should be prepared for urgent delivery and neonatal resuscitation at any time.

OUTCOME AFTER MECHANICAL VENTILATION DURING PREGNANCY

Maternal and neonatal outcomes after mechanical ventilation have not been well studied, and depend on multiple factors including maternal comorbidities, the indication for mechanical ventilation, the duration of ventilation, and the number and severity of organ failures involved. A pre-COVID administrative database study found a maternal mortality of 9% for pregnant women mechanically ventilated for ARDS.[81] Neonatal outcomes are also not well studied and neonatal mortality ranges from 3% to 30%.[42,77] A single study has provided some insight into longer term outcome. A retrospective review of 71 women with gestation greater than 25 weeks ventilated for respiratory failure demonstrated that 20% of the babies required mechanical ventilation, 20% had growth restriction, and 14% demonstrated neurologic impairment at 6 months.[77]

CLINICS CARE POINTS

- Do not alter usual care due to the presence of a pregnancy, unless there is a very good reason to do so
- Best outcomes occur through excellent communication with a multidisciplinary team (critical care, obstetrics/maternal-fetal medicine, anesthesia and obstetric medicine)

DISCLOSURE

The authors have no conflicts of interest relevant to the content of this article.

REFERENCES

1. Elkus R, Popovich J. Respiratory physiology in pregnancy. Clin Chest Med 1992; 13:555–65.
2. Green LJ, Mackillop LH, Salvi D, et al. Gestation-specific vital sign reference ranges in pregnancy. Obstet Gynecol 2020;135:653–64.
3. Lucius H, Gahlenbeck HO, Kleine O, et al. Respiratory functions, buffer system, and electrolyte concentrations of blood during human pregnancy. Respir Physiol 1970;9:311–7.
4. Buss DD, Bisgard GE, Rawlings CA, et al. Uteroplacental blood flow during alkalosis in the sheep. Am J Physiol 1975;228:1497–500.
5. Archer GW, Marx GF. Arterial oxygen tension during apnoea in parturient women. Br J Anaesth 1974;46:358–60.
6. Cole DE, Taylor TL, McCullough DM, et al. Acute respiratory distress syndrome in pregnancy. Crit Care Med 2005;33:S269–78.
7. Aoyama K, Seaward PG, Lapinsky SE. Fetal outcome in the critically ill pregnant woman. Crit Care 2014;18:307.
8. Polvi HJ, Pirhonen JP, Erkkola RU. The hemodynamic effects of maternal hypo- and hyperoxygenation in healthy term pregnancies. Obstet Gynecol 1995;86: 795–9.
9. McHugh A, El-Khuffash A, Bussmann N, et al. Hyperoxygenation in pregnancy exerts a more profound effect on cardiovascular hemodynamics than is observed in the nonpregnant state. Am J Obstet Gynecol 2019;220(4):397.e1–8.
10. Peng AT, Blancato LS, Motoyama EK. Effect of maternal hypocapnia v. eucapnia on the foetus during Caesarean section. Br J Anaesth 1972;44:1173–8.
11. Ivankovic AD, Elam JO, Huffman J. Effect of maternal hypercarbia on the newborn infant. Am J Obstet Gynecol 1970;107:939–46.
12. Elsayegh D, Shapiro JM. Management of the obstetric patient with status asthmaticus. J Intensive Care Med 2008;23:396–402.
13. Lapinsky SE. Pregnancy joins the hit list. Crit Care Med 2012;40:1679–80.
14. Allotey J, Stallings E, Bonet M, et al. Clinical manifestations, risk factors, and maternal and perinatal outcomes of coronavirus disease 2019 in pregnancy: living systematic review and meta-analysis. BMJ 2020;370:m3320.
15. Rowe TF. Acute gastric aspiration: prevention and treatment. Semin Perinatol 1997;21(4):313–9.

16. Abenhaim HA, Azoulay L, Kramer MS, et al. Incidence and risk factors of amniotic fluid embolisms: a population-based study on 3 million births in the United States. Am J Obstet Gynecol 2008;199:49e1–8.
17. Clark SL, Hankins GD, Dudley DA, et al. Amniotic fluid embolism: analysis of the national registry. Am J Obstet Gynecol 1995;172:1158–69.
18. Lao TT. Acute respiratory distress and amniotic fluid embolism in pregnancy. Best Pract Res Clin Obstet Gynaecol 2022;85(Pt A):83–95.
19. Sibai BM, Mabie BC, Harvey CJ, et al. Pulmonary edema in severe preeclampsia-eclampsia: analysis of thirty-seven consecutive cases. Am J Obstet Gynecol 1987;156:1174–9.
20. Masini G, Foo LF, Tay J, et al. Preeclampsia has two phenotypes which require different treatment strategies. Am J Obstet Gynecol 2022;226(2S):S1006–18.
21. Benedetti TJ, Kates R, Williams V. Hemodynamic observation of severe pre-eclampsia complicated by pulmonary edema. Am J Obstet Gynecol 1985; 152:33–4.
22. Siu SC, Sermer M, Colman JM, et al. Prospective multicenter study of pregnancy outcomes in women with heart disease. Circulation 2001;104:515–21.
23. Arany Z, Elkayam U. Peripartum cardiomyopathy. Circulation 2016;133: 1397–409.
24. Pearson GD, Veille JC, Rahimtoola S, et al. Peripartum cardiomyopathy: national heart, lung, and blood institute and office of rare diseases (national Institutes of Health) workshop recommendations and review. JAMA 2000;283:1183–8.
25. Priddy KD. Immunologic adaptations during pregnancy. J Obstet Gynecol Neonatal Nurs 1997;26:388–94.
26. McClymont E, Albert AY, Alton GD, et al. Association of SARS-CoV-2 infection during pregnancy with maternal and perinatal outcomes. JAMA 2022;327(20): 1983–91.
27. Nana M, Hodson K, Lucas N, et al. Diagnosis and management of covid-19 in pregnancy. BMJ 2022;377:e069739.
28. Mosby LG, Rasmussen SA, Jamieson DJ. 2009 pandemic influenza A (H1N1) in pregnancy: a systematic review of the literature. Am J Obstet Gynecol 2011; 205:10–8.
29. Lapinsky SE. Critical illness as a result of influenza A/H1N1 infection in pregnancy. BMJ 2010;340:c1235.
30. Zhang HJ, Patenaude V, Abenhaim HA. Maternal outcomes in pregnancies affected by varicella zoster virus infections: population-based study on 7.7 million pregnancy admissions. J Obstet Gynaecol Res 2015;4:62–8.
31. Lim WS, Macfarlane JT, Colthorpe CL. Pneumonia and pregnancy. Thorax 2001; 56:398–405.
32. Kwon HL, Triche EW, Belanger K, et al. The epidemiology of asthma during pregnancy: prevalence, diagnosis, and symptoms. Immunol Allergy Clin 2006;26: 29–62.
33. Stenius-Aarniala B, Piirilä P, Teramo K. Asthma and pregnancy: a prospective study of 198 pregnancies. Thorax 1988;43:12–8.
34. Elsayegh D, Shapiro JM. Management of the obstetric patient with status asthmaticus. J Intensive Care Med 2008;23:396–402.
35. Miller MA, Chaloub M, Bourjeily G. Peripartum pulmonary embolism. Clin Chest Med 2011;32:147–64.
36. Clark SL, Belfort MA, Dildy GA, et al. Maternal death in the 21st century: causes, prevention, and relationship to cesarean delivery. Am J Obstet Gynecol 2008; 199:36e1–5.

37. Leung AN, Bull TM, Jaeschke R, et al. An official American Thoracic Society/Society of Thoracic Radiology clinical practice guideline: evaluation of suspected pulmonary embolism in pregnancy. Am J Respir Crit Care Med 2011;184:1200–8.

38. Pahade JK, Litmanovich D, Pedrosa I, et al. Quality initiatives: imaging pregnant patients with suspected pulmonary embolism: what the radiologist needs to know. Radiographics 2009;29:639–54.

39. King TA, Adams AP. Failed tracheal intubation. Br J Anaesth 1990;65:400–14.

40. Al-Ansari MA, Hameed AA, Al-Jawder SE, et al. Use of noninvasive positive pressure ventilation in pregnancy: case series. Ann Thorac Med 2007;2:23–5.

41. Allred CC, Matías Esquinas A, Caronia J, et al. Successful use of noninvasive ventilation in pregnancy. Eur Respir Rev 2015;23:142–4.

42. Zhang PJ, Li XL, Cao B, et al. Clinical features and risk factors for severe and critical pregnant women with 2009 pandemic H1N1 influenza infection in China. BMC Infect Dis 2012;12:29.

43. Frassanito L, Draisci G, Pinto R, et al. Successful application of helmet noninvasive ventilation in a parturient with acute respiratory distress syndrome. Minerva Anestesiol 2011;77:1121–3.

44. Acute Respiratory Distress Syndrome Network, Brower RG, Matthay MA, et al. Ventilation with lower tidal volumes as compared with traditional tidal volumes for acute lung injury and the acute respiratory distress syndrome. N Engl J Med 2000;342:1301–8.

45. Serpa Neto A, Cardoso SO, Manetta JA, et al. Association between use of lung-protective ventilation with lower tidal volumes and clinical outcomes among patients without acute respiratory distress syndrome: a meta-analysis. JAMA 2012;308(16):1651–9.

46. LoMauro A, Aliverti A. Respiratory physiology of pregnancy: physiology masterclass. Breathe 2015;11:297–301.

47. Talab HF, Zabani IA, Abdelrahman HS, et al. Intraoperative ventilatory strategies for prevention of pulmonary atelectasis in obese patients undergoing laparoscopic bariatric surgery. Anesth Analg 2009;109:1511–6.

48. Vasquez DN, Giannoni R, Salvatierra A, et al. Ventilatory parameters in obstetric patients with COVID-19 and impact of delivery: a multicenter prospective cohort study. Chest 2022;163:554–66.

49. Ranieri VM, Brienza N, Santostasi S, et al. Impairment of lung and chest wall mechanics in patients with acute respiratory distress syndrome: role of abdominal distension. Am J Respir Crit Care Med 1997;156:1082–91.

50. Akoumianaki E, Maggiore SM, Valenza F, et al. The application of esophageal pressure measurement in patients with respiratory failure. Am J Respir Crit Care Med 2014;189:520–31.

51. Safaee Fakhr B, Wiegand SB, Pinciroli R, et al. High concentrations of nitric oxide inhalation therapy in pregnant patients with severe coronavirus disease 2019 (COVID-19). Obstet Gynecol 2020;136:1109–13.

52. Guérin C, Reignier J, Richard JC, et al. Prone positioning in severe acute respiratory distress syndrome. N Engl J Med 2013;368:2159–68.

53. Nakai Y, Mine M, Nishio J, et al. Effects of maternal prone position on the umbilical arterial flow. Acta Obstet Gynecol Scand 1998;77:967–9.

54. Samanta S, Samanta S, Wig J, et al. How safe is the prone position in acute respiratory distress syndrome at late pregnancy? Am J Emerg Med 2014;32:687e1–3.

55. Kenn S, Weber-Carstens S, Weizsaecker K, et al. Prone positioning for ARDS following blunt chest trauma in late pregnancy. Int J Obstet Anesth 2009;18: 268–71.

56. Tolcher MC, McKinney JR, Eppes CS, et al. Prone positioning for pregnant women with hypoxemia due to coronavirus disease 2019 (COVID-19). Obstet Gynecol 2020;136(2):259–61.

57. Nair P, Davies AR, Beca J, et al. Extracorporeal membrane oxygenation for severe ARDS in pregnant and postpartum women during the 2009 H1N1 pandemic. Intensive Care Med 2011;37:648–54.

58. Barrantes JH, Ortoleva J, O'Neil ER, et al. Successful treatment of pregnant and postpartum women with severe COVID-19 associated acute respiratory distress syndrome with extracorporeal membrane oxygenation. ASAIO J 2021;67(2): 132–6.

59. American College of Obstetricians and Gynecologists' Committee on Obstetric Practice. Committee opinion No. 656: guidelines for diagnostic imaging during pregnancy and lactation. Obstet Gynecol 2016;127:e75–80.

60. Niemann T, Nicolas G, Roser HW, et al. Imaging for suspected pulmonary embolism in pregnancy—what about the fetal dose? A comprehensive review of the literature. Insights Imaging 2010;1:361–72.

61. Tirada N, Dreizin D, Khati NJ, et al. Imaging pregnant and lactating patients. Radiographics 2015;35:1751–65.

62. Briggs GG, Freeman RK, Towers CV, et al. Drugs in pregnancy and lactation: a reference guide to fetal and neonatal risk. 11th edition. Philadelphia: Wolters Kluwer; 2017.

63. Wikner BN, Stiller CO, Bergman U, et al. Use of benzodiazepines and benzodiazepine receptor agonists during pregnancy: neonatal outcome and congenital malformations. Pharmacoepidemiol Drug Saf 2007;16:1203–10.

64. Enato E, Moretti M, Koren G. The fetal safety of benzodiazepines: an updated meta-analysis. J Obstet Gynaecol Can 2011;33:46–8.

65. McElhatton PR. The effects of benzodiazepine use during pregnancy and lactation. Reprod Toxicol 1994;8:461–75.

66. Hilton G, Andrzejowski JC. Prolonged propofol infusions in pregnant neurosurgical patients. J Neurosurg Anesthesiol 2007;19:67–8.

67. Duan M, Lee J, Bittner EA. Dexmedetomidine for sedation in the parturient with respiratory failure requiring noninvasive ventilation. Respir Care 2012;57:1967–9.

68. Yu M, Han C, Jiang X, et al. Effect and placental transfer of dexmedetomidine during caesarean section under general anaesthesia. Basic Clin Pharmacol Toxicol 2015;117:204–8.

69. Guay J, Grenier Y, Varin F. Clinical pharmacokinetics of neuromuscular relaxants in pregnancy. Clin Pharmacokinet 1998;34:483.

70. Jago RH. Arthrogryposis following treatment of maternal tetanus with muscle relaxants. Arch Dis Child 1970;45:277–9.

71. Federal Drug Agency (2016) FDA Drug Safety Communication: FDA review results in new warnings about using general anesthetics and sedation drugs in young children and pregnant women Available at: https://www.fda.gov/drugs/drugsafety/ucm532356.htm. Accessed June 8, 2023.

72. Chanques G, Constantin JM, Devlin JW, et al. Analgesia and sedation in patients with ARDS. Intensive Care Med 2020;46(12):2342–56.

73. Daily WH, Katz AR, Tonnesen A, et al. Beneficial effect of delivery in a patient with adult respiratory distress syndrome. Anesthesiology 1990;72:383–6.

74. Tomlinson MW, Caruthers TJ, Whitty JE, et al. Does delivery improve maternal condition in the respiratory-compromised gravida? Obstet Gynecol 1998;91: 108–11.

75. Mabie WC, Barton JR, Sibai BM. Adult respiratory distress syndrome in pregnancy. Am J Obstet Gynecol 1992;167:950–7.

76. Lapinsky SE, Rojas-Suarez JA, Crozier TM, et al. Mechanical ventilation in critically-ill pregnant women: a case series. Int J Obstet Anesth 2015;24:323–8.

77. Hung CY, Hu HC, Chiu LC, et al. Maternal and neonatal outcomes of respiratory failure during pregnancy. J Formos Med Assoc 2017;117:413–20.

78. Péju E, Belicard F, Silva S, et al. Management and outcomes of pregnant women admitted to intensive care unit for severe pneumonia related to SARS-CoV-2 infection: the multicenter and international COVIDPREG study. Intensive Care Med 2022;48(9):1185–96.

79. Writing Group for the Alveolar Recruitment for Acute Respiratory Distress Syndrome Trial (ART) Investigators. Effect of lung recruitment and titrated positive end-expiratory pressure (PEEP) vs low PEEP on mortality in patients with acute respiratory distress syndrome: a randomized clinical trial. JAMA 2017;318(14): 1335–45.

80. Jenkins TM, Troiano NH, Graves CR, et al. Mechanical ventilation in an obstetric population: characteristics and delivery rates. Am J Obstet Gynecol 2003;188: 549–52.

81. Rush B, Martinka P, Kilb B, et al. Acute respiratory distress syndrome in pregnant women. Obstet Gynecol 2017;129:530–5.

Acute Respiratory Failure in Severe Acute Brain Injury

Zachary Robateau, MD[a],*, Victor Lin, MD[a],
Sarah Wahlster, MD FNCS[a,b,c]

KEYWORDS

- Severe acute brain injury • Traumatic brain injury • Acute ischemic stroke
- Intracranial hemorrhage • Subarachnoid hemorrhage • Cardiac arrest
- Acute respiratory failure • Acute respiratory distress syndrome

KEY POINTS

- Patients with severe acute brain injury have been excluded in most studies guiding mechanical ventilation strategies or acute respiratory distress syndrome management, and there is limited evidence to inform ventilatory strategies in this population.
- Cerebral and pulmonary pathophysiology are intricately intertwined via complex, often bidirectional pathways involving elevated intracranial pressure (ICP), systemic inflammatory pathways and neuroinflammation, hormonal dysregulation, and catecholamine surges.
- Brain-injured patients likely require higher arterial oxygen partial pressure targets than other critically ill patients; however, hyperoxemia is also detrimental. Effects on the cerebral vasculature, ICP, and cerebral perfusion should be considered when determining arterial carbon dioxide partial pressure targets.
- Vigilant monitoring is warranted in patients at risk for elevated ICP with low tidal volume ventilation utilization, positive end-expiratory pressure titration, optimization of plateau pressure and driving pressure, and prone positioning.
- The ability to predict successful extubation in brain-injured patients remains a challenge. There is no benefit of early (<7 days) tracheostomy in stroke, more data are needed in traumatic brain injury.

INTRODUCTION

Severe acute brain injury (SABI) accounts for up to 25% of individuals receiving mechanical ventilation (MV).[1,2] Yet, there are insufficient data to inform ventilatory targets in this population because patients with SABI, in particular those with elevated

a Department of Neurology, University of Washington, Seattle, USA; b Department of Neurological Surgery, University of Washington, Seattle, USA; c Department of Anesthesiology and Pain Medicine, University of Washington, Seattle, USA
* Corresponding author.
E-mail address: zrobateau@gmail.com

Crit Care Clin 40 (2024) 367–390
https://doi.org/10.1016/j.ccc.2024.01.006
0749-0704/24/© 2024 Elsevier Inc. All rights reserved.

intracranial pressure (ICP), have frequently been excluded in landmark trials evaluating MV strategies.[3-6]

SABI refers to sudden onset traumatic or nontraumatic injury to the brain that results in decreased level of consciousness, often in combination with other substantial neurologic deficits. The term SABI encompasses several distinct pathologic conditions, including acute ischemic stroke (AIS), intracerebral hemorrhage (ICH), subarachnoid hemorrhage (SAH), traumatic brain injury (TBI), and hypoxemic-ischemic encephalopathy after cardiac arrest. Current management is focused on minimizing secondary brain injury by optimizing cerebral perfusion and oxygen supply while accounting for ICP, cerebral perfusion pressure (CPP), cerebral oxygen demand and delivery, seizures, and systemic hemodynamics. The long-term neurologic prognosis is often difficult to predict in the acute stage and critical, time-sensitive decisions regarding invasive treatments versus withdrawal of life-sustaining treatment must be made in the face of this prognostic uncertainty.

There are some unique, clinically relevant considerations in managing acute respiratory failure in SABI: (1) Cerebral and pulmonary pathophysiology are intricately intertwined via complex, often bidirectional pathways; (2) The optimal arterial blood gas targets may be different in patients with SABI to optimize ICP, cerebral perfusion, or cerebral oxygen delivery; (3) Lung-protective strategies established in the general critical care population may be harmful in SABI and conflict with neuroprotective measures, especially in patients with elevated ICP; and (4) There are substantial uncertainties around ventilator liberation strategies, gauging adequate airway protection, and predicting the ability to extubate patients with SABI.

The goal of this article is to summarize the relevant evidence in this population, highlight commonly encountered clinical challenges, specifically brain–lung conflict in concomitant SABI and acute respiratory distress syndrome (ARDS), and provide guidance by reviewing important practical considerations in providing care to critically ill brain-injured patients who require MV.

BRAIN–LUNG INTERACTIONS

The interplay between the brain and lungs is intricate, dynamic, and often bidirectional.[7,8] Although not yet fully understood, pathophysiological interactions are thought to be mediated via elevated ICP, neuroinflammatory and systemic inflammatory responses, hormonal dysregulation, catecholamine surges, and dysregulation of central breathing control (Fig. 1). Additional factors commonly encountered in critically ill patients, such as hypotension and shock, sedation and polypharmacy, fever, and delirium, may additionally affect these interactions.

Hypoxemia and inflammation due to acute lung injury can worsen secondary brain injury. ARDS alone has been linked to substantial long-term neurocognitive impairment through various mechanisms, such as acute blood brain barrier (BBB) disruption, altered cerebral blood flow, and hippocampal neuronal damage.[9-11] Conversely, SABI may precipitate secondary lung injury through various mechanisms (see Fig. 1), including neurogenic pulmonary edema (NPE).[8,12] SABI can also induce or worsen ARDS and has been reported in 4% to 48% of patients with SABI.[7,11,13-22]

Clinically, it is challenging to distinguish NPE from ARDS, and there is substantial overlap in pathophysiology between the 2 entities. Current theories suggest distinct underlying mechanisms: NPE is thought to be a consequence of excessive sympathetic activity, resulting in alterations in pulmonary vascular resistance and capillary permeability ultimately causing volume overload, whereas ARDS is mediated by inflammation, resulting in direct intrapulmonary tissue injury.[7,8,12] However, histopathological

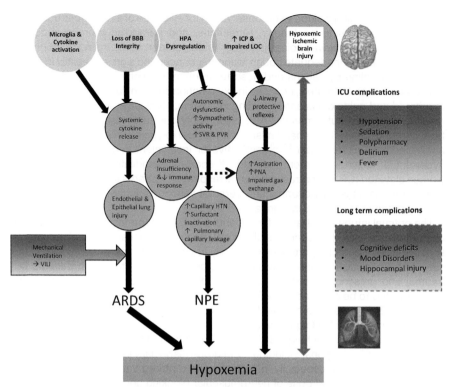

Fig. 1. Brain–lung interactions. ARDS, acute respiratory distress syndrome; HPA, hypothalamic-pituitary-adrenal; HTN, hypertension; ICP, intracranial pressure; ICU, intensive care unit; LOC, level of consciousness; NPE, neurogenic pulmonary edema; PNA, pneumonia; PVR, peripheral vascular resistance; SVR, systemic vascular resistance; VILI, ventilator-induced lung injury.

postmortem analyses suggest similar features, and there are likely bidirectional interactions, and ultimately, clinical management is similar.

INDICATIONS FOR MECHANICAL VENTILATION IN SEVERE ACUTE BRAIN INJURY

Patients with SABI commonly require intubation due to insufficient airway protection in the context of decreased level of consciousness, at times coupled with impaired respiratory drive or cranial nerve dysfunction. Other frequently encountered indications for intubation in SABI include treatment of seizures or status epilepticus, ICP management, to facilitate urgent neuroimaging or procedures, or extreme agitation. Patients with SABI are also at high risk for secondary pulmonary complications including aspiration and/or pneumonia, pulmonary embolism, pulmonary edema, as well as pulmonary contusions or hemothorax/pneumothorax in the context of trauma.

The widely established mantra that a patient with glasgow coma scale (GCS) less than 8 requires immediate intubation was primarily established in trauma populations and is often reflected in published guidelines; however, this practice has since been challenged and may even be harmful in some scenarios, with recent studies suggesting poor outcomes.[23–26] GCS may also be confounded by various sequelae of SABI, such as the presence of aphasia or eyelid opening apraxia, and therefore needs to be interpreted with consideration of affected neuroanatomical structures. When assessing airway protection and the need for intubation, objective signs to suggest compromise of respiratory function include visual observation for evidence of airway obstruction (jaw and tongue prolapsing posteriorly, retractions, and paradoxic thoraco-abdominal movement) or upper airway noises (snoring, stridor, stertor, and gurgling of oropharyngeal secretions). An inadequate cough is another concerning sign, especially in combination with pooling secretions and need for frequent suctioning; the role of the gag reflex is less clear. Ultimately, changes in oxygenation and ventilation should be closely monitored and guide decisions regarding intubation. Hypoxia is widely recognized to result in worsened outcomes in SABI, presumably due to secondary cerebral injury from cerebral metabolic demand mismatch with low oxygen delivery to the hypermetabolic, acutely injured brain.[27–30] Ineffective or insufficient ventilation can result in hypercarbia, which is a potent mediator of cerebral vasodilation and can cause or worsen elevated ICP. In contrast, abnormal respiratory patterns such as central hyperventilation can cause hypocapnia and cerebral vasoconstriction, which may subsequently precipitate cerebral ischemia.[31–33]

The optimal intubation strategy for patients with SABI depends on individual patient characteristics, including concerns about elevated ICP, impaired cerebral autoregulation, insufficient cerebral perfusion (especially in patients with cerebrovascular stenoses, occlusions, dissections, or vasospasm), cervical spine stability in patients with trauma, and presence of concomitant heart failure. Rapid sequence intubation has been reported to be successful in 90%; however, complications have been described in 20% to 25%—most commonly hypotension and hypoxemia—with life-threating complications in 2%.[13] Unique considerations to minimize secondary brain injury in SABI include induction techniques aiming for hemodynamic stability to avoid systemic blood pressure fluctuations, including rapid drops (especially in patients with impaired perfusion) and spikes (especially in patients with ruptured vascular lesions or acute ICH), choosing class and dose of neuromuscular blocking agent, and deliberate utilization of end tidal CO_2 monitoring.[34]

In SABI, propofol is a commonly chosen induction agent because it can blunt cerebral metabolism and therefore decrease cerebral blood flow demand but the clinician must be proactively aware and prepared to treat hypotension. Lidocaine can be used to protect against transient ICP elevations by blunting the sympathetic response, although data supporting its use is limited.[35] Similarly, the use of a nondepolarizing neuromuscular blocking agent can obviate or blunt the cough reflex and minimize ventilator dyssynchrony (VD) for the first ~30 to 90 minutes after administration.

VENTILATOR MANAGEMENT

A recent consensus guideline by the European Society of Intensive Care Medicine (ESICM) emphasizes the lack of evidence to guide ventilator management in SABI, specifically in patients with increased ICP and ARDS.[36] The following sections review the most recent updates and relevant considerations for various ventilator parameters in this population (**Fig. 2**).

Ventilator Mode

To date, it has not been established whether there is an optimal mode of ventilation in SABI, with no major trials directly comparing strategies primarily using controlled versus spontaneous modes. A controlled mode is beneficial to achieve specific arterial carbon dioxide partial pressure ($Paco_2$) and pH targets in the context of elevated ICP. Spontaneous modes can be used in patients with minimal oxygen requirements and intact respiratory drive, and may mimic a more physiologic state, thus increasing patient comfort and requiring decreased levels of sedation. Controlled modes may also exacerbate

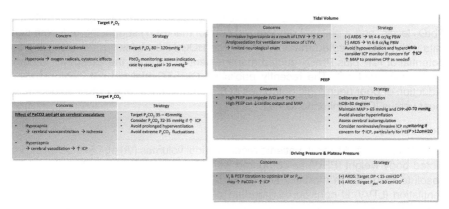

Fig. 2. Ventilatory targets in SABI. ARDS, acute respiratory distress syndrome; CBF, cerebral blood flow; CBV, cerebral blood volume; CPP, cerebral perfusion pressure; DP, driving pressure; HOB, head of bed; ICP, intracranial pressure; JVO, jugular venous outflow; LTVV, low tidal volume ventilation; MAP, mean arterial pressure; Paco₂, arterial carbon dioxide partial pressure; Pao₂, arterial oxygen partial pressure; PbtO₂, brain tissue oxygen pressure; PBW, per body weight; P$_{Plat}$, plateau pressure; PEEP, positive end-expiratory pressure; Vt, tidal volume. [a]Based on ESICM guidelines, [b]Based on BTF guidelines, limited evidence about impact on outcomes, and [c]Thresholds based on ARDS populations, not validated in SABI.

centrally mediated dyssynchronies via increased central stimulation.[37,38] The impact of ventilator mode on paroxysmal sympathetic hyperactivity warrants further investigation.

Arterial Oxygen and Carbon Dioxide Goals

The recent ESICM guidelines strongly recommend targets within generally standard normal physiologic ranges for carbon dioxide (Paco₂ 35–45 mm Hg), as well as slightly higher arterial oxygen partial pressure (Pao₂) goal of 80–120 mm Hg.[36] Paco₂ acts as a fundamental regulator of cerebral blood flow, and both hypercarbia and hypocarbia have been associated with worse clinical outcomes.[39–41] Hypercarbia causes acidosis and cerebral vasodilation, which can result in elevated ICP.[32,33] Hypocarbia causes alkalosis and cerebral vasoconstriction, which can result in cerebral ischemia. Therapeutic hyperventilation can be used as a temporizing measure for reducing acutely elevated ICP but in general is only thought to be effective short-term (for minutes-hours), with risks of cerebral ischemia while hypocapnic (within hours) and rebound ICP spikes on normalization.[30,36] As part of the tiered approach to treat elevated ICP in TBI, slightly lower (Paco₂ 30–35 mm Hg) therapeutic ranges may be prudent in select cases.[42] In contrast, mild hypercapnia may be beneficial in optimizing cerebral blood flow to match cerebral oxygen delivery needs. The recent TAME trial sought to use the cerebral vasodilatory effect of hypercarbia to facilitate improved perfusion following cardiac arrest but found no significant difference in outcomes for patients that were hypercapnic (Paco₂ 50–55 mm Hg) compared with the normocapnic group (Paco₂ 35–45 mm Hg).[43]

Although exact thresholds for Pao₂ remain to be established, both hyperoxia and hypoxia have been associated with worse outcome in SABI, following a U-shaped curve.[28–30,44–46] The ESICM guidelines recommended a higher range than typical Pao₂ goals, with the rationale that the acutely injured, hypermetabolic brain may be more prone to hypoxemia. The value of a brain tissue oxygen pressure (PbtO₂)-guided approach is currently under investigation. For this treatment algorithm, a PbtO₂ probe is inserted in conjunction with an ICP monitor to concurrently monitor these 2 values. PbtO₂ is thought to reflect cerebral perfusion and the diffusion of oxygen across the

BBB. Several studies in TBI and SAH have shown associations between mortality and $PbtO_2$ levels, and a phase 2 randomized control trial (RCT) suggested outcome benefits with $PbtO_2$-directed therapy.[29,47–52] The BOOST-3 trial is further assessing the potential of ICP plus $PbtO_2$-guided management to improve the Glasgow Outcome Scale at 6 months.[53] The recently published OXY-TC trial did not demonstrate a reduction of poor neurologic outcomes at 6-month with ICP and $PbtO_2$-guided treatment versus ICP monitoring alone.[54]

Tidal Volume

In the landmark ARMA trial, patients receiving tidal volumes (Vt) of 4 to 6 cc/kg of predicted body weight (PBW) as compared with 12 cc/kg PBW demonstrated an 8.8% absolute reduction in mortality and fewer MV days.[55] Since then, low tidal volume ventilation (LTVV) is considered standard of care in ARDS, and benefits have also been shown in non-ARDS populations.[55–60] However, patients with elevated ICP were excluded from ARMA. In the ARMA trial, a statistically significant increase in mean P_aCO_2 between the 4 to 6 cc/kg group and 12 cc/kg group was noted. This was thought to be an acceptable trade-off given the improvements in clinical outcomes, leading to the paradigm of permissive hypercapnia in ARDS management. However, higher P_aCO_2 may exacerbate ICP crises in SABI, which may shift the trade off toward potential harm from permissive hypercapnia.

Insufficient knowledge about risks and benefits of LTVV in SABI may result in detrimental outcomes such as herniation in subgroups of patients at risk for elevated ICP; however, these concerns about using LTVV may result in clinicians withholding a therapy with proven benefits. For example, in the recent VENTILO survey, only about half of clinicians were comfortable using 4 to 6 cc/kg PBW in patients with TBI with moderate-to-severe respiratory hypoxemic respiratory failure.[61] However, a secondary analysis of 3 cohort studies showed increasing LTVV utilization between 2004 and 2016 and higher proportion of days spent receiving less than 8 mL/kg PBW. Other studies have also shown that the use of high Vt (>9 mL/kg PBW) is associated with the development of ARDS in various SABI subtypes.[62]

The ESICM guidelines strongly recommend LTVV in brain-injured patients with ARDS without elevated ICP but were unable to make concrete recommendations in patients with ARDS and elevated ICP.[36] In this population, risks and benefits must be weighed carefully based on oxygenation, lung compliance, and neurologic examination plus imaging. Vigilant monitoring of $Paco_2$ is warranted, and an invasive ICP monitor may be considered in high-risk patients to determine individualized $Paco_2$ thresholds and guide use of ICP-lowering therapies. Moreover, a recent small randomized controlled trial suggested that initial ICP, cerebral compliance, and mechanical power (MP) can be predictive of which patients develop elevated ICP with LTVV.[63] Strategies to increase respiratory rate and augment minute ventilation to avoid $Paco_2$ elevations are controversial and warrant further exploration.

Positive End-Expiratory Pressure

Optimal positive end-expiratory pressure (PEEP) titration can promote alveolar expansion, optimize lung recruitment,[64] and enable more homogeneous distribution of MV forces.[65] Several RCTs have showed improved oxygenation with higher PEEP strategies,[66–68] and a meta-analysis of 3 RCTs showed a 5% absolute mortality benefit. However, excessive PEEP can result in impeded venous return due to increased intrathoracic and right atrial pressures, which may subsequently cause elevated ICP by impeding cerebral venous drainage. Higher PEEP may also decrease CPP in patients with impaired cerebral autoregulation, in part due to effects on preload.[7,8,63,69]

Studies investigating the impact of PEEP on ICP in SABI have been smaller single-center studies (<20 patients), included a mix of heterogeneous SABI subtypes with distinct pathophysiology, typically did not assess PEEP greater than 12 to 15 cm H_2O, showed mixed results regarding the impact of PEEP on ICP and CPP, and generally did not assess long-term neurologic outcomes.[63,70–79]

Some reports have suggested that the main mechanism resulting in CPP reductions seems to be a PEEP-dependent decrease in mean arterial pressure (MAP), with ICP and CPP improving once MAP is restored.[74,76] One study found that the impact of PEEP on ICP was substantially higher in patients with alveolar hyperinflation based on static volume–pressure curves.[78] PEEP-mediated ICP elevations have also been shown to occur preferentially in patients with decreased respiratory compliance.[61,70,80]

To date, there is insufficient data to predict the impact of PEEP titration on ICP and ultimately, neurologic outcome. What is becoming more recognized is tolerability of higher PEEP in a subpopulation with intact cerebral autoregulation and preserved lung compliance. PEEP titration in patients with SABI should be deliberate and carefully monitored, with special attention toward maintaining MAP and avoiding alveolar hyperdistention. Invasive and noninvasive techniques to monitor ICP and cerebral perfusion should be considered in patients at high risk for herniation, especially at higher PEEP (>12 cm H_2O). The simultaneous use of lung and brain ultrasound to guide PEEP titration in SABI has been described.[73]

Plateau Pressure and Driving Pressure

The ARMA trial demonstrated lower mortality and fewer MV days in patients with plateau pressure (P_{Plat}) of 25 to 30 cm H_2O, compared with those receiving P_{Plat} 45 to 50 cm H_2O.[55] The optimal P_{Plat} for patients with SABI remains unknown. A special consideration, again, is the special risk of elevated ICP when adjusting Vt or titrating PEEP to reduce P_{Plat}. In addition, high P_{plat} may result in ICP elevations due to decreased cerebral venous return. Until further evidence is available, it is reasonable to avoid P_{Plat} greater than 30 cm H_2O to reduce the risk of barotrauma and ventilator-induced lung injury (VILI). Patients with concomitant ARDS and elevated ICP should be managed with an individualized strategy, with gradual adjustments of Vt and PEEP while observing ICP effects and treating elevated ICP as needed. It is also important to recognize and address other potential contributors to elevated P_{Plat} independent of Vt, including alveolar overdistention, pulmonary congestion, pneumothorax, or migration of the endotracheal tube.

Driving pressure (ΔP), measured as the difference between P_{plat} and PEEP, was the ventilatory variable most strongly associated with mortality in a secondary analysis of 9 RCTs, independent of Vt.[81] This association has been confirmed in other ARDS cohorts.[82–85] As such, some have proposed that ΔP should be used as a physiologic target in patients with ARDS.[86] In SABI, an observational study of 986 patients showed that higher ΔP was associated with an increased risk of ARDS, whereas this association was not seen with Vt and PEEP.[62] Moreover, a preplanned secondary analysis of the TTM2-trial demonstrated associations between ΔP and mortality as well as neurologic outcome at 6 months in patients with postanoxic encephalopathy.[87] More data from RCTs directly examining the effects of ΔP is needed to establish as causal relationship. Clinically, ΔP can be modified by gradually lowering Vt and adjusting PEEP to optimize alveolar recruitment, while considering the impact on ICP.

Mechanical Power

The concept of MP as a determinant of VILI has gained increasing attention. MP is defined as the total energy transferred by the ventilator to the respiratory system per each respiratory cycle, which is derived from several ventilator variables including pressure, volume, flow, and respiratory rate.[87–89] MP has been associated with mortality in ARDS populations,[90,91] and recently in several SABI cohorts.[92,93] A retrospective single-center study including 529 patients with mixed SABI subtypes demonstrated an association between MP in the first 24 hours and ICU mortality, with MP being a stronger predictor of mortality than GCS.[92] A secondary analysis of the TTM2-trial demonstrated associations between MP and mortality but not neurologic outcomes.[94] Another recent secondary analysis of a prospective, observational multicenter study including 1512 patients with SABI showed associations between MP at hospital day 1, 3, and 7 with mortality, reintubation, and development of ARDS.[93]

A causal relationship between MP and outcomes remains to be further evaluated in RCTs, and ventilatory strategies to limit MP should be viewed as exploratory. Further important areas of research include establishing critical MP thresholds in SABI versus other ICU populations, comparing the impact of MP in different SABI subtypes with distinct pathophysiology, and accounting for interactions between MP and ICP.

RESCUE MANEUVERS
Prone Positioning

The PROSEVA trial demonstrated a 17% absolute mortality reduction in patients with a ratio of partial pressure of arterial oxygen to the fraction of inspired oxygen (P/F ratio) less than 150 who were prone for greater than 16 hours per day[95]; however, patients with ICP greater than 30 were excluded. There are several important considerations and logistical challenges when proning patients with SABI, such as cervical spine instability in trauma, positioning in patients with cranial bone flaps, dislodgment of ICP monitors, or inadequate cerebrospinal fluid (CSF) flow from external ventricular drain (EVDs). A main concern is also the potential for ICP elevations due to increased abdominal pressure, decreased head elevation, and compression of neck veins affecting cerebral venous drainage. Studies investigating effects of prone positioning on ICP are all limited to date due to small sample size, mixed subtypes of brain injuries, various degrees of head elevation, and short proning durations (which was a key criticism of negative proning trials before PROSEVA).[96–99] A recent systematic review summarizing these studies showed that many demonstrated statistically significant transient elevations in ICP by 5 to 15 mm Hg, with mixed effects on CPP, while also showing substantial improvement of Pao_2 and $PbtO_2$.[96] The clinical relevance of these findings is not clear because long-term outcomes are not reported. Given the substantial mortality benefit in ARDS and potential impacts on cerebral oxygen delivery, proning should be strongly considered in patients with SABI and concomitant moderate-to-severe ARDS. In cases with concerns about ICP, invasive monitoring can be used to guide adjunct ICP treatments such as hyperosmolar therapy or CSF diversion. Other measures to mitigate ICP elevations include aggressive bowel regimens, padding to decrease abdominal pressure, and modifying the prone angle to improve cerebral venous return. In addition, CPP can be supported via MAP augmentation with vasopressors. In cases where proning is thought to be contraindicated, supine chest wall compression with the use of anterior chest weights can be considered.

Venovenous Extracorporeal Membrane Oxygenation

Venovenous extracorporeal membrane oxygenation (VV-ECMO) can be an effective rescue therapy in severe refractory ARDS. The CESAR trial demonstrated lower mortality in patients with ARDS who were transferred to an extracorporeal membrane oxygenation (ECMO) center,[100] and the EOLIA trial showed a nonsignificant trend toward improved outcome with VV-ECMO.[6] Historically, SABI had been considered a relative contraindication for ECMO due to concerns about hematoma expansion or hemorrhagic conversion with the use of therapeutic anticoagulation, decreased cerebral venous return with large venous cannulas placed in the internal jugular vein, and hesitations around resource utilization in patients with anticipated poor neurologic outcomes. However, there have been significant advances in the past years and increasing utilization of ECMO in SABI.[101] Heparin-bonded circuits and polymethyl pentene oxygenators have allowed for extended VV-ECMO support with low-dose or no systemic anticoagulation without premature oxygenator failure or excessive thrombotic complications.[101,102] Femoral-femoral cannula configurations avoid impairments in cerebral venous drainage. In general, rapid $Paco_2$ correction or extreme fluctuations in $Paco_2$ should be avoided by using low initial sweep gas rates and slow titration in general to minimize ischemic or hemorrhagic complications.[103] Overall, ECMO is feasible in highly selected patients with SABI and should be considered on a case-by-case basis with nuanced consideration of anticipated neurologic outcome.

DYSSYNCHRONY AND BREATHING PATTERNS

The full examination of management of VD and interpretation of ventilator waveforms to assist with such is beyond the scope of this article; however, we will highlight some key considerations specific to SABI. VD develops when there is a mismatch between patient and ventilator inspiratory and expiratory times. Respiratory drive and rhythm are controlled via the brainstem with cortical input, thus patients with SABI are at an increased risk for VD. This can develop due to issues with triggering breaths, oxygen flow, and improper cycling. Various types of centrally mediated VD are depicted in **Table 1**. Separately, agitation and patient discomfort may also lead to VD.

VD can result in inadequate oxygenation and ventilation, increased work of breathing, agitation, and patient discomfort, leading to increasing sedation requirements, which may result in increased MV days. VD can also impede venous return via increased intrathoracic pressure, which can lead to increased ICP, decreased brain perfusion and brain tissue oxygenation. In such severe clinically significant cases of VD, neuromuscular blockade (NMB) can be used to effectively eliminate any patient-initiated efforts. This, however, limits the ability for clinicians to track the patient's neurologic status. Another strategy is to blunt the respiratory drive using sedative medications.[104] With both NMB and sedation, careful titration of ventilator settings will need to be used to avoid inadvertent hypercapnia from decreased respiratory drive. With heavy sedation, patients may experience "paradoxic VD" termed reverse triggering, where the ventilator delivered breath triggers diaphragmatic effort.[105] Depending on the timing of this diaphragmatic effort, this may result in additional tidal volume being delivered or triggering a second breath. In patients with impaired intracranial compliance, this may lead to impaired venous return and increased ICP, which can counteract decreased cerebral metabolic demand from sedation.

In patients with SABI, often the need for MV may continue despite resolution of acute lung injury due to impaired airway protection. For such patients, spontaneous ventilator modes may minimize the development of VD or improve VD compared with a controlled mode, without requiring heavy sedation. In patients with a Cheyne-Stokes breathing pattern, this may result in triggering a backup control mode ventilation particularly during prolonged apneic pauses or periods of lower respiratory effort. This can be modulated by extending the apnea alarm times or decreasing the pressure or flow trigger sensitivities. In centrally mediated tachypnea,

Table 1
Centrally mediated breathing patterns and neuroanatomical correlates

Breathing Patterns	Definition	Neuroanatomy	Prognosis	Wave form	Anatomy
Cheyne-Stokes	Oscillation between hyperventilation and hypoventilation	Bilateral or diencephalic insult typically but may occur anywhere between forebrain and pons	Typically portends good prognosis in stable patient however new onset could indicate impending herniation		
Short cycle periodic breathing	Faster Cheyne-Stokes pattern w/1–2 waxing breaths followed by 3–4 rapid breaths	Increased ICP, expanding posterior fossa lesion or lower pontine lesion			

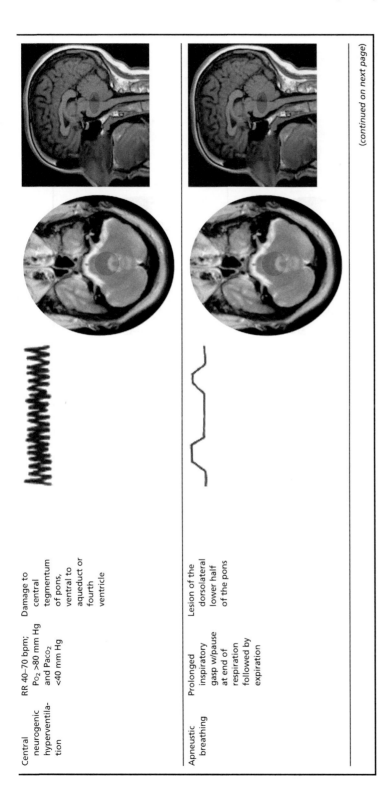

| Central neurogenic hyperventilation | RR 40–70 bpm; Po_2 >80 mm Hg and $Paco_2$ <40 mm Hg | Damage to central tegmentum of pons, ventral to aqueduct or fourth ventricle | | |
| Apneustic breathing | Prolonged inspiratory gasp w/pause at end of respiration followed by expiration | Lesion of the dorsolateral lower half of the pons | | |

(continued on next page)

Table 1
(continued)

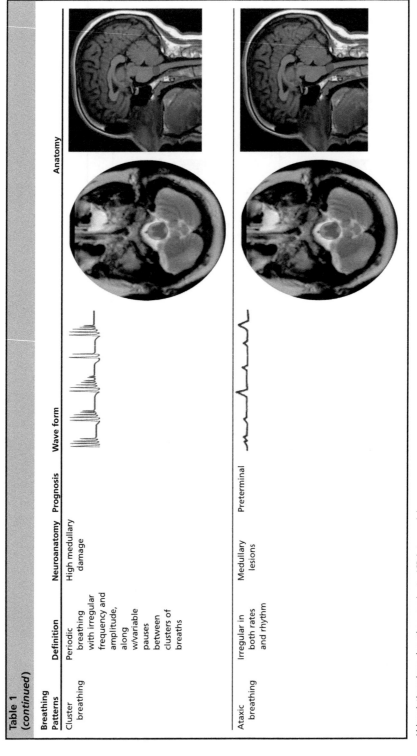

Breathing Patterns	Definition	Neuroanatomy	Prognosis	Wave form	Anatomy
Cluster breathing	Periodic breathing with irregular frequency and amplitude, along w/variable pauses between clusters of breaths	High medullary damage			
Ataxic breathing	Irregular in both rates and rhythm	Medullary lesions	Preterminal		

Abbreviations: bpm, breaths per minute; ICP, intracranial pressure.

pressure support ventilation may be helpful in minimizing inadvertent hypocapnia from hyperventilation with static tidal volumes.

OTHER AREAS OF BRAIN–LUNG CONFLICT
Hemodynamic and Fluid Strategy

The FACTT trial demonstrated that conservative fluid management in ARDS decreased MV duration and ICU stay; however, there was no improvement in overall mortality.[106] In general, volume overload is strictly avoided in patients with ARDS,[107] and several studies have found reduced mortality with early diuresis.[108–110] In SABI, the mantra "dry lungs are happy lungs" and aggressive diuresis may pose a challenge in patients with acutely impaired brain perfusion. In particular, patients with acute proximal occlusions of the cerebral or cervical vasculature, those with a large ischemic penumbra, and those with SAH in cerebral vasospasm are at high risk for secondary brain injury due to cerebral ischemia.

Hypotension is associated with higher mortality and worse outcomes in all SABI subtypes.[28,111–113] Studies about the optimal volume status are often limited by crude modalities of volume status assessment such as total body balance. Both hypovolemia and hypervolemia in TBI and SAH have been associated with mortality.[114–117] Hyperosmolar therapies to treat elevated ICP can also affect volume and respiratory status. Mannitol causes an osmotic diuresis and may lead to decreased preload and cardiac output but can also exacerbate acute kidney injury. Hypertonic saline may increase preload and worsen pulmonary edema. It should be noted that both cause a transient shift of fluids to the intravascular compartment, which may affect cardiopulmonary physiology. Overall, volume management of patients with concurrent ARDS and SABI requires a tailored approach, using daily multimodal volume status assessments during critical time windows (eg, vasospasm period or while preserving an ischemic penumbra), and frequent reassessment of blood pressure and fluid targets. Additional imaging modalities such as CT-angiogram, CT-perfusion, or transcranial Dopplers may prove useful in stratifying the risk of cerebral ischemia, assessing cerebrovascular flow dynamics, and guiding cerebral physiology-based targets.

Steroids

After several negative trials of steroids in the treatment of ARDS, DEXA-ARDS was the first major RCT showing lower mortality and reduced MV days in patients with moderate-to-severe ARDS,[118] and multiple studies followed in COVID-ARDS populations demonstrating outcome benefits of steroids.[118–121] The use of steroids in SABI is controversial. Corticosteroids can reduce cerebral vasogenic edema by decreasing BBB permeability[122] and have shown benefits in subtypes of bacterial meningitis or brain tumors. However, studies in AIS,[123] SAH,[124,125] and ICH[126] did not show beneficial effects on outcomes but increased medical complications have been reported.[123–128] Corticosteroids in the postcardiac arrest population have been shown to improve return of spontaneous circulation rates when simultaneously infused with vasopressors but no improvement in neurologic outcomes has been shown.[129–131] In TBI, high-dose corticosteroids are contraindicated (Brain Trauma Foundation guidelines, level 1 recommendation)[42] based on the MRC CRASH trial, which demonstrated higher mortality at 2 weeks[128] and 6 months[127] with use of high-dose methylprednisolone.[127,128] With insufficient data to guide decisions about steroids in concomitant ARDS and SABI, more research is needed to establish which ARDS and SABI subpopulations may benefit or be harmed by steroids. Meanwhile, decisions about steroids in this population need to be made on a case-by case basis; generally, they would be avoided in TBI, and other indications and contraindications for steroids in critically ill patients should be considered.

EXTUBATION DECISIONS AND TRACHEOSTOMY

The optimal strategy to liberate patients with SABI from MV is not known. The unique challenge in SABI is how to determine "extubation readiness" in patients with decreased level of consciousness and potentially impaired airway protective reflexes.

In several recent SABI extubation cohorts, rates of extubation failure within 2 to 7 days ranged between 15% and 40%; factors such as younger age, type of brain injury, higher GCS, intact gag or cough reflex, deglutition, prophylactic physical therapy, and lower frequency of suctioning were associated with successful extubation.[132–138] The role of GCS has been controversial, with mixed findings across studies. In the largest study to date, a prospective, observational multicenter trial including 1512 across 73 ICUs (ENIO), 19.4% of patients required reintubation within 5 days, and extubation failure rates ranged from 0% to 28.6% between countries. A predictive model with 20 variables predictors was derived from this cohort; however, its area under the curve (AUC) and predictive power were low.[138] A secondary analysis of ENIO found that extubation to noninvasive devices did not increase extubation success.[135] A prospective study in brain-injured patients with decreased levels of consciousness who met "extubation readiness" otherwise showed higher rates of pneumonia, MV, ICU length of stay, and cost of care in those who remained intubated for greater than 48 hours, suggesting that "waiting" is not necessarily beneficial.[139] However, it is always important to optimize quickly reversible factors, such as elevated ICP or seizures.

The question about ideal timing of tracheostomy also remains controversial but highly relevant. In ENIO, 21% of patients received a tracheostomy without an extubation attempt. Rates for tracheostomy are generally higher in mechanically ventilated patients with SABI (15%–35%) compared with the general ICU populations (10%–15%).[2,140,141] The SET score and Trach score were developed to anticipate the need for tracheostomy in patients[142,143] and to account for relevant factors such as subcortical or infratentorial location and SABI size, hydrocephalus, and midline shift. A meta-analysis of 10 studies including 503 patients with stroke and TBI found lower ICU length of stay and lower long-term mortality in patients with early tracheostomy (defined as <7 days) but the mortality benefit was no longer observed when excluding one study with high risk of bias.[134] A recent multicenter RCT in German and US Centers assessing early (within 3–5 days) versus late (10–14 days) tracheostomy in patients with stroke (AIS, ICH, and SAH) did not find any differences in long-term neurologic outcomes, mortality, ICU length of stay, sedation, or MV duration; however, 22% of patients who were randomized to the late tracheostomy group did not require a tracheostomy.[144] Benefits of early tracheostomy are insufficiently explored in the TBI population, where stimulation by the endotracheal tube may precipitate or exacerbate paroxysmal sympathetic hyperactivity or contribute to ICP crises. A prospective observational study from the CENTER-TBI cohort showed tracheostomy rates between 8% and 50% between countries and early tracheostomy rates between 0% and 17%, reflecting the variations in practice and lack of definite knowledge on this topic.[144]

Finally, information on long-term outcomes after tracheostomy in SABI is valuable to guide goals of care discussions. Current studies have shown that up to 80% of survivors with SABI who undergo tracheostomy placement are eventually decannulated[145;

however, mortality is as high as 30% to 40% at 1 year, and 30% to 50% are in a functionally dependent state at 6 to 12 months.[144,145] Neurologic disability, mortality, and decannulation rates vary based on type of brain injury, with SAH and TBI generally showing more favorable outcomes compared with AIS, ICH, and cardiac arrest.[146,147] More data are needed to further inform neuroprognostication and nuanced decisions about resuming life-sustaining treatments.[148]

SUMMARY

Acute respiratory failure is common in SABI, yet there is insufficient evidence to guide MV strategies as patients with SABI have been underrepresented in landmark studies. The relationship between brain–lung pathophysiology is complex and bidirectional, and at times management strategies between the lung and brain may conflict. Potential conflicts include utilization of LTVV, PEEP titration, P_{Plat} and ΔP optimization, and prone positioning in patients at risk for elevated ICP. Additional challenges include balancing the needs for sedation to ensure ventilator tolerance/synchrony with the importance of preserving the neurologic examination, volume status management in patients who may benefit from diuresis from a respiratory standpoint but are at risk for impaired cerebral perfusion, and treatment with corticosteroids, with some benefits shown in ARDS subpopulations but increased mortality in TBI. These concerns may be mitigated by close invasive and noninvasive neuromonitoring and require considerations of risks and benefits in the individual patient. More evidence is needed to guide optimal strategies in various SABI subpopulations. Our ability to predict successful extubation in this population remains limited but recent larger cohort studies have identified associations to inform clinical decisions. A recent RCT did not show benefits of early tracheostomy in stroke, and more data are needed in TBI. An important but understudied area is the interplay between extubation/tracheostomy decisions and neurologic prognostication.

DISCLOSURE

The authors declare no conflicts of interest or financial disclosures relevant to this article.

REFERENCES

1. Pham T, Heunks L, Bellani G, et al. Weaning from mechanical ventilation in intensive care units across 50 countries (WEAN SAFE): a multicentre, prospective, observational cohort study. Lancet Respir Med 2023;11(5):465–76.
2. Pelosi P, Ferguson ND, Frutos-Vivar F, et al. Management and outcome of mechanically ventilated neurologic patients. Crit Care Med 2011;39(6):1482–92.
3. Papazian L, Forel J-M, Gacouin A, et al. Neuromuscular blockers in early acute respiratory distress syndrome. N Engl J Med 2010;363(12):1107–16.
4. National Heart Lung, Blood Institute PETAL Clinical Trials Network, Moss M, Huang DT, et al. Early neuromuscular blockade in the acute respiratory distress syndrome. N Engl J Med 2019;380(21):1997–2008.
5. Peek GJ, Clemens F, Elbourne D, et al. CESAR: conventional ventilatory support vs extracorporeal membrane oxygenation for severe adult respiratory failure. BMC Health Serv Res 2006;6:163.
6. Combes A, Hajage D, Capellier G, et al. Extracorporeal membrane oxygenation for severe acute respiratory distress syndrome. N Engl J Med 2018;378(21):1965–75.

7. Matin N, Sarhadi K, Crooks CP, et al. Brain-lung crosstalk: management of concomitant severe acute brain injury and acute respiratory distress syndrome. Curr Treat Options Neurol 2022;24(9):383–408.

8. Mrozek S, Constantin J-M, Geeraerts T. Brain-lung crosstalk: implications for neurocritical care patients. World J Crit Care Med 2015;4(3):163–78.

9. Aisiku IP, Yamal J-M, Doshi P, et al. The incidence of ARDS and associated mortality in severe TBI using the Berlin definition. J Trauma Acute Care Surg 2016; 80(2):308–12.

10. Pitoni S, D'Arrigo S, Grieco DL, et al. Tidal volume lowering by instrumental dead space reduction in brain-injured ARDS patients: effects on respiratory mechanics, gas exchange, and cerebral hemodynamics. Neurocritical Care 2021;34(1):21–30.

11. Johnson NJ, Caldwell E, Carlbom DJ, et al. The acute respiratory distress syndrome after out-of-hospital cardiac arrest: incidence, risk factors, and outcomes. Resuscitation 2019;135:37–44.

12. Zhao J, Xuan N-X, Cui W, et al. Neurogenic pulmonary edema following acute stroke: the progress and perspective. Biomed Pharmacother 2020;130:110478.

13. Rajajee V, Riggs B, Seder DB. Emergency neurological life support: airway, ventilation, and sedation. Neurocritical Care 2017;27(Suppl 1):4–28.

14. Pitts T. Airway protective mechanisms. Lung 2014;192(1):27–31.

15. Taran S, Wahlster S, Robba C. Ventilatory targets following brain injury. Curr Opin Crit Care 2023;29(2):41–9.

16. Holland MC, Mackersie RC, Morabito D, et al. The development of acute lung injury is associated with worse neurologic outcome in patients with severe traumatic brain injury. J Trauma 2003;55(1):106–11.

17. Rincon F, Ghosh S, Dey S, et al. Impact of acute lung injury and acute respiratory distress syndrome after traumatic brain injury in the United States. Neurosurgery 2012;71(4):795–803.

18. Kahn JM, Caldwell EC, Deem S, et al. Acute lung injury in patients with subarachnoid hemorrhage: incidence, risk factors, and outcome. Crit Care Med 2006;34(1):196–202.

19. Solenski NJ, Haley EC, Kassell NF, et al. Medical complications of aneurysmal subarachnoid hemorrhage: a report of the multicenter, cooperative aneurysm study. Participants of the Multicenter Cooperative Aneurysm Study. Crit Care Med 1995;23(6):1007–17.

20. Gruber A, Reinprecht A, Illievich UM, et al. Extracerebral organ dysfunction and neurologic outcome after aneurysmal subarachnoid hemorrhage. Crit Care Med 1999;27(3):505–14.

21. Elmer J, Hou P, Wilcox SR, et al. Acute respiratory distress syndrome after spontaneous intracerebral hemorrhage. Crit Care Med 2013;41(8):1992–2001.

22. Rincon F, Maltenfort M, Dey S, et al. The prevalence and impact of mortality of the acute respiratory distress syndrome on admissions of patients with ischemic stroke in the United States. J Intensive Care Med 2014;29(6):357–64.

23. Jakob DA, Lewis M, Benjamin ER, et al. Isolated traumatic brain injury: routine intubation for Glasgow Coma Scale 7 or 8 may be harmful. J Trauma Acute Care Surg 2021;90(5):874–9.

24. Irvin CB, Szpunar S, Cindrich LA, et al. Should trauma patients with a Glasgow Coma Scale score of 3 be intubated prior to hospital arrival? Prehospital Disaster Med 2010;25(6):541–6.

25. Gentleman D, Dearden M, Midgley S, et al. Guidelines for resuscitation and transfer of patients with serious head injury. BMJ 1993;307(6903):547–52.

26. Hatchimonji JS, Dumas RP, Kaufman EJ, et al. Questioning dogma: does a GCS of 8 require intubation? Eur J Trauma Emerg Surg 2021;47(6):2073–9.
27. Doerfler S, Faerber J, McKhann GM, et al. The incidence and impact of secondary cerebral insults on outcome after aneurysmal subarachnoid hemorrhage. World Neurosurg 2018;114:e483–94.
28. Manley G, Knudson MM, Morabito D, et al. Hypotension, hypoxia, and head injury: frequency, duration, and consequences. Arch Surg 2001;136(10): 1118–23.
29. Lazaridis C, Ajith A, Mansour A, et al. Prediction of intracranial hypertension and brain tissue hypoxia utilizing high-resolution data from the BOOST-II clinical trial. Neurotrauma Reports 2022;3(1):473–8.
30. Siwicka-Gieroba D, Robba C, Gołacki J, et al. Cerebral oxygen delivery and consumption in brain-injured patients. J Personalized Med 2022;12(11).
31. Sharma D. Perioperative management of aneurysmal subarachnoid hemorrhage. Anesthesiology 2020;133(6):1283–305.
32. Roberts BW, Kilgannon JH, Chansky ME, et al. Association between postresuscitation partial pressure of arterial carbon dioxide and neurological outcome in patients with post-cardiac arrest syndrome. Circulation 2013;127(21):2107–13.
33. Roberts BW, Karagiannis P, Coletta M, et al. Effects of PaCO2 derangements on clinical outcomes after cerebral injury: a systematic review. Resuscitation 2015; 91:32–41.
34. Miller JD. Early insults to the injured brain. JAMA, J Am Med Assoc 1978;240(5): 439–42.
35. Robinson N. In patients with head injury undergoing rapid sequence intubation, does pretreatment with intravenous lignocaine/lidocaine lead to an improved neurological outcome? A review of the literature. Emerg Med J 2001;18(6): 453–7.
36. Robba C, Poole D, McNett M, et al. Mechanical ventilation in patients with acute brain injury: recommendations of the European Society of Intensive Care Medicine consensus. Intensive Care Med 2020;46(12):2397–410.
37. Luo X-Y, He X, Zhou Y-M, et al. Patient-ventilator asynchrony in acute brain-injured patients: a prospective observational study. Ann Intensive Care 2020; 10(1):144.
38. Epstein SK. How often does patient-ventilator asynchrony occur and what are the consequences? Respir Care 2011;56(1):25–38.
39. Davis DP, Meade W, Sise MJ, et al. Both hypoxemia and extreme hyperoxemia may be detrimental in patients with severe traumatic brain injury. J Neurotrauma 2009;26(12):2217–23.
40. Helmerhorst HJF, Schultz MJ, van der Voort PHJ, et al. Bench-to-bedside review: the effects of hyperoxia during critical illness. Crit Care 2015;19(1):284.
41. Alali AS, Temkin N, Vavilala MS, et al. Matching early arterial oxygenation to long-term outcome in severe traumatic brain injury: target values. J Neurosurg 2019;132(2):537–44.
42. Carney N, Totten AM, O'Reilly C, et al. Guidelines for the management of severe traumatic brain injury, fourth edition. Neurosurgery. 2017;80(1):6-15. doi:10.1227/NEU.0000000000001432.
43. Eastwood G, Nichol AD, Hodgson C, et al. Mild hypercapnia or normocapnia after out-of-hospital cardiac arrest. N Engl J Med 2023;389(1):45–57.
44. Menon DK, Coles JP, Gupta AK, et al. Diffusion limited oxygen delivery following head injury. Crit Care Med 2004;32(6):1384–90.

45. Okonkwo DO, Shutter LA, Moore C, et al. Brain oxygen optimization in severe traumatic brain injury phase-II: a phase II randomized trial. Crit Care Med 2017;45(11):1907–14.

46. Sheinberg M, Kanter MJ, Robertson CS, et al. Continuous monitoring of jugular venous oxygen saturation in head-injured patients. J Neurosurg 1992;76(2): 212–7.

47. Maloney-Wilensky E, Gracias V, Itkin A, et al. Brain tissue oxygen and outcome after severe traumatic brain injury: a systematic review. Crit Care Med 2009; 37(6):2057–63.

48. Xie Q, Wu H-B, Yan Y-F, et al. Mortality and outcome comparison between brain tissue oxygen combined with intracranial pressure/cerebral perfusion pressure-guided therapy and intracranial pressure/cerebral perfusion pressure-guided therapy in traumatic brain injury: a meta-analysis. World Neurosurg 2017;100: 118–27.

49. Narotam PK, Morrison JF, Nathoo N. Brain tissue oxygen monitoring in traumatic brain injury and major trauma: outcome analysis of a brain tissue oxygen-directed therapy. J Neurosurg 2009;111(4):672–82.

50. Gouvea Bogossian E, Diaferia D, Ndieugnou Djangang N, et al. Brain tissue oxygenation guided therapy and outcome in non-traumatic subarachnoid hemorrhage. Sci Rep 2021;11(1):16235.

51. Lubillo ST, Parrilla DM, Blanco J, et al. Prognostic value of changes in brain tissue oxygen pressure before and after decompressive craniectomy following severe traumatic brain injury. J Neurosurg 2018;128(5):1538–46.

52. Spiotta AM, Stiefel MF, Gracias VH, et al. Brain tissue oxygen-directed management and outcome in patients with severe traumatic brain injury. J Neurosurg 2010;113(3):571–80.

53. Bernard F, Barsan W, Diaz-Arrastia R, et al. Brain Oxygen Optimization in Severe Traumatic Brain Injury (BOOST-3): a multicentre, randomised, blinded-endpoint, comparative effectiveness study of brain tissue oxygen and intracranial pressure monitoring versus intracranial pressure alone. BMJ Open 2022;12(3): e060188.

54. Payen J-F, Launey Y, Chabanne R, et al. Intracranial pressure monitoring with and without brain tissue oxygen pressure monitoring for severe traumatic brain injury in France (OXY-TC): an open-label, randomised controlled superiority trial. Lancet Neurol 2023;22(11):1005–14.

55. Acute Respiratory Distress Syndrome Network, Brower RG, Matthay MA, et al. Ventilation with lower tidal volumes as compared with traditional tidal volumes for acute lung injury and the acute respiratory distress syndrome. N Engl J Med 2000;342(18):1301–8.

56. Futier E, Constantin J-M, Paugam-Burtz C, et al. A trial of intraoperative low-tidal-volume ventilation in abdominal surgery. N Engl J Med 2013;369(5): 428–37.

57. Mascia L, Pasero D, Slutsky AS, et al. Effect of a lung protective strategy for organ donors on eligibility and availability of lungs for transplantation: a randomized controlled trial. JAMA 2010;304(23):2620–7.

58. Serpa Neto A, Cardoso SO, Manetta JA, et al. Association between use of lung-protective ventilation with lower tidal volumes and clinical outcomes among patients without acute respiratory distress syndrome: a meta-analysis. JAMA 2012; 308(16):1651–9.

59. Asehnoune K, Mrozek S, Perrigault PF, et al. A multi-faceted strategy to reduce ventilation-associated mortality in brain-injured patients. The BI-VILI project: a nationwide quality improvement project. Intensive Care Med 2017;43(7):957–70.

60. Roquilly A, Cinotti R, Jaber S, et al. Implementation of an evidence-based extubation readiness bundle in 499 brain-injured patients. a before-after evaluation of a quality improvement project. Am J Respir Crit Care Med 2013;188(8): 958–66.

61. Picetti E, Pelosi P, Taccone FS, et al. VENTILatOry strategies in patients with severe traumatic brain injury: the VENTILO Survey of the European Society of Intensive Care Medicine (ESICM). Crit Care 2020;24(1):158.

62. Tejerina E, Pelosi P, Muriel A, et al. Association between ventilatory settings and development of acute respiratory distress syndrome in mechanically ventilated patients due to brain injury. J Crit Care 2017;38:341–5.

63. Beqiri E, Smielewski P, Guérin C, et al. Neurological and respiratory effects of lung protective ventilation in acute brain injury patients without lung injury: brain vent, a single centre randomized interventional study. Crit Care 2023;27(1):115.

64. Briel M, Meade M, Mercat A, et al. Higher vs lower positive end-expiratory pressure in patients with acute lung injury and acute respiratory distress syndrome: systematic review and meta-analysis. JAMA 2010;303(9):865–73.

65. Gattinoni L, Carlesso E, Brazzi L, et al. Positive end-expiratory pressure. Curr Opin Crit Care 2010;16(1):39–44.

66. Meade MO, Cook DJ, Guyatt GH, et al. Ventilation strategy using low tidal volumes, recruitment maneuvers, and high positive end-expiratory pressure for acute lung injury and acute respiratory distress syndrome: a randomized controlled trial. JAMA 2008;299(6):637–45.

67. Nishikimi M, Ohshimo S, Hamaguchi J, et al. High versus low positive end-expiratory pressure setting in patients receiving veno-venous extracorporeal membrane oxygenation support for severe acute respiratory distress syndrome: study protocol for the multicentre, randomised ExPress SAVER Trial. BMJ Open 2023;13(10):e072680.

68. Mercat A, Richard J-CM, Vielle B, et al. Positive end-expiratory pressure setting in adults with acute lung injury and acute respiratory distress syndrome: a randomized controlled trial. JAMA 2008;299(6):646–55.

69. Neto AS, Simonis FD, Barbas CSV, et al. Lung-protective ventilation with low tidal volumes and the occurrence of pulmonary complications in patients without acute respiratory distress syndrome: a systematic review and individual patient data analysis. Crit Care Med 2015;43(10):2155–63.

70. Boone MD, Jinadasa SP, Mueller A, et al. The effect of positive end-expiratory pressure on intracranial pressure and cerebral hemodynamics. Neurocritical Care 2017;26(2):174–81.

71. Videtta W, Villarejo F, Cohen M, et al. Effects of positive end-expiratory pressure on intracranial pressure and cerebral perfusion pressure. Acta Neurochir Suppl 2002;81:93–7.

72. Caricato A, Conti G, Della Corte F, et al. Effects of PEEP on the intracranial system of patients with head injury and subarachnoid hemorrhage: the role of respiratory system compliance. J Trauma 2005;58(3):571–6.

73. Robba C, Ball L, Battaglini D, et al. Effects of positive end-expiratory pressure on lung ultrasound patterns and their correlation with intracranial pressure in mechanically ventilated brain injured patients. Crit Care 2022;26(1):31.

74. Georgiadis D, Schwarz S, Baumgartner RW, et al. Influence of positive end-expiratory pressure on intracranial pressure and cerebral perfusion pressure in patients with acute stroke. Stroke 2001;32(9):2088–92.

75. Huynh T, Messer M, Sing RF, et al. Positive end-expiratory pressure alters intracranial and cerebral perfusion pressure in severe traumatic brain injury. J Trauma 2002;53(3):488–92, discussion 492.

76. Muench E, Bauhuf C, Roth H, et al. Effects of positive end-expiratory pressure on regional cerebral blood flow, intracranial pressure, and brain tissue oxygenation. Crit Care Med 2005;33(10):2367–72.

77. McGuire G, Crossley D, Richards J, et al. Effects of varying levels of positive end-expiratory pressure on intracranial pressure and cerebral perfusion pressure. Crit Care Med 1997;25(6):1059–62.

78. Mascia L, Grasso S, Fiore T, et al. Cerebro-pulmonary interactions during the application of low levels of positive end-expiratory pressure. Intensive Care Med 2005;31(3):373–9.

79. Corradi F, Robba C, Tavazzi G, et al. Combined lung and brain ultrasonography for an individualized "brain-protective ventilation strategy" in neurocritical care patients with challenging ventilation needs. Crit Ultrasound J 2018;10(1):24.

80. Shapiro HM, Marshall LF. Intracranial pressure responses to PEEP in head-injured patients. J Trauma 1978;18(4):254–6.

81. Amato MBP, Meade MO, Slutsky AS, et al. Driving pressure and survival in the acute respiratory distress syndrome. N Engl J Med 2015;372(8):747–55.

82. Bellani G, Laffey JG, Pham T, et al. Epidemiology, patterns of care, and mortality for patients with acute respiratory distress syndrome in intensive care units in 50 countries. JAMA 2016;315(8):788–800.

83. Baedorf Kassis E, Loring SH, Talmor D. Mortality and pulmonary mechanics in relation to respiratory system and transpulmonary driving pressures in ARDS. Intensive Care Med 2016;42(8):1206–13.

84. Coppola S, Caccioppola A, Froio S, et al. Effect of mechanical power on intensive care mortality in ARDS patients. Crit Care 2020;24(1):246.

85. Aoyama H, Pettenuzzo T, Aoyama K, et al. Association of driving pressure with mortality among ventilated patients with acute respiratory distress syndrome: a systematic review and meta-analysis. Crit Care Med 2018;46(2):300–6.

86. Pelosi P, Ball L, Barbas CSV, et al. Personalized mechanical ventilation in acute respiratory distress syndrome. Crit Care 2021;25(1):250.

87. Robba C, Badenes R, Battaglini D, et al. Oxygen targets and 6-month outcome after out of hospital cardiac arrest: a pre-planned sub-analysis of the targeted hypothermia versus targeted normothermia after Out-of-Hospital Cardiac Arrest (TTM2) trial. Crit Care 2022;26(1):323.

88. Gattinoni L, Tonetti T, Cressoni M, et al. Ventilator-related causes of lung injury: the mechanical power. Intensive Care Med 2016;42(10):1567–75.

89. Cressoni M, Gotti M, Chiurazzi C, et al. Mechanical power and development of ventilator-induced lung injury. Anesthesiology 2016;124(5):1100–8.

90. Costa ELV, Slutsky AS, Brochard LJ, et al. Ventilatory variables and mechanical power in patients with acute respiratory distress syndrome. Am J Respir Crit Care Med 2021;204(3):303–11.

91. Serpa Neto A, Deliberato RO, Johnson AEW, et al. Mechanical power of ventilation is associated with mortality in critically ill patients: an analysis of patients in two observational cohorts. Intensive Care Med 2018;44(11):1914–22.

92. Jiang X, Zhu Y, Zhen S, et al. Mechanical power of ventilation is associated with mortality in neurocritical patients: a cohort study. J Clin Monit Comput 2022; 36(6):1621–8.
93. Wahlster S, Sharma M, Taran S, et al. Utilization of mechanical power and associations with clinical outcomes in brain injured patients: a secondary analysis of the extubation strategies in neuro-intensive care unit patients and associations with outcome (ENIO) trial. Crit Care 2023;27(1):156.
94. Robba C, Badenes R, Battaglini D, et al. Ventilatory settings in the initial 72 h and their association with outcome in out-of-hospital cardiac arrest patients: a preplanned secondary analysis of the targeted hypothermia versus targeted normothermia after out-of-hospital cardiac arrest (TTM2) trial. Intensive Care Med 2022;48(8):1024–38.
95. Guérin C, Reignier J, Richard J-C, et al. Prone positioning in severe acute respiratory distress syndrome. N Engl J Med 2013;368(23):2159–68.
96. Wright JM, Gerges C, Shammassian B, et al. Prone position ventilation in neurologically ill patients: a systematic review and proposed protocol. Crit Care Med 2021;49(3):e269–78.
97. Reinprecht A, Greher M, Wolfsberger S, et al. Prone position in subarachnoid hemorrhage patients with acute respiratory distress syndrome: effects on cerebral tissue oxygenation and intracranial pressure. Crit Care Med 2003;31(6): 1831–8.
98. Roth C, Ferbert A, Deinsberger W, et al. Does prone positioning increase intracranial pressure? A retrospective analysis of patients with acute brain injury and acute respiratory failure. Neurocritical Care 2014;21(2):186–91.
99. Thelandersson A, Cider A, Nellgård B. Prone position in mechanically ventilated patients with reduced intracranial compliance. Acta Anaesthesiol Scand 2006; 50(8):937–41.
100. Peek GJ, Mugford M, Tiruvoipati R, et al. Efficacy and economic assessment of conventional ventilatory support versus extracorporeal membrane oxygenation for severe adult respiratory failure (CESAR): a multicentre randomised controlled trial. Lancet 2009;374(9698):1351–63.
101. Kurihara C, Walter JM, Karim A, et al. Feasibility of venovenous extracorporeal membrane oxygenation without systemic anticoagulation. Ann Thorac Surg 2020;110(4):1209–15.
102. Fina D, Matteucci M, Jiritano F, et al. Extracorporeal membrane oxygenation without therapeutic anticoagulation in adults: a systematic review of the current literature. Int J Artif Organs 2020;43(9):570–8.
103. Gajkowski EF, Herrera G, Hatton L, et al. ELSO guidelines for adult and pediatric extracorporeal membrane oxygenation circuits. ASAIO J 2022;68(2):133–52.
104. Mellott KG, Grap MJ, Munro CL, et al. Patient-ventilator dyssynchrony: clinical significance and implications for practice. Crit Care Nurse 2009;29(6):41–55, quiz 1 p following 55.
105. Antonogiannaki E-M, Georgopoulos D, Akoumianaki E. Patient-ventilator dyssynchrony. Korean J Crit Care Med 2017;32(4):307–22.
106. Silversides JA, McAuley DF, Blackwood B, et al. Fluid management and deresuscitation practices: a survey of critical care physicians. J Intensive Care Soc 2020;21(2):111–8.
107. National Heart, Lung, and Blood Institute Acute Respiratory Distress Syndrome (ARDS) Clinical Trials Network, Wiedemann HP, Wheeler AP, et al. Comparison of two fluid-management strategies in acute lung injury. N Engl J Med 2006; 354(24):2564–75.

108. Seitz KP, Caldwell ES, Hough CL. Fluid management in ARDS: an evaluation of current practice and the association between early diuretic use and hospital mortality. J Intensive Care 2020;8:78.
109. Zhang R, Chen H, Gao Z, et al. The effect of loop diuretics on 28-day mortality in patients with acute respiratory distress syndrome. Front Med 2021;8:740675.
110. Griffiths MJD, McAuley DF, Perkins GD, et al. Guidelines on the management of acute respiratory distress syndrome. BMJ Open Respir Res 2019;6(1):e000420.
111. Stead LG, Gilmore RM, Decker WW, et al. Initial emergency department blood pressure as predictor of survival after acute ischemic stroke. Neurology 2005; 65(8):1179–83.
112. Vemmos KN, Tsivgoulis G, Spengos K, et al. U-shaped relationship between mortality and admission blood pressure in patients with acute stroke. J Intern Med 2004;255(2):257–65.
113. Wohlfahrt P, Krajcoviechova A, Jozifova M, et al. Low blood pressure during the acute period of ischemic stroke is associated with decreased survival. J Hypertens 2015;33(2):339–45.
114. Zhao Z, Wang D, Jia Y, et al. Analysis of the association of fluid balance and short-term outcome in traumatic brain injury. J Neurol Sci 2016;364:12–8.
115. Clifton GL, Miller ER, Choi SC, et al. Fluid thresholds and outcome from severe brain injury. Crit Care Med 2002;30(4):739–45.
116. Wijdicks EF, Vermeulen M, ten Haaf JA, et al. Volume depletion and natriuresis in patients with a ruptured intracranial aneurysm. Ann Neurol 1985;18(2):211–6.
117. Wiegers EJA, Lingsma HF, Huijben JA, et al. Fluid balance and outcome in critically ill patients with traumatic brain injury (CENTER-TBI and OzENTER-TBI): a prospective, multicentre, comparative effectiveness study. Lancet Neurol 2021; 20(8):627–38.
118. Villar J, Ferrando C, Martínez D, et al. Dexamethasone treatment for the acute respiratory distress syndrome: a multicentre, randomised controlled trial. Lancet Respir Med 2020;8(3):267–76.
119. Yoshihro S, Taito S, Yatabe T. The influence of steroid type on outcomes in patients with acute respiratory distress syndrome. J Intensive Care 2023;11(1):32.
120. Khilnani GC, Hadda V. Corticosteroids and ARDS: a review of treatment and prevention evidence. Lung India 2011;28(2):114–9.
121. Ma S, Xu C, Liu S, et al. Efficacy and safety of systematic corticosteroids among severe COVID-19 patients: a systematic review and meta-analysis of randomized controlled trials. Signal Transduct Targeted Ther 2021;6(1):83.
122. Witt KA, Sandoval KE. Steroids and the blood-brain barrier: therapeutic implications. Adv Pharmacol 2014;71:361–90.
123. Sandercock PA, Soane T. Corticosteroids for acute ischaemic stroke. Cochrane Database Syst Rev 2011;2011(9):CD000064.
124. Feigin VL, Anderson N, Rinkel GJE, et al. Corticosteroids for aneurysmal subarachnoid haemorrhage and primary intracerebral haemorrhage. Cochrane Database Syst Rev 2005;3:CD004583.
125. Mistry AM, Mistry EA, Ganesh Kumar N, et al. Corticosteroids in the management of hyponatremia, hypovolemia, and vasospasm in subarachnoid hemorrhage: a meta-analysis. Cerebrovasc Dis 2016;42(3–4):263–71.
126. Poungvarin N, Bhoopat W, Viriyavejakul A, et al. Effects of dexamethasone in primary supratentorial intracerebral hemorrhage. N Engl J Med 1987;316(20): 1229–33.

127. Edwards P, Arango M, Balica L, et al. Final results of MRC CRASH, a randomised placebo-controlled trial of intravenous corticosteroid in adults with head injury-outcomes at 6 months. Lancet 2005;365(9475):1957–9.

128. Roberts I, Yates D, Sandercock P, et al. Effect of intravenous corticosteroids on death within 14 days in 10008 adults with clinically significant head injury (MRC CRASH trial): randomised placebo-controlled trial. Lancet 2004;364(9442): 1321–8.

129. Mentzelopoulos SD, Malachias S, Chamos C, et al. Vasopressin, steroids, and epinephrine and neurologically favorable survival after in-hospital cardiac arrest: a randomized clinical trial. JAMA 2013;310(3):270–9.

130. Andersen LW, Granfeldt A. Vasopressin and methylprednisolone vs placebo and return of spontaneous circulation in patients with in-hospital cardiac arrest—reply. JAMA 2022;327(5):487.

131. Shah K, Mitra AR. Use of corticosteroids in cardiac arrest-A systematic review and meta-analysis. Crit Care Med 2021;49(6):e642–50.

132. Jaber S, Quintard H, Cinotti R, et al. Risk factors and outcomes for airway failure versus non-airway failure in the intensive care unit: a multicenter observational study of 1514 extubation procedures. Crit Care 2018;22(1):236.

133. Godet T, Chabanne R, Marin J, et al. Extubation failure in brain-injured patients: risk factors and development of a prediction score in a preliminary prospective cohort study. Anesthesiology 2017;126(1):104–14.

134. McCredie VA, Ferguson ND, Pinto RL, et al. Airway management strategies for brain-injured patients meeting standard criteria to consider extubation. A prospective cohort study. Ann Am Thorac Soc 2017;14(1):85–93.

135. Taran S, Diaz-Cruz C, Perrot B, et al. Association of non-invasive respiratory support with extubation outcomes in brain-injured patients receiving mechanical ventilation: a secondary analysis of ENIO. Am J Respir Crit Care Med 2023. https://doi.org/10.1164/rccm.202212-2249OC.

136. Anderson CD, Bartscher JF, Scripko PD, et al. Neurologic examination and extubation outcome in the neurocritical care unit. Neurocritical Care 2011;15(3): 490–7.

137. Castro AAM, Cortopassi F, Sabbag R, et al. Respiratory muscle assessment in predicting extubation outcome in patients with stroke. Arch Bronconeumol 2012; 48(8):274–9.

138. Cinotti R, Pelosi P, Schultz MJ, et al. Extubation strategies in neuro-intensive care unit patients and associations with outcomes: the ENIO multicentre international observational study. Ann Transl Med 2020;8(7):503.

139. Coplin WM, Pierson DJ, Cooley KD, et al. Implications of extubation delay in brain-injured patients meeting standard weaning criteria. Am J Respir Crit Care Med 2000;161(5):1530–6.

140. Alsherbini K, Goyal N, Metter EJ, et al. Predictors for tracheostomy with external validation of the stroke-related early tracheostomy score (SETscore). Neurocritical Care 2019;30(1):185–92.

141. Kurtz P, Fitts V, Sumer Z, et al. How does care differ for neurological patients admitted to a neurocritical care unit versus a general ICU? Neurocritical Care 2011;15(3):477–80.

142. Schönenberger S, Al-Suwaidan F, Kieser M, et al. The SETscore to predict tracheostomy need in cerebrovascular neurocritical care patients. Neurocritical Care 2016;25(1):94–104.

143. Szeder V, Ortega-Gutierrez S, Ziai W, et al. The TRACH score: clinical and radiological predictors of tracheostomy in supratentorial spontaneous intracerebral hemorrhage. Neurocritical Care 2010;13(1):40–6.

144. Bösel J, Niesen W-D, Salih F, et al. Effect of early vs standard approach to tracheostomy on functional outcome at 6 months among patients with severe stroke receiving mechanical ventilation: the SETPOINT2 randomized clinical trial. JAMA 2022;327(19):1899–909.

145. Wahlster S, Sharma M, Chu F, et al. Outcomes after tracheostomy in patients with severe acute brain injury: a systematic review and meta-analysis. Neurocritical Care 2021;34(3):956–67.

146. Wabl R, Williamson CA, Pandey AS, et al. Long-term and delayed functional recovery in patients with severe cerebrovascular and traumatic brain injury requiring tracheostomy. J Neurosurg 2018;131(1):114–21.

147. Avesani R, Dambruoso F, Formisano R, et al. Considerations about status of severe acquired brain injuries in Italy. Int J Neurorehabilitation Eng 2017;04(02).

148. Lou W, Granstein JH, Wabl R, et al. Taking a chance to recover: families look back on the decision to pursue tracheostomy after severe acute brain injury. Neurocritical Care 2022;36(2):504–10.

Ventilator Weaning and Extubation

Karen E.A. Burns, MD, FRCPC, MSc[a,b,c,d],*, Bram Rochwerg[d,e,f],
Andrew J.E. Seely[g,h,i]

KEYWORDS

- Ventilator weaning • Noninvasive ventilation • High flow nasal cannulae • Extubation

KEY POINTS

- Increasing evidence supports specific approaches to liberate patients from invasive ventilation including the use of liberation protocols, inspiratory assistance during spontaneous breathing trials (SBTs), early extubation of patients with chronic obstructive pulmonary disease to noninvasive ventilation, and prophylactic use of noninvasive support strategies after extubation.
- Additional research is needed to elucidate the best criteria to identify patients who are ready to undergo an SBT and to inform optimal screening frequency, the best SBT technique and duration, extubation assessments, and extubation decision-making.
- Additional clarity is also needed regarding the optimal timing to measure and report extubation success and to standardize reporting of weaning (SBT outcome) and extubation outcomes.

INTRODUCTION

For critically ill patients who are recovering from critical illness requiring invasive ventilation, *liberation from mechanical ventilation* refers to the processes of weaning and

[a] Interdepartmental Division of Critical Care Medicine, University of Toronto, Toronto, Ontario, Canada; [b] Department of Medicine and Division of Critical Care, Unity Health Toronto, St. Michaels Hospital, Toronto, Ontario, Canada; [c] Li Ka Shing Knowledge Institute, Unity Health Toronto, St. Michael's Hospital, Toronto, Ontario, Canada; [d] Department of Health Research Methods, Evidence and Impact, McMaster University, Hamilton, Ontario, Canada; [e] Department of Medicine, Hamilton Health Sciences, Juravinski Hospital, Hamilton, Ontario, Canada; [f] Department of Critical Care, Hamilton Health Sciences, Juravinski Hospital, Hamilton, Ontario, Canada; [g] Department of Critical Care, Ottawa Hospital, Ottawa, Ontario, Canada; [h] Division of Thoracic Surgery, Department of Surgery, University of Ottawa, Ottawa, Ontario, Canada; [i] Clinical Epidemiology Program, Ottawa Hospital Research Institute, University of Ottawa, Ottawa, Ontario, Canada
* Corresponding author. Unity Health Toronto, St. Michael's Hospital, 30 Bond Street, Office 4-045 Donnelly Wing, Toronto, Ontario M5B 1W8, Canada.
E-mail address: Karen.burns@unityhealth.to
Twitter: @KarenBurnsK (K.E.A.B.); @Bram_Rochwerg (B.R.)

Crit Care Clin 40 (2024) 391–408
https://doi.org/10.1016/j.ccc.2024.01.007
0749-0704/24/© 2024 Elsevier Inc. All rights reserved.

extubation and includes efforts made by clinicians to reduce and ultimately remove the need for invasive or noninvasive ventilation (NIV). The liberation process includes reversal or improvement of the factors that precipitated respiratory failure and identification of the earliest time that patients can resume the work of breathing (liberation from the ventilator) and maintain a patent airway (liberation from the artificial airway). Extubation is the act of endotracheal tube removal. Patients with acute respiratory failure spend approximately 40% of the time on invasive mechanical ventilation in the liberation phase.[1] Timely and successful liberation has been identified as a key priority for critical care.[2] An inherent trade-off exists in liberating critically ill patients from invasive ventilation. Premature failed attempts at liberation may result in airway compromise, ineffective gas exchange, aspiration, nosocomial respiratory infections, respiratory muscle fatigue,[3] and increase the risk for ventilator-associated pneumonia (VAP).[4] Conversely, delayed and prolonged attempts at liberation may contribute to patient harm related to ventilator-associated lung injury, diaphragmatic dysfunction, development of VAP and neuromuscular weakness, and increase costs of care.[5] In this article, we summarize how to identify, test, and optimize patients for liberation from mechanical ventilation. Additionally, we highlight the use of NIV and high flow nasal cannulae (HFNC) in liberation and summarize evidence related to assessments for extubation readiness.

DISCUSSION
Identifying Candidates for Liberation from Mechanical Ventilation

Liberation from invasive ventilation ideally begins when the underlying cause of acute respiratory failure that led to the need for invasive ventilation has improved or resolved and the patient is able to initiate spontaneous breaths.[2,6] Clinicians aim to use spontaneous modes of ventilation as early as possible in the course of recovery from critical illness provided that patients do not demonstrate insufficient or excessive effort during weaning attempts.[7] The multistep process typically includes ascertaining patient's readiness to undergo a spontaneous breathing trial (SBT), conduct of an SBT, and extubation after successful completion of an SBT[8] (Fig. 1).

Assessing Readiness to Undergo Spontaneous Breathing Trials

Invasively ventilated patients should be screened once daily to determine whether they meet selected criteria to undergo a SBT[9,10] or a test of their capacity to breathe spontaneously for up to 120 minutes. Compared with physician judgment, weaning protocols have been shown to reduce the duration of mechanical ventilation by 25 hours (95% confidence interval [CI], 12.5–35.5 hours) and intensive care unit (ICU) length of stay by approximately 1 day (95% CI, 0.24–1.7 days; low certainty evidence).[9,10] Similarly, a Cochrane Review found that protocolized weaning reduced the mean duration of ventilation especially in medical, surgical, and mixed ICUs but not in neurosurgical ICUs, as well as, weaning, and ICU length of stay.[11] The American Thoracic Society (ATS)/American College of Chest physicians (ACCP) guidelines provided a conditional recommendation for the use of a ventilator liberation protocol for the management for acutely hospitalized patients who have been mechanically ventilated for more than 24 hours.[9,10]

The parameters used in screening protocols to identify patients who are ready to undergo an SBT vary across studies and with regard to their positive and negative predictive values. Parameters often include objective parameters (ie, the respiratory rapid shallow breathing index [RSBI],[12] tidal volume [V_T], respiratory rate (RR), inspiratory effort and maximal pressures, and blood gas and hemodynamic measurements);

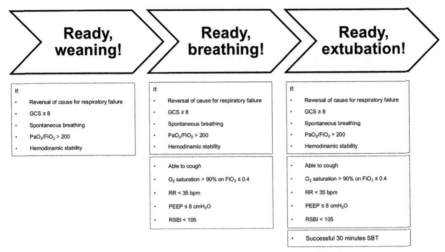

Fig. 1. The process of liberation from invasive ventilation. The weaning path. Fio_2, fractional inspired concentration of oxygen; GCS, Glasgow comas scale; O_2 saturation, oxygen saturation; Pao_2/Fio_2, partial pressure of oxygen/fractional inspired concentration of oxygen; PEEP, positive end-expiratory pressure; RR, respiratory rate; RSBI, rapid shallow breathing index; SBT, spontaneous breathing trial.

subjective parameters that may evaluate weaning and extubation readiness (ie, reversal of the underlying cause of respiratory failure, cough strength, and secretion volume); and other parameters (ie, hemodynamic status, no or minimal vasopressor or inotropic support required, and so forth).[13]

The RSBI evaluates whether patients can avoid rapid shallow breathing as ventilator support is reduced. The RSBI is the ratio of the patient's breathing frequency (f or RR) divided by the patient's V_T in liters measured during 1 minute of unassisted, spontaneous breathing.[12] As originally described by Yang and Tobin, an RSBI less than 105 breaths/min/L, measured using a Wright's spirometer attached to the end of an endotracheal tube without ventilator support, had a sensitivity of 97% and specificity of 64% for predicting extubation success.[12] Subsequent studies have brought into question the utility of the RSBI to predict extubation success recognizing that this outcome confounds both liberation from the ventilator and the artificial airway.[14,15] A meta-analysis found that the RSBI had limited value in predicting successful extubation (positive likelihood ratio of 1.49).[14] A more recent meta-analysis of 48 studies found that the RSBI had a sensitivity of 83% and a specificity of 58% for predicting extubation success.[15] In sensitivity analyses, RSBI sensitivity and specificity did not vary significantly with the use of different thresholds (<80 vs <105 breaths/min/L), ventilator support used during RSBI measurement (T-piece, Pressure Support [PS]), or the timing of RSBI measurement.[15]

The RSBI has also been assessed as a permissive criterion to decide whether invasively ventilated patients area ready to undergo an SBT (RSBI <105 breaths/min/L along with other safety criteria). An international survey of intensivist's stated practices in liberating critically ill adults from invasive ventilation identified that only one-third of respondents reported using an RSBI threshold of 105 breaths/min/L to determine patient readiness to undergo an SBT.[16] In a randomized trial, Tanios and colleagues found that inclusion of the RSBI in an SBT protocol delayed successful extubation and did not reduce the rate of extubation failure.[17]

Criteria to determine SBT outcome (pass/fail) have largely been derived from clinical trials and clinical practice guidelines.[18–21] Additional research is needed to elucidate the best combination of criteria for clinicians to identify patients who are ready to undergo an SBT and the optimal screening frequency, SBT technique, and SBT duration. Moreover, the impact of specific interventions on both liberation from the ventilator (time to first successful SBT) and the endotracheal tube (time to successful extubation) require clarification and standardization. Additional clarity is also needed regarding the optimal timing to measure and report extubation success (48 hours vs 72 hours vs 7 days).

Conduct of Spontaneous Breathing Trials

SBTs represent a formal assessment of extubation readiness performed using reduced or no ventilator support as a test of a patient's capacity to breathe spontaneously for 30 to 120 minutes. SBTs may be conducted using a variety of techniques including T-piece, low levels of PS with or without positive end-expiratory pressure (PEEP), continuous positive airway pressure (CPAP), automatic tube compensation, and other less frequently used techniques.[16,22]

Data regarding the optimal SBT technique for clinicians to use are conflicting. A physiologic systematic review that examined effort to breathe using alternative SBT techniques found that SBTs conducted with PS decreased work of breathing more than SBTs conducted with other techniques including T-piece or CPAP.[23] Conversely, a meta-analysis of randomized trials that compared alternative SBT techniques and reported clinical outcomes found that although patients were not more likely to pass an SBT using PS with or without PEEP SBTs versus T-piece SBTs, they were 6% more likely to remain successfully extubated with PS SBTs (number needed to treat of 22).[22] Aligned with these findings, the ATS/ACCP guidelines made a conditional recommendation for the conduct of SBTs with augmentation of inspiratory pressure.[9,24]

More recently, Subira and colleagues[25] conducted an RCT that compared 30-minute SBTs with PS 8 cm H_2O without PEEP (less-demanding technique) to a 2-hour SBT with T-piece (more demanding technique) for patients who received invasive ventilation for at least 24 hours in 18 Spanish ICUs. The authors found that the less-demanding SBT technique had an 8.2% absolute increase in the rate of successful extubation, defined as remaining free of mechanical ventilation 72 hours after first SBT, without an increase in the rate of reintubation.[25] In this trial, participants received the assigned SBT technique during the first SBT. Subsequently, Thille and colleagues compared PS (without PEEP) versus T-piece SBTs for patients who were invasively ventilated for more than 24 hours and deemed to be at "high risk" for reintubation (>65 years of age or with any underlying chronic cardiac or lung disease) in 31 ICUs in France.[26] The authors found no differences between the alternative SBT techniques in the median number of ventilator-free days at day 28, and in the rates of extubation (within 24 hours and within 7 days) and reintubation.[26] A large-scale observational study found that initial SBTs are most commonly conducted using PS with PEEP (457/930 [49.1%]) or T-piece (236/930 [25.4%]) and less frequently with CPAP (100/930 [10.8%]) or PS without PEEP (88/930 [9.5%]).[27] Four trials, including the aforementioned trial by Subira and colleagues have compared shorter (20 or 30 minute) versus longer (120 minute) SBTs and found no important differences in SBT outcome, extubation outcome, and reintubation rates.[25,28–30]

Important study design features including the use of daily screening and incorporation of extubation criteria among criteria to identify SBT candidates, whether SBT techniques were applied once or repeated until a trial end-point was achieved, and the reporting of weaning (ie, time to successful SBT) versus extubation (ie, time to successful extubation) outcomes remain poorly characterized. In addition, no trial comparing alternative SBT techniques was powered to assess equivalency. Uncertainty remains regarding the role for more frequent screening to identify SBT candidates and the best SBT technique and duration for clinicians to use. Additionally, we do not know which patients may benefit from longer SBTs and whether certain patients (ie, chronic obstructive pulmonary disease [COPD], congestive heart failure, or neuromuscular disease) may benefit from the use of specific SBT techniques.

Optimizing Patients for Liberation from Invasive Ventilation

Analgesics and sedatives are frequently used to enhance patient comfort and prevent self-extubation. Trials examining the effects of sedation strategies have shown that sedation protocols focused on minimizing sedation in mechanically ventilated patients result in shorter duration of ICU stay and a trend toward reduced duration of mechanical ventilation and received a conditional recommendation for patients invasively ventilated for more than 24 hours in a clinical practice guideline.[24] Conflicting evidence exists regarding the benefits associated with sedation interruption for critically ill patients. A trial of 336 invasively ventilated patients randomized to either a daily spontaneous awakening trial (SAT) followed by an SBT or with sedation as per usual care plus a daily SBT found that patients in the combined SAT plus SBT (vs usual care plus SBT) group spent more days breathing without assistance during the 28-day study period and were discharged from ICU and hospital earlier. Although more patients in the intervention group self-extubated compared with the control group, a similar number of patients in both groups required reintubation.[31] Conversely, a trial of 430 invasively ventilated patients randomly allocated to either protocolized sedation plus daily sedation interruption or protocolized sedation alone did not find between-group differences in the median time to successful extubation, ICU and hospital lengths of stay. Daily sedation interruption was associated with higher mean daily doses of fentanyl and midazolam and more daily boluses of opiates and benzodiazepines.[32] In a secondary analysis of this trial, the authors found that patients received higher doses of benzodiazepines and opioids at night and higher nighttime doses were associated with more SBT failures and delayed extubation.[33]

Critically ill patients, especially those who are severely ill and those who receive protracted ventilation, are at high risk for the development of ICU-acquired weakness[34] and sequelae of immobility may contribute to delayed weaning and extubation failure. For patients who are invasively ventilated for more than 24 hours, a conditional recommendation (low certainty evidence) supports the use of protocolized rehabilitation directed toward early mobilization.[9]

Laryngeal edema is also associated with postextubation stridor and an increased risk for reintubation. Although a cuff leak test may help to identify laryngeal edema before extubation and decrease the risk of postextubation stridor,[35,36] this approach may also delay extubation due to false-positive test results.[9,10] Guidelines provide a conditional recommendation to perform a cuff leak test for patients who meet extubation criteria and are deemed to be at high risk for postextubation stridor (traumatic intubation, large endotracheal tubes, women, and those ventilated for 1 week or more).[9,10] For patients who have failed a cuff leak test and who are at high risk for postextubation stridor, a conditional recommendation supports administration of systemic steroids 4 hours before extubation.[9]

Use of Noninvasive Positive Pressure Ventilation for Weaning

Although life-saving, invasive ventilation is associated with ventilator-related complications, especially VAP. VAP, in turn, is associated with morbidity and an attributable mortality of approximately 13%.[37] Cumulative exposure to invasive ventilation is also associated with the development of long-term sequelae including muscle weakness,[38,39] reduced health-related quality of life,[40,41] depression,[42] delirium,[43] posttraumatic stress disorder,[44,45] and cognitive impairment.[46] For these reasons, minimizing patients' exposure to invasive ventilation has been identified as a key research priority by critical care and respiratory societies.[2]

Investigators have studied the use of NIV as a method to reduce patients' exposure to invasive ventilation during weaning by prematurely extubating selected patients to NIV. NIV, administered with a patient–ventilator interface, provides partial ventilator support and preserves patients' ability to cough, swallow, and speak[47] but does not provide airway protection. NIV can augment tidal volumes, reduces RRs, enable application of PEEP, and improve gas exchange.[48,49] Studies demonstrate that patients who are treated with NIV receive less-invasive monitoring and sedation[50] and experience less psychological distress.[51] In the periextubation period, NIV can be used to facilitate weaning (direct extubation to NIV for the purpose of weaning); applied prophylactically for patients who are at risk for extubation failure; or applied after post-extubation respiratory failure has developed. When NIV is used to facilitate earlier extubation and weaning, patients who do not meet conventional criteria for extubation (ie, *fail* an SBT or are *too early* to undergo an SBT) are extubated directly to NIV. In pressure mode, noninvasive support (the difference between inspiratory positive airway pressure and expiratory positive airway pressure [EPAP]) and EPAP are reduced over time in a manner similar to reductions in invasive PS in intubated patients. As such, NIV replaces invasive PS and reduces patients' exposure to invasive ventilation and its associated complications.

Noninvasive weaning may be ideally suited to patients with COPD because failure to wean in this population is characterized by respiratory muscle weakness, gas trapping, and increased intrinsic PEEP. With NIV, clinicians can administer oxygen, augment inhaled volume, and apply extrinsic PEEP to counteract intrinsic PEEP.[49] NIV has been shown to augment V_T, reduce breathing frequency, improve gas exchange, and rest the muscles of respiration.[48] An international survey of self-reported practices in liberating critically ill patients from invasive ventilation found that many intensivists (>50% of respondents in most regions) reported using noninvasive weaning in patients with COPD but were less likely to use NIV for other indications such as cardiogenic pulmonary edema or in the postoperative setting.[16]

A recent systematic review and meta-analysis, including 28 trials (n = 2066) compared extubation with NIV for the purpose of weaning versus continued invasive weaning in critically ill patients.[52] Compared with invasive weaning, noninvasive weaning reduced mortality (**Fig. 2**), VAP (**Fig. 3**), and weaning failures—all with high-quality evidence. Compared with invasive weaning, noninvasive weaning also reduced length of stay in the ICU and hospital, and rates of tracheostomy. Moreover, the noninvasive (vs invasive) approach to weaning significantly reduced the duration of invasive (endo-tracheal) ventilation, total duration of ventilation, and the duration of ventilation related to weaning. Subgroup analysis suggested that the benefits of noninvasive weaning were greater in COPD versus mixed patient populations, with significant between-group differences in mortality, ICU length of stay, and reintubation favoring patients with COPD.[52] In this review, patients with COPD were the focus of half of the included trials and 44.6% of the patients.[52] The lack of blinding and inconsistent use of standardized weaning protocols in both treatment arms and the absence of a sedation protocol in the invasive weaning arms raises the possibility that control patients may not have received optimal care in some trials, biasing in favor of the noninvasive approach to weaning.

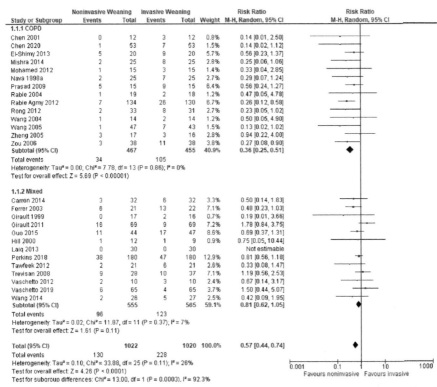

Fig. 2. Effect of noninvasive weaning (vs invasive weaning) on mortality. COPD, chronic obstructive pulmonary disease; M-H, Mantel-Haenszel. (Granton, David MD, et al., High-Flow Nasal Cannula Compared With Conventional Oxygen Therapy or Noninvasive Ventilation Immediately Postextubation: A Systematic Review and Meta-Analysis. Critical Care Medicine 48(11):p e1129-e1136, November 2020. https://doi.org/10.1097/CCM.0000000000004576.)

In the largest single trial conducted to date comparing the alternative weaning strategies, Perkins and coworkers found significant differences in the duration of invasive ventilation and total duration of ventilation.[53] In contrast to the aforementioned meta-analysis, the authors of this trial did not find differences in rates of mortality or tracheostomy.[53] It is important to note 2 key differences in the design of this trial. First, the trial by Perkins and colleagues enrolled patients with various reasons for acute respiratory failure and only 4% of their participants included patients with COPD. Second, the authors were diligent in using protocolized weaning strategies in both groups and thereby may have reduced performance bias. The difference in duration of invasive ventilation is, in part, directed by the protocol and early extubation of patients in the NIV arm. Similarly, the total duration of ventilation is of greatest interest when it is restricted to the postrandomization period because the prerandomization period does not reflect the interventions being studied. These factors, may in part, explain the discordant findings between the results of this large trial and the meta-analysis.

Compared with a prior meta-analysis conducted by Yeung and colleagues published in 2018,[54] the more recent meta-analysis[52] included more trials and documented similar beneficial effects of NIV on mortality, VAP, duration of invasive ventilation, and ICU stay. In a sensitivity analysis of 9 trials involving 788 patients who failed an initial SBT, Yeung

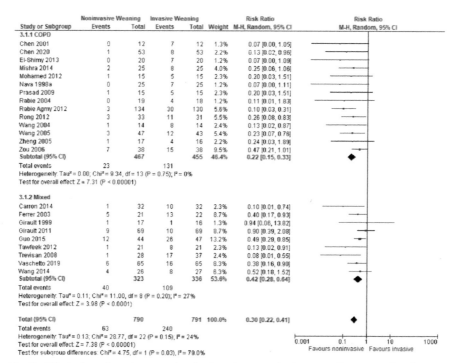

Fig. 3. Effect of noninvasive weaning (vs invasive weaning) on ventilator-associated pneumonia. COPD, chronic obstructive pulmonary disease; M-H, Mantel-Haenszel. (Burns KEA, Stevenson J, Laird M, et al. Non-invasive ventilation versus invasive weaning in critically ill adults: a systematic review and meta-analysis Thorax 2022;77:752-761. https://doi.org/10.1136/thoraxjnl-2021-216993.)

and coworkers also identified beneficial effects of noninvasive weaning on hospital mortality but wide "highest posterior density intervals," from Bayesian estimates, precluded a definitive statement regarding the effect of NIV on this outcome.[54] The more recent meta-analysis also identified beneficial effects of noninvasive (vs invasive) weaning on the proportion of weaning failures and tracheostomies, as well as, hospital length of stay and the duration of ventilation related to weaning; however, these summary estimates had considerable heterogeneity.[52] Aligned with these findings, a recent systematic review and individual patient meta-analysis of 6 trials highlighted the potential beneficial effect of NIV after early extubation in reducing the total days spent on invasive ventilation, although this was not associated with a significant reduction in ICU mortality.[55]

The ATS/ACCP guidelines provided a strong recommendation (moderate certainty evidence) in favor of extubation to preventative NIV for patients who received mechanical ventilation for more than 24 hours and *passed* an SBT but were considered to be at high risk of extubation failure.[9] The guidelines; however, did *not* address early extubation to NIV for patients who *failed* an initial SBT or were *too early* to undergo an SBT. On balance, the above findings support beneficial effects of noninvasive (vs invasive) weaning on important clinical outcomes especially for patients with COPD. Notwithstanding, the benefits of noninvasive weaning are unclear in non-COPD patients and represents an area for future investigation. Enthusiasm for noninvasive weaning should be tempered by local considerations including the need for standalone noninvasive ventilators or ventilators capable of providing both forms of ventilation, and the experience of physicians, nurses, and respiratory therapists to safely implement noninvasive weaning and perform reintubation if required.

Extubation Decision-Making and Extubation

An international survey found that diverse health-care providers participate in various aspects of weaning and extubation; however, intensivists are largely responsible for extubation decision-making.[16] During extubation decision-making, clinicians aim to avoid extubation failure (ie, need for reintubation within hours to days) because it has been associated with an increased risk of death, ICU length of stay, need for rehabilitation following ICU discharge, and hospital costs (US$34,000 per failed extubation).[56–64] Although few studies have examined how extubation decisions are made, clinicians should use a patient-centered, stepwise to extubation decision-making including (1) dynamic evaluation of individual patient's extubation readiness and his/her risks and consequences of extubation failure, (2) establishing a plan should extubation fail, and (3) mitigating the risk for extubation failure with strategic interventions performed preextubation or postextubation.

Determining the risk for extubation failure (ie, estimation of future prevalence) involves the science of prediction of extubation outcomes. Readiness for extubation usually but not always involves an SBT. Surgical patients who are intubated for procedural general anesthesia and undergo a short period of ventilation may not need a formal SBT because the likelihood of success is exceptionally high and an SBT may unnecessarily prolong ventilation.[22] However, for acutely hospitalized patients invasively ventilated for less than 24 hours, current guidelines suggest that an SBT be performed with inspiratory pressure augmentation (conditional recommendation) as part of the liberation assessment.[9,24] In this manner, an SBT not only aids clinicians to assess patient's capacity to assume spontaneous breathing but also informs clinician's prediction of extubation outcome. Clinicians may perceive that some patients are at greater risk for the consequences of failed extubation. For example, patients with advanced coronary artery disease and documented myocardial ischemia, or frail patients recovering from respiratory failure may suffer greater potential harm following a failed attempt at extubation. In contrast, other patients may be at lower risk for the consequences of a failed attempt at extubation (eg, surgical patients). The balance of the risks and consequences of a failed extubation aids clinicians in determining when a trial of extubation should *not* be attempted, and a tracheostomy may be considered. Tracheostomy without a trial of extubation is a feasible option when both the risk and consequences of extubation failure are prohibitive. Identifying patients who benefit from direct tracheostomy remains an important area of investigation.[27]

Several of the previously discussed parameters used in screening protocols to identify SBT candidates (ie, RSBI) are also used to predict extubation outcome, in addition to, other routinely performed, bedside assessments, and more novel approaches to prediction. Bedside assessments, typically performed by respiratory therapists and nurses, include a patient's handgrip strength, cough strength, lift his/her head off the pillow, and ability to follow commands. Although an active area of investigation, several studies have demonstrated that loss of respiratory variability is associated with[65–71] and is predictive of extubation failure.[72–74] In this field of investigation, loss of respiratory and heart rate variability represent diminished physiologic reserve and/or increased illness severity.[75]

Although extubation decisions are made by ICU clinicians daily in practice, few studies have examined physician's ability to predict extubation outcomes. A survey of 45 intensivists in the United States identified only fair agreement between physicians in extubation decision-making but with low accuracy (receiver operating characteristic area under the curve of 0.35, sensitivity [57%], and specificity [31%]).[76] Additionally, a single-center longitudinal study found that protocolized assessments of extubation readiness decreased extubation failure rates.[77]

Postextubation management must be planned before extubation to ensure clarity of action in the event of patient deterioration. Prompt reintubation is warranted for patients who demonstrate signs of impending respiratory failure postextubation. However, reintubation and prolonged life-support with a tracheostomy may not be aligned with the goals of care of some patients. Therefore, a discussion with the patient's family and legally authorized representatives to clarify goals of care is warranted before extubation. Occasionally, based on the patient's preexpressed wishes or values, optimal care may include extubation with full care while optimizing conditions for success; yet with a clear plan not to pursue reintubation in the event that the patient deteriorates or is unable to tolerate breathing on his/her own. A "one-way extubation" may be used for patients who want an opportunity to recover and regain their prior functional status but do not wish for prolonged life support, hospitalization, tracheostomy, and rehabilitation.

Risk mitigation of extubation failure involves recognizing specific risk factors and targeting therapies to address modifiable factors. Risk factors may be airway-related (eg, airway obstruction, excessive secretions, impaired cough, aspiration, and decreased level of consciousness) or breathing-related (eg, congestive heart failure, hypoxemia, hypoventilation, pulmonary disease, and impaired consciousness).[78] Once identified these factors should be addressed, where feasible, before extubation. For example, patients with hypertension, especially in the presence of left ventricular systolic function, should undergo afterload reduction before and after extubation.[79] Diuresis is commonly used to mitigate risk of extubation failure in the setting of a positive cumulative fluid balance.[80] Delirium may increase the risk for extubation failure and should be treated based on clinical judgment. Instituting risk mitigation strategies before extubation is appropriate, and it is reasonable to delay extubation if the risk of extubation failure may be meaningfully reduced.[59] Finally, for patients who are at an increased risk for extubation failure, clinicians must decide whether to apply HFNC[81] or NIV[82,83] prophylactically after extubation.

Use of High Flow Nasal Cannula After Extubation

HFNC uses a single-limb inspiratory setup and is able to deliver humidified oxygen at flows much higher than traditional soft plastic nasal cannula. This high flow oxygen, as high as 60 to 70 L/min, is able to achieve reliably high Fio_2 delivery and also more adequately match the inspiratory demands of a dyspneic patient. Previous randomized controlled trials and systematic reviews[84] have demonstrated the benefit of HFNC in patients with acute hypoxemic respiratory failure and newer data have shown similar benefit in hypercarbic respiratory failure.[85] As compared with bilevel NIV, HFNC is better tolerated by patients, more comfortable, and usually allows patients to eat and speak during treatment.

Because HFNC is a relatively new oxygen-delivery strategy in adults, the evidence base is less well developed compared with that of NIV. Few studies have examined HFNC as a tool for weaning or to facilitate early extubation and, as opposed to NIV. However, there are some data to support delivery of high flow oxygen in tracheostomized patients to increase airway pressure and reduce work of breathing during tracheostomy collar trials; however, these data are limited to small physiology-based crossover trials.[86] Use of high flow for these indications remains variable given the sparse evidence supporting its use.

HFNC is more widely used to help with the transition off invasive mechanical ventilation after extubation. The sudden loss of positive pressure during extubation may be abrupt, and many patients experience postextubation dyspnea with a smaller proportion require reintubation. NIV is used in this setting but is associated with limitations, especially related to patient comfort and delivery of care. When considering oxygen support in the postextubation period, prophylaxis is key because data suggest once postextubation respiratory failure develops, the use of noninvasive supports may just delay reintubation and worsen patient outcomes.[87] When used for prophylaxis following extubation, data demonstrate that HFNC probably reduces the need for reintubation (pooled RR, 0.46; 95% CI, 0.30–0.70; moderate certainty, **Fig. 4**) although with no effect on mortality (RR, 0.93; 95% CI, 0.57–1.52; moderate certainty). Based on this, a recent guideline suggested that the use of HFNC as opposed to conventional oxygen therapy (COT) for patients who are intubated more than 24 hours and have any high-risk feature (conditional recommendation, moderate certainty evidence).[84] The data underpinning these recommendations were derived from 5 trials[81,88–91] that compared HFNC to COT and 3 trials[92–94] that compared HFNC with NIV (bilevel or CPAP). The definition for high risk varied with the largest trial[92] defining high risk as at least one of the following: age older than 65 years, congestive heart failure, moderate–severe COPD, Acute Physiology and Chronic Health Evaluation II score greater than 12, body mass index greater than 30, airway patency or secretion problems, difficulty weaning, 2 or more comorbidities, or duration of ventilation greater than 7 days. The guideline panel also suggested continued use of NIV as opposed to HFNC (conditional recommendation, low certainty evidence) for patients who clinicians would normally extubate to NIV, especially those with COPD. This practice is supported by recently updated meta-analysis that demonstrated a reduction in mortality (RR, 0.57; 95% CI, 0.44–0.74; high certainty), weaning failure (RR, 0.59; 95% CI, 0.43–0.81; high certainty), and ICU/hospital length of stay when using NIV to facilitate weaning from invasive mechanical ventilation in selected patients, mostly those with underlying structural lung disease such as COPD.[52]

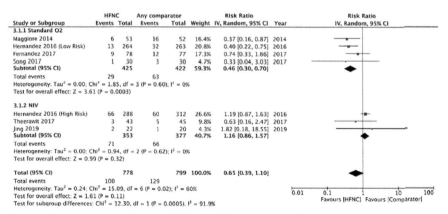

Fig. 4. Effect of postextubation HFNC on risk of reintubation. df, degrees of freedom; HFNC, high flow nasal cannula; NIV, noninvasive ventilation. (Burns KEA, Stevenson J, Laird M, et al. Non-invasive ventilation versus invasive weaning in critically ill adults: a systematic review and meta-analysisThorax 2022;77:752-761. https://doi.org/10.1136/thoraxjnl-2021-216993.)

SUMMARY

Increasing evidence supports specific approaches to liberate patients from invasive ventilation including the use of liberation protocols, inspiratory assistance during SBTs, early extubation of patients with COPD to NIV, and prophylactic use of noninvasive support strategies after extubation. Additional research is needed to elucidate the best criteria to identify patients who are ready to undergo an SBT and to inform optimal screening frequency, the best SBT technique and duration, extubation assessments, and extubation decision-making. Additional clarity is also needed regarding the optimal timing to measure and report extubation success (48 hours vs 72 hours vs 7 days) and to standardize reporting of weaning (SBT outcome) and extubation outcomes.

CLINICS CARE POINTS

- Clinicians should use a protocolized approach to weaning and extubation with individualized consideration of patient's goals and values, as well as, the risks and consequences of extubation failure. Liberation from invasive ventilation is a multistep process involving optimizing patients for liberation from invasive ventilation, screening to identify candidates who are ready to undergo a breathing trial (SBT), conduct of an SBT, assessment for extubation, and extubation where feasible.

- An updated meta-analysis supports the beneficial effects of early extubation to NIV (vs continued invasive weaning) on important clinical outcomes especially for patients with COPD. The benefits of noninvasive weaning are unclear in non-COPD patients. Application of noninvasive weaning in practice should be tempered by local considerations.

- A patient-centered, stepwise approach to extubation decision-making involves (1) dynamic evaluation of individual patient's extubation readiness and his/her risks and consequences of extubation failure, (2) establishing a plan should extubation fail, and (3) mitigating the risk for extubation failure with strategic interventions performed before or after extubation.

- HFNC is a noninvasive oxygenation strategy that can aid in transitioning patients off of invasive ventilation.

DISCLOSURE

K.E.A. Burns holds a Canadian Institutes of Health Research grant to investigate weaning strategies and Physician Services Incorporated Mid Career Research Award. A.J. Seely is the founder and CEO of Therapeutic Monitoring Systems, which holds global licensing rights for intellectual property related to Extubation Advisor (a tool designed to aid extubation assessment) and tools being developed in the Ottawa Hospital Research Institute Dynamical Analysis Laboratory that require regulatory approval and commercialization for bedside application. B. Rochwerg has no conflicts of interest to declare.

REFERENCES

1. Esteban A, Alia I, Ibanez J, et al. Modes of mechanical ventilation and weaning. A national survey of Spanish hospitals. the Spanish lung failure collaborative group. Chest 1994;106:1188–93.
2. MacIntyre NR, Cook DJ, Ely EW, et al. Evidence-based guidelines for weaning and discontinuing ventilatory support. A collective task force facilitated by the American College of chest physicians; the American association for respiratory

care; and the American College of critical care medicine. Chest 2001;6(Suppl): 375–95.

3. Zein H, Baratloo A, Negida A, et al. Ventilator weaning and spontaneous breathing trials; an educational review. Emerg (Tehran) 2016;4:65–71.

4. Torres A, Gatell JM, Aznar E, et al. Re-intubation increases the risk of nosocomial pneumonia in patients needing mechanical ventilation. Am J Respir Crit Care Med 1995;152:137–41.

5. Wunsch H, Linde-Zwirble WT, Angus DC, et al. The epidemiology of mechanical ventlilation use in the United States. Crit Care Med 2010;38(10):1947–53.

6. Goligher EC, Jonkman AH, Dianti J, et al. Clinical strategies for implementing lung and diaphragm-protective ventilation: avoiding insufficient and excessive effort. Intensive Care Med 2020;46(12):2314–26.

7. Vetrugno L, Guadagnin GM, Brussa A, et al. Mechanical ventilation weaning issues can be counted on the fingers of just one hand: part 1. Ultrasound J 2020;12:9. https://rdcu.be/dhxza.

8. Vallverdu I, Calaf N, Subirana M, et al. Clinical characteristics, respiratory functional parameters, and outcome of a two-hour T-piece trial in patients weaning from mechanical ventilation. Am J Respir Crit Care Med 1998;158:1855–62.

9. Schmidt GA, Girard TD, Kress JP, et al. Official executive summary of an American Thoracic Society/American College of Chest Physicians clinical practice guideline: liberation from mechanical ventilation in critically ill adults. Am J Respir Crit Care Med 2017;195:115–9.

10. Girard TD, Alhazzani W, Kress JP, et al. An official American Thoracic Society/ American College of Chest Physicians clinical practice guideline: liberation from mechanical ventilation in critically ill adults. Rehabilitation protocols, ventilator liberation protocols, and cuff leak tests. Am J Respir Crit Care Med 2017; 195:120–33.

11. Blackwood B, Burns KE, Cardwell CR, et al. Protocolized versus non-protocolized weaning for reducing the duration of mechanical ventilation in critically ill adult patients. Cochrane Database Syst Rev 2014;2014:CD006904.

12. Yang KL, Tobin MJ. A prospective study of indexes predicting the outcome of trials of weaning from mechanical ventilation. N Engl J Med 1991;324:1445–50.

13. Baptistella AR, Sarmento FJ, da Silva KR, et al. Predictive factors of weaning from mechanical ventilation and extubation outcome: a systematic review. J Crit Care 2018;48:56–62.

14. Meade M, Guyatt G, Cook D, et al. Predicting success in weaning from mechanical ventilation. Chest 2001;120:400S–24S.

15. Trivedi V, Chaudhuri D, Jinah R, et al. The usefulness of the Rapid Shallow Breathing Index in predicting successful extubation: a systematic review and meta-analysis. Chest 2022;161:97–111.

16. Burns KE, Raptis SR, Nisenbaum R, et al. International practice variation in weaning critically ill adults from invasive mechanical ventilation. Ann Am Thorac Soc 2018;15(4):494–502.

17. Tanios MA, Nevins ML, Hendra KP, et al. A randomized, controlled trial of the role of weaning predictors in clinical decision making. Crit Care Med 2006;34:2530–5.

18. Esteban A, Frutos F, Tobin MJ, et al. A comparison of four methods of weaning patients from mechanical ventilation. Spanish Lung Failure Collaborative Group. N Engl J Med 1995;332:345–50.

19. Brochard L, Rauss A, Benito S, et al. Comparison of three methods of gradual withdrawal from ventilatory support during weaning from mechanical ventilation. Am J Respir Crit Care Med 1994;150:896–903.

20. Ely EW, Baker AM, Dunagan DP, et al. Effect on the duration of mechanical ventilation of identifying patients capable of breathing spontaneously. N Engl J Med 1996;335:1864–9.

21. Girard TD, Kress JP, Fuchs BD, et al. Efficacy and safety of a paired sedation and ventilator weaning protocol for mechanically ventilated patients in intensive care (Awakening and Breathing Controlled trial): a randomised controlled trial. Lancet 2008;371:126–34.

22. Burns KE, Soliman I, Adhikari NKJ, et al. Trials directly comparing alternative spontaneous breathing trial techniques: a systematic review and meta-analysis. Crit Care 2017;21(1):127.

23. Sklar MC, Burns K, Rittayamai N, et al. Effort to breathe with various spontaneous breathing trial techniques. A physiologic meta-analysis. Am J Respir Crit Care Med 2017;195:1477–85.

24. Ouellette DR, Patel S, Girard TD, et al. Liberation from mechanical ventilation in critically ill adults: an official American College of Chest Physicians/American Thoracic Society clinical practice guideline: inspiratory pressure augmentation during spontaneous breathing trials, protocols minimizing sedation, and noninvasive ventilation immediately after extubation. Chest 2017;151:166–80.

25. Subira C, Hernández G, Vazquez A, et al. Effect of pressure support vs T-piece ventilation strategies during spontaneous breathing trials on successful extubation among patients receiving mechanical ventilation: a randomized clinical trial. JAMA 2019;321(22):2175–82.

26. Thille AW, Gacouin A, Coudroy R, et al, REVA Research Network. Spontaneous breathing trials with pressure support ventilation or T-piece. N Engl J Med 2022;387(20):1843–54.

27. Burns KEA, Rizvi L, Cook DJ, et al, Canadian Critical Care Trials Group. Meade MO for the Canadian critical care trials group. International practices in discontinuing mechanical ventilation. JAMA 2021;325(12):1173–84.

28. Esteban A, Alia I, Tobin MJ, et al. Effect of spontaneous breathing trial duration on outcome of attempts to discontinue mechanical ventilation. Spanish Lung Failure Collaborative Group. Am J Respir Crit Care Med 1999;159:512–8.

29. Chawla K, Kupfer Y, Goldman I, et al. The spontaneous breathing trial: how long? Am J Respir Crit Care Med 2001;163:A892.

30. Perren A, Domenighetti G, Mauri S, et al. Protocol-directed weaning from mechanical ventilation: clinical outcome in patients randomized for a 30-min or 120-min trial with pressure support ventilation. Intensive Care Med 2002;28:1058–63.

31. Girard TD, Kress JP, Fuchs BD, et al. Efficacy and safety of a paired sedation and ventilator weaning protocol for mechanically ventilated patients in intensive care (Awakening and Breathing Controlled trial): a randomized controlled trial. Lancet 2008;371:126–34.

32. Mehta S, Burry L, Cook DJ, et al, SLEAP Investigators, Canadian Critical Care Trials Group. SLEAP Investigators Canadian Critical Care Trials Group. Daily sedation interruption in mechanically ventilated criticallly ill patients cared for with a sedation protocol: a randomized controlled trial. JAMA 2012;308(19):1985–92.

33. Mehta S, Meade MO, Burry L, et al, SLEAP Investigators and the Canadian Critical Care Trials Group. Cook DJ for the SLEAP Investigators and the Canadian Critical Care Trials Group. Variation in diurnal sedation of mechanically ventilated patients who are managed with a sedation protocol alone or a sedation protocol and daily interruption. Crit Care 2016;20(1):233.

34. Yang T, Li Z, Jiang L, et al. Risk factors for intensive care unit-acquired weakness: a systematic review and meta-analysis. Acta Neurol Scand 2018;138:104–14.

35. Ochoa ME, Marin Mdel C, Frutos-Vivar F, et al. Cuff-leak test for the diagnosis of upper airway obstruction in adults: a systematic review and meta-analysis. Intensive Care Med 2009;35:1171–9.

36. Zhou T, Zhang HP, Chen WW, et al. Cuff-leak test for predicting postextubation airway complications: a systematic review. J Evid Based Med 2011;4:242–54.

37. Melsen WG, Rovers MM, Groenwold RHH, et al. Attributable mortality of ventilator-associated pneumonia: a meta-analysis of individual patient data from randomized prevention studies. Lancet Infect Dis 2013;13(8):665–71.

38. Farhan H, Moreno-Duarte I, Latronico N, et al. Acquired muscle weakness in the surgical intensive care unit: nosology, epidemiology, diagnosis, and prevention. Anesthesiology 2016;124:207–34.

39. Herridge MS, Tansey CM, Matté A, et al, Canadian Critical Care Trials Group. Canadian Critical Care Trials Group. Functional disability 5 years after acute respiratory distress syndrome. N Engl J Med 2011;364:1293–304.

40. Dowdy DW, Eid MP, Sedrakyan A, et al. Quality of life in adult survivors of critical illness: a systematic review of the literature. Intensive Care Med 2005;31:611–20.

41. Combes A, Costa MA, Trouillet JL, et al. Morbidity, mortality, and quality-of-life outcomes of patients requiring > or = 14 days of mechanical ventilation. Crit Care Med 2003;31:1373–81.

42. Jubran A, Lawm G, Kelly J, et al. Depressive disorders during weaning from prolonged mechanical ventilation. Intensive Care Med 2010;36:828–35.

43. Ely EW, Gautam S, Margolin R, et al. The impact of delirium in the intensive care unit on hospital length of stay. Intensive Care Med 2001;27:1892–900.

44. Cuthbertson BH, Hull A, Strachan M, et al. Post-traumatic stress disorder after critical illness requiring general intensive care. Intensive Care Med 2004;30: 450–5.

45. Jubran A, Lawm G, or +Duffner L, Collins EG, Lanuza DM, Hoffman LA, Tobin MJ. Post-traumatic stress disorder after weaning from prolonged mechanical ventilation. Intensive Care Med 2010;36:2030–7.

46. Pandharipande PP, Girard TD, Jackson JC, Morandi A, Thompson JL, Pun BT, I et a, Hughes CG, Vasilevskis EE, Shintani AK, Moons KG, Geevarghese SK, Canonico A, Hopkins RO, Bernard GR, Dittus RS, Ely EW, BRAIN-ICU Study InvestigatorsBRAIN-ICU Study InvestigatorsLong-term. Cognitive impairment after critical illness. N Engl J Med 2013;369(14):1306–16.

47. Mehta S, Hill NS. Noninvasive ventilation. Am J Respir Crit Care Med 2001;163: 540–77.

48. Nava S, Ambrosino N, Rubini F, Fracchia C, Rampulla C, Torri G, Calderini E. Effect of nasal pressure support ventilation and external positive end expiratory pressure on diaphragmatic function in patients with severe stable COPD. Chest 1993;103:143–50.

49. Appendini L, Patessio A, Zanaboni S, Carone M, Gukov B, Donner CF, Rossi A. Physiological effects of positive end expiratory pressure and mask pressure support during exacerbations of chronic obstructive pulmonary disease. Am J Respir Crit Care Med 1994;149:1069–76.

50. Rathgeber J, Schorn B, Falk V, Kazmaier S, Spiegel T, Burchardi H. The influence of controlled mechanical ventilation (CMV), intermittent mandatory ventilation (IMV) and biphasic intermittent positive airway pressure (BIPAP) on duration of intubation and consumption of analgesics and sedatives. A prospective analysis

of in 596 patients following adult cardiac surgery. Eur J Anaesthesiol 1997;14: 576–82.

51. Criner GJ, Tzouanakis A, Kreimer DT. Overview of improving tolerance of long-term mechanical ventilation. Crit Care Clin 1994;10:845–66.

52. Burns KEA, Stevenson J, Laird J, Adhikari NKJ, Li Y, Lu C, He X, Wang W, Liang Z, Chen L, Zhang H, Friedrich JO. Noninvasive ventilation versus invasive weaning in critically ill adults: a systematic review and meta-analysis. Thorax 2021;77(8):752–61.

53. Perkins GD, Mistry D, Gates S, Gao F, Snelson C, Hart N, Comporota L, Varley J, Carle C, Paramasivam E, Hoddell B, McAuley DF, Walsh TS, Blackwood B, Rose L, Lamb SE, Petrou S, Young D, Lall R, for the BREATHE Collaborators. Effect of protocolizedweaning with early extubation to noninvasive ventilation vs invasive-weaning on time to liberation from mechanical ventilation among patients with respiratory failure: the breathe randomized clinical trial. JAMA 2018;320(18):1881–8.

54. Yeung J, Couper K, Ryan EG, Gates S, Hart N, Perkins GD. Non-invasive ventilation as a weaning strategy from mechanical ventilation: a systematic review and Bayesian meta-analysis. Intensive Care Med 2018;44:2192–204.

55. Vaschetto R, Pecere A, Perkins GD, Mistry D, Cammarota G, Longhini F, Ferrer M, Pletsch-Assuncao R, Carron M, Moretto F, Qiu H, Della Corte F, Barone-Adesi F, Navalesi P. Effects of early extubation followed by noninvasive ventilation versus standard extubation on the duration of invasive mechanical ventilation in hypoxemic non-hypercapnic patients: a systematic review and individual patient data meta-analysis of randomized controlled trials. Crit Care 2021;25(1):189.

56. Seymour CW, Martinez A, Christie JD, Fuchs BD. The outcome of extubation failure in a community hospital intensive care unit: a cohort study. Crit Care 2004; 8(5):R322–7.

57. Epstein SK, Ciubotaru RL, Wong JB. Effect of failed extubation on the outcome of mechanical ventilation. Chest 1997;112(1):186–92.

58. Demling RH, Read T, Lind LJ, Flanagan HL. Incidence and morbidity of extubation failure in surgical intensive care patients. Crit Care Med 1988;16(6):573–7.

59. Epstein SK. Extubation failure: an outcome to be avoided. Crit Care 2004;8(5): 310–2.

60. Frutos-Vivar F, Esteban A, Apezteguia C, et al. Outcome of reintubated patients after scheduled extubation. J Crit Care 2011;26(5):502–9.

61. Thille AW, Harrois A, Schortgen F, Brun-Buisson C, Brochard L. Outcomes of extubation failure in medical intensive care unit patients. Crit Care Med 2011;39(12): 2612–8.

62. Epstein SK. Decision to extubate. Intensive Care Med 2002;28(5):535–46.

63. Quintard H, l'Her E, Pottecher J, et al. Intubation and extubation of the ICU patient. Anaesth Crit Care Pain Med 2017;36(5):327–41.

64. Thille AW, Boissier F, Ben Ghezala H, Razazi K, Mekontso-Dessap A, Brun-Buisson C. Risk factors for and prediction by caregivers of extubation failure in ICU patients: a prospective study. Crit Care Med 2015;43(3):613–20.

65. Brack T, Jubran A, Tobin MJ. Dyspnea and decreased variability of breathing in patients with restrictive lung disease. Am J Respir Crit Care Med 2002;165(9): 1260–4.

66. Shen HN, Lin LY, Chen KY, et al. Changes of heart rate variability during ventilator weaning. Chest 2003;123(4):1222–8.

67. Wysocki M, Cracco C, Teixeira A, et al. Reduced breathing variability as a predictor of unsuccessful patient separation from mechanical ventilation.[see comment]. Crit Care Med 2006;34(8):2076–83.

68. Bien MY, Hseu SS, Yien HW, et al. Breathing pattern variability: a weaning predictor in postoperative patients recovering from systemic inflammatory response syndrome. Intensive Care Med 2004;30(2):241–7.
69. Orini M, Giraldo BF, Bailon R, et al. Time-frequency analysis of cardiac and respiratory parameters for the prediction of ventilator weaning. Conf Proc IEEE Eng Med Biol Soc 2008;2008:2793–6.
70. Engoren M, Blum JM. A comparison of the rapid shallow breathing index and complexity measures during spontaneous breathing trials after cardiac surgery. J Crit Care 2013;28(1):69–76.
71. Huang CT, Tsai YJ, Lin JW, Ruan SY, Wu HD, Yu CJ. Application of heart rate variability in patients undergoing weaning from mechanical ventilation. Crit Care 2014;18(1):R21.
72. Seely AJ, Bravi A, Herry C, et al. Do heart and respiratory rate variability improve prediction of extubation outcomes in critically ill patients? Crit Care 2014; 18(2):R65.
73. Ahmad S, Ramsay T, Huebsch L, et al. Continuous multi-parameter heart rate variability analysis heralds onset of sepsis in adults. PLoS One 2009;4(8):e6642.
74. Green GC, Bradley B, Bravi A, Seely AJ. Continuous multiorgan variability analysis to track severity of organ failure in critically ill patients. J Crit Care 2013; 28(5):e871–9.
75. Seely AJ, Macklem PT. Complex systems and the technology of variability analysis. Crit Care 2004;8(6):R367–84.
76. Tulaimat A, Mokhlesi B. Accuracy and reliability of extubation decisions by intensivists. Respir Care 2011;56(7):920–7.
77. Nitta K, Okamoto K, Imamura H, et al. A comprehensive protocol for ventilator weaning and extubation: a prospective observational study. J Intensive Care 2019;7:50.
78. Epstein SK, Ciubotaru RL. Independent effects of etiology of failure and time to reintubation on outcome for patients failing extubation. Am J Respir Crit Care Med 1997;158(2):489–93.
79. Vignon P. Cardiovascular failure and weaning. Ann Transl Med 2018;6(18):354.
80. Ghosh S, Chawla A, Mishra K, Jhalani R, Salhotra R, Singh A. Cumulative fluid balance and outcome of extubation: a prospective observational study from a general intensive care unit. Indian J Crit Care Med 2018;22(11):767–72.
81. Hernandez G, Vaquero C, Gonzalez P, et al. Effect of postextubation high-flow nasal cannula vs conventional oxygen therapy on reintubation in low-risk patients: a randomized clinical trial. JAMA 2016;315(13):1354–61.
82. Ferrer M, Valencia M, Nicolas JM, Bernadich O, Badia JR, Torres A. Early noninvasive ventilation averts extubation failure in patients at risk: a randomized trial. Am J Respir Crit Care Med 2006;173(2):164–70.
83. Nava S, Gregoretti C, Fanfulla F, et al. Noninvasive ventilation to prevent respiratory failure after extubation in high-risk patients. Crit Care Med 2005;33(11): 2465–70.
84. Rochwerg B, Granton D, Wang DX, Helviz Y, Einav S, Frat JP, Mekontso-Dessap A, Schreiber A, Azoulay E, Mercat A, Demoule A, Lemiale V, Pesenti A, Riviello ED, Mauri T, Mancebo J, Brochard L, Burns K. High flow nasal cannula compared with conventional oxygen therapy for acute hypoxemic respiratory failure: a systematic review and meta-analysis. Intensive Care Med 2019;45(5):563–72.
85. Ovtcharenko N, Ho E, Alhazzani W, Cortegiani A, Ergan B, Scala R, Sotgiu G, Chaudhuri D, Oczkowski S, Lewis K. High-flow nasal cannula versus non-

invasive ventilation for acute hypercapnic respiratory failure in adults: a systematic review and meta-analysis of randomized trials. Crit Care 2022;26(1):348.

86. Natalini D, Grieco DL, Santantonio MT, et al. Physiological effects of high-flow oxygen in tracheostomized patients. Ann Intensive Care 2019;9:114.

87. Esteban A, Frutos-Vivar F, Ferguson ND, Arabi Y, Apezteguía C, González M, Epstein SK, Hill NS, Nava S, Soares MA, D'Empaire G, Alía I, Anzueto A. Noninvasive positive-pressure ventilation for respiratory failure after extubation. N Engl J Med 2004;350(24):2452–60.

88. Maggiore SM, Idone FA, Vaschetto R, et al. Nasal high-fow versus Venturi mask oxygen therapy after extubation. Efects on oxygenation, comfort, and clinical outcome. Am J Respir Crit Care Med 2014;190(3):282–8.

89. Rittayamai N, Tscheikuna J, Rujiwit P. High-fow nasal cannula versus conventional oxygen therapy after endotracheal extubation: a randomized crossover physiologic study. Respir Care 2014;59(4):485–90.

90. Fernandez R, Subira C, Frutos-Vivar F, et al. High-fow nasal cannula to prevent postextubation respiratory failure in high-risk non-hypercap- nic patients: a randomized multicenter trial. Ann Intensive Care 2017;7(1):47.

91. Song HZ, Gu JX, Xiu HQ, Cui W, Zhang GS. The value of high-fow nasal cannula oxygen therapy after extubation in patients with acute respiratory failure. Clin (Sao Paulo) 2017;72(9):562–7.

92. Hernandez G, Vaquero C, Colinas L, et al. Efect of postextubation high-fow nasal cannula vs noninvasive ventilation on reintubation and postextubation respiratory failure in high-risk patients: a randomized clinical trial. JAMA 2016;316(15): 1565–74.

93. Theerawit PN, Sutherasan Y. The efcacy of the Whispherfow CPAP system versus high fow nasal cannula in patients at high risk for postex- tubation failure. Intensive Care Med Exp 2017;5:206.

94. Jing G, Li J, Hao D, et al. Comparison of high fow nasal cannula with noninvasive ventilation in chronic obstructive pulmonary disease patients with hypercapnia in preventing postextubation respiratory failure: a pilot randomized controlled trial. Res Nurs Health 2019;42(3):217–25.

Prolonged Mechanical Ventilation, Weaning, and the Role of Tracheostomy

Louise Rose, RN, PhD[a,b,*], Ben Messer, MBChB[c]

KEYWORDS

- Prolonged mechanical ventilation • Difficult weaning • Chronic critical illness
- Rehabilitation • Tracheostomy • Nutrition • Occupational therapy
- Psychological services

KEY POINTS

- Depending on the definitional criteria used, approximately 5% to 10% of critically adults will require PMV with longer-term outcomes that are worse than those ventilated for a shorter duration.
- Outcomes are affected by patient characteristics before critical illness and its severity but also by organizational characteristics and care models.
- Definitive trials of interventions to inform care activities, such as ventilator weaning, upper airway management, rehabilitation, and nutrition specific to the PMV patient population, are lacking.
- Given the heterogeneity in this patient population a structured and individualized approach developed by the multiprofessional team in discussion with the patient and their family is warranted.

INTRODUCTION

Given the aging population with increasing morbidity but also importantly scientific and technological advances that prolong the ability to support survival in intensive care, the number of patients that require prolonged mechanical ventilation (PMV) is rising. This has consequences to health care systems. In the United States, the cost of PMV patients are estimated to be $25 billion annually.[1] Furthermore, hospital and longer term mortality remain high for these patients with many patients unable to return home.[2,3] Patient burden is substantial because of an uncertain disease trajectory; numerous symptoms causing discomfort; and profound physical, neuropsychological,

---

[a] Florence Nightingale Faculty of Nursing, Midwifery and Palliative Care, King's College London, 57 Waterloo Road, London SE1 8WA, UK; [b] Department of Critical Care and Lane Fox Unit, Guy's & St Thomas' NHS Foundation Trust, King's College London, 57 Waterloo Road, London SE1 8WA, UK; [c] Royal Victoria Infirmary, Newcastle-Upon-Tyne NHS Hospitals NHS Foundation Trust, Queen Victoria Road, Newcastle upon Tyne NE1 4LP, UK
* Corresponding author. 57 Waterloo Road, London SE1 8WA, UK.
E-mail address: louise.rose@kcl.ac.uk

Crit Care Clin 40 (2024) 409–427
https://doi.org/10.1016/j.ccc.2024.01.008
0749-0704/24/© 2024 Elsevier Inc. All rights reserved.

criticalcare.theclinics.com

and cognitive deficits.[4,5] Patients requiring PMV require a change in clinical management with a greater focus on rehabilitation, symptom relief, and discharge planning.[6]

In this review we outline definitional considerations for PMV and difficult weaning in the setting of acute respiratory failure and patient prevalence, important factors to understanding the epidemiology of these patients. We then discuss the evidence around processes of care important to these patients including weaning methods, managing the upper airway (tracheostomy timing; cuff deflation and its role in weaning, as a communication adjunct, and for dysphagia management; secretion management), the role of physiotherapy in weaning (mobilization and rehabilitation, airway clearance, management of respiratory muscle dysfunction), the role of nutrition in weaning, the role of other therapies including occupational therapy and psychological services, and the role of specialized weaning centers (SWC).

DEFINITION OF PROLONGED MECHANICAL VENTILATION

The way PMV is defined in the current evidence base varies, which is problematic in terms of understanding the epidemiology and designing research to inform optimal care delivery. Commonly a definition of PMV includes mechanical ventilation (MV) duration. Yet the reported MV duration within this definition ranges from 5 hours in a surgical population to up to 1 year.[7] A consensus conference held more than 18 years ago by the US Association for Medical Direction of Respiratory Care defined PMV as greater than or equal to 21 consecutive days of MV for greater than or equal to 6 hours.[8] However, given the average duration of MV is between 4 to 5 days depending on case mix and region, MV greater than or equal to 7 days could be considered to represent a patient requiring PMV. The terms persistent or chronic critical illness may also be applied to this patient cohort given that most require PMV and tracheostomy.[1]

Frequently MV is prolonged because of failure to wean. Using the Joint Task Force on Weaning from Mechanical Ventilation definition,[9] prolonged weaning is the need for more than 7 days of weaning after the first spontaneous breathing trial (SBT). The WIND (Weaning according to a New Definition) classification[10] further extends this definition to weaning that is not achieved (either by successful separation or death) by 7 days after the first separation attempt.

PREVALENCE

The prevalence of PMV in any intensive care unit (ICU) patient cohort is dependent on the definition used, but generally ranges between 5% and 10%. For example, in the recently published WEANSAFE study enrolling 5869 patients from 481 ICUs in 50 countries, 433 (9.6%) of the 4523 patients that underwent at least one attempt to separate from the ventilator required prolonged weaning that is, greater than or equal to 7 days.[11] Previous population based studies report PMV prevalence as 5.4% (1594/11,594; Canada)[12] and 6.3% (349/5552; UK)[13] when defined as greater than or equal to 21 days of MV. In the United States, the prevalence of chronically critically ill patients defined as greater than or equal to 8 days in ICU plus one of five eligible conditions (MV for >96 hours, tracheostomy, sepsis, severe wounds, and multiple organ failure or neurologic injury) was 7.6% (246,151/3,235,741).[1] In Japan, using a similar definition, prevalence was 9.0% (216,434/2,395,016).[14]

FACTORS ASSOCIATED WITH DEVELOPING PROLONGED MECHANICAL VENTILATION

Numerous factors contributing to the development of a requirement for PMV have been investigated and factors associated with the longer-term mortality in this patient group. A recent single-center observational study of 195 patients found predictors of prolonged weaning were MV duration before SBTs were commenced, tracheostomy, Pao_2/FiO_2 ratio, and requirement for renal-replacement therapy.[15] A systematic review examining risk factors for PMV, weaning failure, and prolonged weaning identified 23 studies recruiting a total of 23,418 patients.[16] Of these, the 14 studies investigating risk factors for developing PMV had substantial heterogeneity in terms definitions for PMV and weaning failure as described previously. Risk factors for PMV included markers of severity of critical illness reflecting acute organ dysfunction, such as the SOFA score. Comorbid factors, such as age, body mass index (high and low), chronic obstructive pulmonary disease (COPD), neuromuscular disease, and previous requirement for home ventilation, were more predictive of weaning failure than markers of severity of acute illness.

Development of PMV may not just be caused by patient characteristics. Two studies from the United States suggest organizational factors may contribute to the development of PMV and subsequent risk-adjusted mortality. Using the Veteran Affairs database containing data from 100 US hospitals, Viglianti and colleagues[17] found higher number of patients developing PMV in hospitals with higher risk- and reliability-adjusted 30-day mortality rates. An ethnographic study of eight US long-term acute care hospitals (LTACH) found care delivery and organizational processes that actively promoted interdisciplinary communication and coordination differentiated high versus low performing hospitals in terms of risk-adjusted mortality.[18] Therefore care processes and structures are important to consider when optimizing the management of this patient group.

OUTCOMES

In a review of long-term survival of patients requiring PMV among cohort studies (124 studies representing 16 countries), pooled 1-year mortality was approximately 60%.[3] Furthermore, the proportion of patients able to return home after PMV was only 19%.[3] In a Canadian administrative database study identifying 11,594 patients who underwent PMV for more than 21 days, 1- and 5-year mortality was higher for PMV patients versus patients who required a shorter MV duration (17% vs 11% and 42% vs 30%, respectively).[12] A recent retrospective Taiwanese single-center study of 296 patients requiring PMV (>21 days) admitted to a weaning center demonstrated 1- and 5-year mortality of 80% and 89%, respectively. Five-year survival was associated with the absence of comorbidities, age younger than 75 years, and successful weaning.[19] Another recent retrospective study of 80 patients requiring PMV and undergoing tracheostomy found that hospital mortality or hospital discharge with a tracheostomy still in situ were associated with older age and higher body mass index.[20] Before this, a 2017 systematic review of patients receiving PMV for greater than 14 days identified 14 studies investigating 19 factors associated with 6-month mortality. As with variables associated with the need for PMV, those associated with 6-month mortality commonly reflected the severity of acute critical illness including thrombocytopenia, acute kidney injury, and vasopressor dependence with other risk factors being advanced age, preexisting kidney injury, and failure to wean.[21]

WEANING METHODS

There is limited empiric evidence for the optimal weaning method evaluated specifically for patients requiring PMV. An early multicenter randomized controlled trial (RCT) enrolling patients with COPD experiencing weaning difficulty compared tracheostomy mask trials with low-level pressure support ventilation (PSV) and found no difference in weaning duration or success.[22] A subsequent seminal RCT recruiting 316 patients from a single US LTACH demonstrated increased weaning success and a shorter weaning time using a once-daily tracheostomy mask trial, with progressive extension based on tolerance, compared with PSV.[23] Of note, 37% of the patients referred to the LTACH for weaning and screened for trial inclusion were excluded. This was because of successful weaning in the 5-day screening window during which unassisted breathing with humidified oxygen was delivered through a tracheostomy collar. This finding emphasizes the need for a daily focused assessment of weaning and extubation readiness, whichever weaning method is used.

More recently Wu and colleagues[24] report a retrospective cohort study of 403 patients receiving MV greater than 21 days admitted to an SWC in Taiwan. Because of concerns around virus transmission during the COVID-19 pandemic, this SWC switched from a 5-day weaning screen comprising unassisted breathing as used in the previously mentioned trial to the use of 5 days of automatic tube compensation. Automatic tube compensation is designed to compensate for tube-related additional work of breathing. It uses closed loop monitoring of the nonlinear flow-dependent pressure drop during inspiration and expiration.[25] When comparing outcomes of patients who received an automatic tube compensation 5-day screen compared with the former usual screening method, those screened using automatic tube compensation had better predictive ability for weaning success and in-hospital survival.[24]

Neurally adjusted ventilatory assist delivers inspiratory pressures proportional to diaphragm electrical activity detected via a specialized nasogastric feeding catheter (Getinge, Solna, Sweden).[26] Three RCTs that compared neurally adjusted ventilatory assist with PSV in patients at risk of PMV demonstrate reduced dyssynchrony[27] and MV duration.[28,29] Therefore neurally adjusted ventilatory assist may have a role in preventing PMV or shortening its overall duration; however, further trials are needed.

Although not specifically recruiting a PMV patient population there is evidence to suggest noninvasive ventilatory strategies following extubation may reduce the risk of developing PMV. In a multicenter RCT of 641 patients conducted by Thille and colleagues[30] a combination of high-flow nasal oxygen alternating with noninvasive ventilation was found to decrease reintubation rates compared with high-flow nasal oxygen alone in patients at high risk for extubation failure (ie, >65 years or any underlying chronic cardiac or lung disease).

A recent systematic review[31] of 28 trials (2066 participants) compared early extubation with noninvasive ventilation for patients who failed or were not ready for an SBT with ongoing invasive ventilation. This review found early extubation to noninvasive ventilation improved in mortality, ventilator-associated pneumonia (VAP) incidence, hospital and ICU length of stay, and MV duration. Improved outcomes were particularly seen for patients with COPD who accounted for almost half of the trial participants.

Despite evidence of effectiveness in patients with an overall shorter MV duration,[32] to-date there are no studies of weaning protocols specific to PMV patients. Furthermore, current guidelines for weaning and ventilator liberation provide little guidance on the management of this patient population.[33,34] However, PMV patients are most likely to benefit from a structured approach to weaning incorporating trials of unsupported weaning with adequate support during periods of ventilation, and consideration of strategies to manage the upper airway that are discussed next.[8,23] Furthermore an individualized weaning plan should be developed by the interprofessional team in discussion with the patient and their family, with regular review and update as required.[35]

MANAGING THE UPPER AIRWAY
Tracheostomy Timing

Tracheostomy insertion is frequently undertaken in intensive care with the main advantages being enabling the ability to vocalize, allowing oral intake, improving comfort[36] with reduced sedation, and improving oral hygiene.[37] TracMan was the largest RCT published to-date investigating early versus late tracheostomy, recruiting 909 patients from 72 hospital in the United Kingdom.[38] This trial did not demonstrate a mortality advantage of early (within 4 days) compared with late (after 10 days) tracheostomy at any measurement time point (30 days up to 2 years). Of note, more than half of the patients randomized to late tracheostomy did not require a tracheostomy, primarily because of discharge from intensive care or no longer requiring MV.[38]

Three recent systematic reviews[39–41] support the lack of effect on mortality finding of the TracMan trial. However, the effect on other patient outcomes of early tracheostomy (defined as insertion within 10 days after intubation) compared with prolonged intubation is less certain. Chorath and colleagues[40] conducted a systematic review including 17 trials recruiting 3145 participants. Early tracheostomy was defined as no more than 7 days after MV initiation and late as placement after 7 days or no tracheostomy. Their meta-analyses identified a reduction in VAP, and ICU length of stay with more ventilator-free days with early tracheostomy. Similarly Deng and colleagues[39] reported a shorter ICU length of stay and reduced MV duration but no effect on VAP rates (15 trials, 3003 participants with early tracheostomy defined using the original study definition). The most recent systematic review by Villemure-Poliquin and colleagues[41] defining early tracheostomy as within 10 days of intubation (9 trials, 2457 patients) found no differences in ICU length of stay, MV duration, or VAP rates. Despite also identifying no mortality difference, these authors cautioned that their analyses were likely underpowered with only moderate certainty evidence. Conversely, a fourth review (19 trials, 3508 patients)[42] using a Bayesian analysis suggests early tracheostomy demonstrates benefit on all clinical outcomes including mortality. Importantly, the RCTs included in all meta-analyses that we describe excluded patients with neurologic disease who have a different prognosis and different reasons for tracheostomy (ie, airway protection) compared with other patient groups requiring PMV.

Although the evidence surrounding the effect of early tracheostomy on the previously mentioned outcomes remains somewhat uncertain, tracheostomy is a commonly undertaken procedure and appropriate tracheostomy management has important implications for weaning from PMV. Earlier tracheostomy benefits other patient-centric outcomes, such as participation in activities important to rehabilitation at an earlier timepoint. These include talking, out-of-bed mobility, and eating/drinking.[43] These benefits are caused by important features of tracheostomy management that include cuff deflation and the use of a one-way speaking valve (**Fig. 1**). However, the decision to perform earlier tracheostomy needs to be carefully considered on an individual basis to avoid the possibility of an unnecessary tracheostomy in some cases.

Tracheostomy Cuff Deflation and Its Role in Weaning

Tracheostomy cuff deflation and tracheostomy downsizing facilitates an increased airway diameter leading to reduced airway resistance and work of breathing. This can improve airflows and end-expiratory lung volume.[44] Use of a one-way speaking valve in conjunction with cuff deflation also improves lung recruitment during weaning.[45,46] Cuff deflation may reduce complications associated with prolonged use of an endotracheal tube and improve patient outcomes including reducing weaning and MV duration, although the evidence base is limited.[47] One RCT recruiting 195

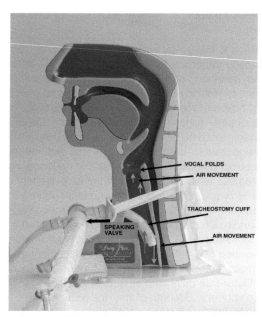

Fig. 1. Passy Muir one-way speaking valve. (Image courtesy of Passy Muir, Inc. Irvine, CA.)

patients using tracheostomy cuff deflation during T-piece SBTs reported a reduced weaning duration with fewer respiratory infections and improved swallow compared with T-piece SBTs with an inflated cuff.[48]

Few studies report predictors of successful cuff deflation to guide patient selection criteria; however, one retrospective cohort found 95% of patients tolerated cuff deflation on the first attempt.[49] Medical and respiratory stability and above-cuff secretions of less than 1 mL/h are predictive of success. There are no published evidenced-based protocols or guidelines on how best to perform early cuff deflation and establish use of a one-way speaking valve, although specialized services use locally developed protocols and decision tools.[50]

Cuff Deflation as a Communication Adjunct

Early cuff deflation helps to promote vocalization alleviating patient distress and frustration associated with inability to communicate.[51] ICU survivors frequently identify the inability to communicate using speech because of an advanced airway as one of the most negative experiences of an ICU admission.[52] Cuff deflation, combined with a one-way speaking valve, directs expiratory gas flow through the vocal cords to restore phonation. Importantly, it is used safely during invasive MV, thereby restoring phonation more quickly compared with use only when a patient is self-ventilating.[53] If cuff deflation and use of a speaking valve is not feasible (eg, in the presence of excessive oral secretions[54]) as assessed by a speech and language therapist, other communication options that include above-cuff vocalization can be explored.[55]

Cuff Deflation for Dysphagia Management

Dysphagia is highly prevalent in the critically ill and associated with PMV and tracheostomy.[56] Indeed, the incidence of swallowing dysfunction in patients requiring PMV and receiving a tracheostomy is estimated at 40%.[57] Breathing and swallowing are interdependent processes with shared anatomy and neurophysiologic regulation.[58] Early tracheostomy cuff deflation and use of a one-way speaking valve may reduce the frequency of aspiration events during swallowing.[59]

Secretion Management

Excessive oral secretions are the result of dysphagia or sialorrhea, common in patients with neurologic disease and brain injury.[60] Excess oral secretions/saliva is associated with adverse outcomes including aspiration pneumonia and delayed weaning.[61] Secretions may be managed via upright positioning; oral suctioning; and subglottic suctioning and pharmacotherapy, such as sublingual atropine, glycopyrronium, hyoscine, and intrasalivary gland botulinum toxin injections.[54] Few studies describe management of sialorrhea in patients requiring PMV. Evidence is limited to cohort studies in other settings, such as home and long-term ventilation centers.[62]

Other reasons for excessive secretions common to patients requiring PMV include bronchorrhea, VAP, and ventilator-associated tracheobronchitis. Potential pharmacotherapies include mucolytics, prophylactic antibiotics, and nebulized antibiotics. However, a systematic review of 13 RCTs recruiting 1712 patients investigating mucolytics including N-acetylcysteine, nebulized heparin, and nebulized hypertonic saline found no effect on mortality, MV duration, ventilator-free days, or duration of hospital stay, but a reduction in ICU length of stay (very low evidence certainty).[63] As a prophylactic antibiotic with anti-inflammatory properties, azithromycin may also have a role in the management of bronchorrhea. It has been investigated extensively in patients with COPD, with one RCT recruiting 1142 patients demonstrating a 27% reduction in exacerbation frequency.[64] However, as yet, no studies have investigated its use for managing bronchorrhea in patients requiring PMV. A meta-analysis of azithromycin use in an outpatient setting demonstrated an increase in macrolide resistance. However, it is unclear whether this has an adverse effect on any clinical outcomes particularly when used for short time periods, such as during weaning.[65]

Prophylactic nebulized colistin has been investigated as a potential intervention for VAP prevention. One RCT recruiting 168 patients compared nebulized colistin of 0.5 million units three times daily with nebulized normal saline but did not show a reduction in VAP incidence.[66] However, further definitive RCTs are required. Nebulized antibiotics have also been investigated for VAP. A systematic review with a Bayesian meta-analysis demonstrated that nebulized tobramycin and colistin were associated with high rates of recovery and also microbiologic eradication.[67]

PHYSIOTHERAPY AND ITS ROLE IN WEANING
Mobilization and Rehabilitation

Loss of muscle mass and muscle function occurs early in critical illness with resultant loss of functional capacity in patients requiring PMV.[68] ICU-acquired muscle weakness is highly prevalent, with maintenance of bed rest an important contributor.[69] Mobilization, incorporating functional training and exercise, promotes recovery through improved muscle strength. It also reduces limitations to movements that are required to perform functional activities of daily living important for returning home.[70] It may also reduce the overall duration of MV.[71] Professional society endorsed practice guidelines advocate for mobilization commencing 24 hours after ICU admission, if safe to do so.[33,71,72] In most cases, mobilization would be safe well before the patient meets criteria for PMV. RCTs informing these guidelines advocate for an interprofessional team approach to mobilization and a protocolized, standardized, or structured approach.[72]

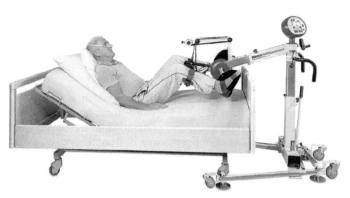

Fig. 2. Cycle ergometer (With permission from Reck-Technik, Gmbh & Co. Kg, Betzenweiler, Germany.)

Other interventions that may reduce loss of muscle mass and improve muscle strength are neuromuscular electrical stimulation and cycle ergometry (**Fig. 2**). Neuromuscular electrical stimulation involves application of local surface electrodes to deliver an electrical impulse that generates muscle contraction.[73,74] One RCT of neuromuscular electrical stimulation used in conjunction with an early mobilization protocol recruiting 74 patients with a median MV duration of 12 days demonstrated improved short-term functional outcomes as compared with the early mobilization protocol alone.[30] Cycle ergometry enables mobilization of the upper and lower extremities that can be individualized to a patient's needs and has been shown to be feasible and safe to deliver in the ICU setting.[75]

As with ventilator weaning, few trials of rehabilitation interventions focus specifically on the PMV patient population. A small number of observation studies[76–79] demonstrate improvements in functional outcomes when examining the effect of various rehabilitation interventions in patients ventilated for greater than 21 days. One German cohort[80] described 150 patients who received an intensive rehabilitation intervention comprising physiotherapy and occupational therapy (?60 minutes each, five times per week) based on individualized goal-driven treatment plans with better mobilization outcomes in those patients spending longer periods practicing walking. Verceles and colleagues[81] conducted a 33-participant RCT that evaluated a progressive and patient-specific multimodal rehabilitation program combining muscular strength and endurance training with functional retraining compared with usual rehabilitation practice. They reported greater weaning success and discharge to home in those patients receiving this multimodal approach.

More recently, an RCT recruiting PMV patients (inclusion criterion of >72 hours of ventilation with mean intubation duration of >8 days) found improved diaphragmatic function and reduced MV duration with a progressive six-stage rehabilitative exercise program compared with usual care.[82] Therefore as with optimal strategies for weaning patients requiring PMV, a strategy that mostly likely is of benefit is an individualized and structured approach with a rehabilitation plan developed by the interprofessional team in collaboration with the patient and their family members as appropriate.

Airway Clearance

Patients requiring PMV often experience airway secretion retention because of ineffective cough, reduced mucociliary transport, and respiratory muscle weakness.[83] Retained secretions can lead to atelectasis, VAP, and can prolong weaning. Airway clearance techniques include manually assisted cough, lung volume recruitment maneuvers, and mechanically assisted cough using a mechanical insufflation-exsufflation device. Manually assisted cough consists of a cough that is timed with an abdominal or lateral costal compression. Mechanical insufflation-exsufflation uses a positive insufflation pressure to expand the lungs to approximately 90% of capacity[84] rapidly alternated with a negative exsufflation pressure. This rapid alternation between positive and negative pressures promotes air flow rates, improves sputum mobilization, and stimulates a cough.[85] Mechanical insufflation-exsufflation is used as a noninvasive technique using a mask or is delivered via an endotracheal or tracheostomy tube as an adjunct to ventilator weaning. Although limited, the evidence in the critically ill patient population suggests these techniques are safe with few adverse events.[86,87] Further studies are required to ascertain their effect when used to promote ventilator weaning in patients requiring PMV.

Treatment of Respiratory Muscle Dysfunction

Respiratory muscle weakness is a consequence of PMV. Rapid atrophy of the diaphragm and other respiratory muscles results in an imbalance between the respiratory load and reduced muscle capacity.[88] Strategies that promote spontaneous breathing

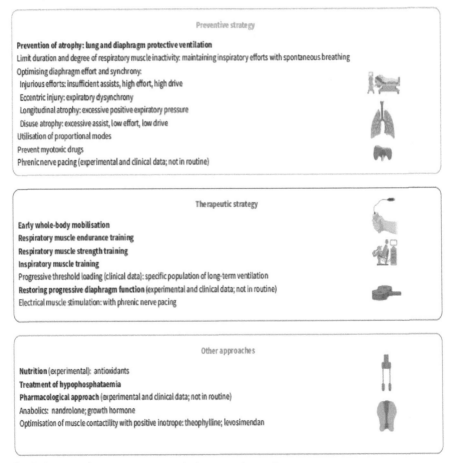

Fig. 3. Intervention to manage respiratory muscle weakness.

early in patients with PMV are key to preserving respiratory muscle activity.[89] Such strategies are seen as preventative or therapeutic (**Fig. 3**).

Inspiratory muscle training is designed to improve strength and endurance of the diaphragm and accessory inspiratory muscles through the application of resistance during inspiration. Inspiratory muscle training includes either strength or endurance training using resistive and threshold loading. Resistive loading involves placement of a resistor that increases the pressure for respiratory muscles to generate a given flow. Threshold loading uses a valve that requires a certain pressure to be generated by the respiratory muscles before it opens to allowing inspiratory flow. Threshold loading is not dependent on patient effort and therefore more commonly used in ventilated patients.[90] A 2018 systematic review and meta-analysis identified a total of 28 studies of inspiratory muscle training with 14 conducted in difficult-to-wean patients. Although subgroup analyses were not performed on these 14 studies, overall improvements in maximal inspiratory pressure and maximal expiratory pressure were found with an uncertain effect on patient outcomes, such as MV and weaning duration.[91]

NUTRITION AND ITS ROLE IN WEANING

Although multifactorial, catabolism is a contributing mechanism of respiratory and other muscle weakness and therefore associated with PMV and weaning failure.[89,92] Patients can lose up to 30% of their quadriceps skeletal muscle mass within 10 days of MV.[68] Malnutrition and insufficient food intake are common, and have been associated with worse patient outcomes.[93] International clinical nutrition guidelines define phases of metabolism as (1) acute-early (days 1–2), (2) acute-late (days 3–7), and (3) recovery (>7) days.[94] In the acute phases, metabolism is catabolic and in the adaptive stress state. At this time nutrient metabolism is likely to be impaired.[93] In the later phases, which coincides with the definition of PMV, metabolism switches to anabolism and is likely a more appropriate time for nutritional interventions used in combination with rehabilitation activities.

Recommendations for feeding in guidelines for the provision of nutrition support therapy in the critically ill,[94,95] although not specific to PMV patients, are shown in **Box 1**. Importantly, although early feeding is recommended, harm is likely to be associated with feeding to full estimated energy expenditure.[96] PMV are likely to benefit most from an individualized and personalized approach to nutrition.[97,98]

OTHER THERAPIES AND THEIR ROLE IN WEANING
Occupational Therapy

Occupational therapy includes assessments and provision of interventions to treat physical, cognitive, emotional, or psychological domains targeting impairments, activity limitations, and participation restrictions (**Fig. 4**).[99] Given the loss of functional and

---

Box 1
Guidance for feeding patients requiring PMV

- Target feed between 12 and 25 kcal/kg in the first 7 to 10 days of the ICU stay
- Target protein intake of 1.2 to 2.0 g/kg/day
- Commence feeding early with either enteral or if not feasible with parenteral nutrition
- Do not start supplemental parenteral nutrition before Day 7 of ICU admission
- Use either mixed-oil or 100% soybean oil intravenous lipid emulsions or fish-oil or non–fish oil intravenous lipid emulsions for patients requiring parenteral nutrition

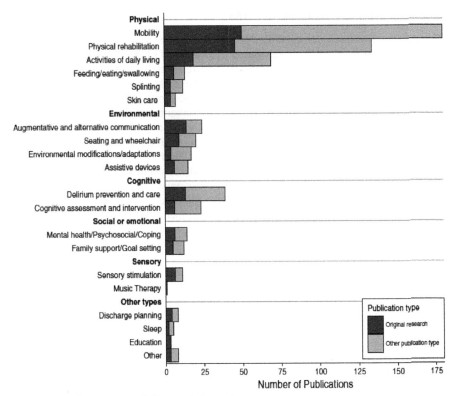

Fig. 4. Role of occupational therapy in intensive care.

cognitive capacity resulting in inability to perform activities of daily living common to patients requiring PMV, occupational therapy can assist with helping to achieve rehabilitation and basic self-care goals.[100] Furthermore, occupational therapists can provide cognitive interventions that prevent delirium, again highly prevalent in PMV patients, and to improve attention and concentration, memory, executive functioning, processing speed, and language skills.[101] As such, occupational therapists are important members of the ICU interprofessional team contributing to the planning and delivery of a range of rehabilitative interventions. However, the inclusion of occupational therapists in the ICU team is highly variable within and across regions internationally.[100,102,103]

Psychology Services

Patients experiencing PMV and difficulty weaning experience several psychological symptoms that warrant psychology input. Fear and anxiety are commonly reported and may be exacerbated with repeated failure of weaning attempts or SBTs.[104] Anxiety may be compounded into panic-like symptoms caused by increased sympathetic arousal and accompanying dyspnea, ultimately resulting in SBT failure.[105] Agitation is also common and may contribute to the need for PMV and to weaning failure.[106] Cognitive behavioral therapy for acute stress may be a useful tool for managing profound anxiety and agitation in difficult-to-wean patients.[105] Dexmedetomidine, a central α_2-receptor agonist, may have a role in promoting weaning success in PMV patients experiencing delirium, agitation, or anxiety.[107,108] Undiagnosed depression or delirium may be other reasons for lack of engagement in rehabilitation interventions that promote weaning, which may benefit from input from psychological services.[109]

ROLE OF SPECIALIZED WEANING CENTERS

Care location has been demonstrated to improve outcomes for several patient populations. Improvement in outcomes related to location of care has been demonstrated in coronary care units,[110] stroke units,[111] and respiratory support units for COPD exacerbation.[112] Volume-outcome relationships have also been demonstrated in major trauma systems,[113] critical care,[114] and surgical specialties.[115] Therefore care located within an SWC also may be important for patients with PMV experiencing difficult weaning. In the United States, an SWC may be colocated in an LTACH. In the systematic review we refer to earlier reporting outcomes of patients requiring PMV from 16 countries, 12-month mortality of patients admitted to a SWCs was better than those remaining in an ICU (48% vs 59%).[3] Mortality outcomes were worse in US hospitals compared with other countries (12-month mortality, 73% vs 47%). Outcomes in UK SWUs compare favorably with the international data presented previously. A single-center cohort study published in 2017 recruiting 458 patients demonstrated hospital and 12-month mortality of 9% and 35%, respectively, with 82% returning home, which is substantially higher than the aforementioned 19% reported in a systematic review of cohort studies.[116]

In the United Kingdom, professional society–endorsed guidance has been recently published to guide the SWU development and care models.[117] This guidance discusses governance structures, patient pathways, service models, and the multiprofessional staffing required to deliver high-quality care to patients requiring PMV. Importantly, there is the recommendation that SWUs be colocated with complex long-term ventilation centers because in the United Kingdom up to 60% of patients are discharged on long-term ventilation (either invasive or noninvasive).[116]

SUMMARY

Depending on the definitional criteria used, approximately 5% to 10% of critically adults will require PMV with longer-term outcomes that are worse than those ventilated for a shorter duration. Outcomes are affected by patient characteristics before critical illness and its severity but also by organizational characteristics and care models. Definitive trials of interventions to inform care activities, such as ventilator weaning, upper airway management, rehabilitation, and nutrition specific to the PMV patient population, are lacking. However, given the heterogeneity in this patient population a structured and individualized approach developed by the interprofessional team in discussion with the patient and their family is warranted.

CLINICS CARE POINTS

- A standardized yet individualized approach is required for weaning for PMV patients comprising progressive lengthening of tracheostomy collar trials with adequate ventilatory support developed by the interprofessional team with the patient and family members involved.

- Management of the upper airway involves consideration of tracheostomy timing and early cuff deflation to promote weaning, enable vocalization, and restore oral intake.

- Interventions focused on rehabilitation, mobilization, and nutrition are important to the recovery of patients requiring PMV.

- Speech language therapists, physiotherapists, dieticians, occupational therapists, psychologists, and pharmacists have important roles in the recovery of this patient group.

DISCLOSURE

The authors have no potential conflicts of interest to declare relevant to this publication.

REFERENCES

1. Kahn J, Le T, Angus D, et al. The epidemiology of chronic critical illness in the United States. Crit Care Med 2015;43:282–7.
2. Kahn J, Davis B, Le T, et al. Variation in mortality rates after admission to long-term acute care hospitals for ventilator weaning. J Crit Care 2018;46:6–12.
3. Damuth E, Mitchell J, Bartock J, et al. Long-term survival of critically ill patients treated with prolonged mechanical ventilation: a systematic review and meta-analysis. Lancet Respir Med 2015;3:544–53.
4. Carson S, Kahn J, Hough C, et al. A multicenter mortality prediction model for patients receiving prolonged mechanical ventilation. Crit Care Med 2012;40: 1171–6.
5. Maguire J, Carson S. Strategies to combat chronic critical illness. Curr Opin Crit Care 2013;19:480–7.
6. Rose L, Fowler R, Goldstein R, et al. Patient transitions relevant to individuals requiring ongoing ventilatory assistance: a Delphi study. Can Respir J 2014; 21:287–92.
7. Rose L, McGinlay M, Amin R, et al. Variation in definition of prolonged mechanical ventilation: a scoping review. J Crit Care 2017;62:1324–32.
8. MacIntyre NR, Epstein SK, Carson S, et al, National Association for Medical Direction of Respiratory Care. Management of patients requiring prolonged mechanical ventilation: report of a NAMDRC consensus conference. Chest 2005; 128:3937–54.
9. Boles J-M, Bion J, Connors A, et al. Weaning from mechanical ventilation. Eur Respir J 2007;29:1033–56.
10. Béduneau G, Pham T, Schortgen F, et al. Epidemiology of weaning outcome according to a new definition. The WIND Study. Am J Respir Crit Care Med 2017; 195:772–83.
11. Pham T, Heunks L, Bellani G, et al. Weaning from mechanical ventilation in intensive care units across 50 countries (WEAN SAFE): a multicentre, prospective, observational cohort study. Lancet Respir Med 2023;11:465–76.
12. Hill A, Fowler R, Burns K, et al. Long-term outcomes and health care utilization after prolonged mechanical ventilation. Ann Am Thorac Soc 2017;14:355–62.
13. Lone N, Walsh T. Prolonged mechanical ventilation in critically ill patients: epidemiology, outcomes and modelling the potential cost consequences of establishing a regional weaning unit. Crit Care 2011;15:R102.
14. Ohbe H, Matsui H, Fushimi K, et al. Epidemiology of chronic critical illness in Japan: a nationwide inpatient database study. Crit Care Med 2021;49:70–8.
15. Na S, Ko R, Nam J, et al. Factors associated with prolonged weaning from mechanical ventilation in medical patients. Ther Adv Respir Dis 2022;16. 1753466 6221117005.
16. Trudzinski F, Neetz B, Bornitz F, et al. Risk factors for prolonged mechanical ventilation and weaning failure: a systematic review. Respiration 2022;101:959–69.
17. Viglianti E, Bagshaw S, Bellomo R, et al. Hospital-level variation in the development of persistent critical illness. Intensive Care Med 2020;46:1567–75.

18. Rak K, Ashcraft L, Kuza C, et al. Effective care practices in patients receiving prolonged mechanical ventilation. an ethnographic study. Am J Respir Crit Care Med 2020;201:823–31.

19. Huang C. Five years follow up of patient receiving prolonged mechanical ventilation: data for a single center in Taiwan. Front Med 2022;9:1038915.

20. Cabrio D, Vesin T, Lupieri E, et al. Early prediction of hospital outcomes in patients tracheostomized for complex mechanical ventilation weaning. Ann Intensive Care 2022;12:73.

21. Dettmer M, Damuth E, Zarbiv S, et al. Prognostic factors for long-term mortality in critically ill patients treated with prolonged mechanical ventilation: a systematic review. Crit Care Med 2017;45:69–74.

22. Vitacca M, Vianello A, Colombo D, et al. Comparison of two methods for weaning patients with chronic obstructive pulmonary disease requiring mechanical ventilation for more than 15 days. Am J Respir Crit Care Med 2001;164:225–30.

23. Jubran A, Grant B, Duffner L, et al. Effect of pressure support vs unassisted breathing through a tracheostomy collar on weaning duration in patients requiring prolonged mechanical ventilation: a randomized trial. JAMA 2013; 309:671–7.

24. Wu C, Lin F, Jerng J, et al. Automatic tube compensation for liberation from prolonged mechanical ventilation in tracheostomized patients: a retrospective analysis. J Formos Med Assoc 2023;S0929-6646(23):00146–8.

25. Guttmann J, Haberthür C, Mols G, et al. Automatic tube compensation (ATC). Minerva Anestesiol 2002;68:369–77.

26. Sinderby C, Navalesi P, Beck J, et al. Neural control of mechanical ventilation in respiratory f ailure. Nat Med 1999;5:1433–6.

27. Kuo NY, Tu ML, Hung TY, et al. A randomized clinical trial of neurally adjusted ventilatory assist versus conventional weaning mode in patients with COPD and prolonged mechanical ventilation. Int J COPD 2016;11:945–51.

28. Hadfield DJ, Rose L, Reid F, et al. Neurally adjusted ventilatory assist versus pressure support ventilation: a randomized controlled feasibility trial performed in patients at risk of prolonged mechanical ventilation. Crit Care 2020;24:220.

29. Liu L, Xu X, Sun Q, et al. Neurally adjusted ventilatory assist versus pressure support ventilation in difficult weaning. Anesthesiol 2020;132:1482–93.

30. Thille A, Muller G, Gacouin A, et al. Effect of postextubation high-flow nasal oxygen with noninvasive ventilation vs high-flow nasal oxygen alone on reintubation among patients at high risk of extubation failure: a randomized clinical trial. JAMA 2019;322:1465–75.

31. Burns K, Stevenson J, Laird M, et al. Non-invasive ventilation versus invasive weaning in critically ill adults: a systematic review and meta-analysis. Thorax 2022;77:752–61.

32. Blackwood B, Burns K, Cardwell C, et al. Protocolized versus non-protocolized weaning for reducing the duration of mechanical ventilation in critically ill adult patients. Cochrane Database Syst Rev 2014;11:CD006904.

33. Girard T, Alhazzani W, Kress J, et al. An official American Thoracic Society/American College of Chest Physicians clinical practice guideline: liberation from mechanical ventilation in critically ill adults. Rehabilitation protocols, ventilator liberation protocols, and cuff leak tests. Am J Respir Crit Care Med 2017; 195:120–33.

34. Ouellette D, Patel S, Girard T, et al. Liberation from mechanical ventilation in critically ill adults: an official American College of Chest Physicians/American Thoracic Society clinical practice guideline: inspiratory pressure augmentation

during spontaneous breathing trials, protocols minimizing sedation, and noninvasive ventilation immediately after extubation. Chest 2017;151:166–80.

35. Rose L, Istanboulian L, Amaral A, et al. Co-designed and consensus based development of a quality improvement checklist of patient and family-centered actionable processes of care for adults with persistent critical illness. J Crit Care 2022;72:154153.

36. Blot F, Similowski T, Trouillet J, et al. Early tracheotomy versus prolonged endotracheal intubation in unselected severely ill ICU patients. Intensive Care Med 2008;34:1779–87.

37. Mussa C, Gomaa D, Rowley D, et al. AARC clinical practice guideline: management of adult patients with tracheostomy in the acute care setting. Respir Care 2021;66:156–69.

38. Young D, Harrison D, Cuthbertson B, et al, TracMan Collaborators. Effect of early vs late tracheostomy placement on survival in patients receiving mechanical ventilation: the TracMan randomized trial. JAMA 2013;309:2121–9.

39. Deng H, Fang Q, Chen K, et al. Early versus late tracheotomy in ICU patients: a meta-analysis of randomized controlled trials. Medicine 2021;100:e24329.

40. Chorath K, Hoang A, Rajasekaran K, et al. Association of early vs late tracheostomy placement with pneumonia and ventilator days in critically ill patients: a meta-analysis. JAMA Otolaryngol Head Neck Surg 2021;147:450–9.

41. Villemure-Poliquin N, Lessard Bonaventure P, Costerousse O, et al. Impact of early tracheostomy versus late or no tracheostomy in nonneurologically injured adult patients: a systematic review and meta-analysis. Crit Care Med 2023;51:310–8.

42. Quinn L, Veenith T, Bion J, et al. Bayesian analysis of a systematic review of early versus late tracheostomy in ICU patients. Br J Anaesth 2022;129:693–702.

43. Sutt A, Tronstad O, Barnett A, et al. Earlier tracheostomy is associated with an earlier return to walking, talking, and eating. Aust Crit Care 2020;33:213–8.

44. Hernandez G, Ortiz R, Pedrosa A, et al. The indication for tracheostomy is the main determinant in predicting timing for tracheostomy decannulation. Med Intensiva 2012;36:531–9.

45. Sutt A, Caruana L, Dunster K, et al. Speaking valves in tracheostomised ICU patients weaning off mechanical ventilation: do they facilitate lung recruitment? Crit Care 2016;20:91.

46. Sutt A, Anstey C, Caruana L, et al. Ventilation distribution and lung recruitment with speaking valve use in tracheostomised patient weaning from mechanical ventilation in intensive care. J Crit Care 2017;164–70.

47. Whitmore K, Townsend S, Laupland K. Management of tracheostomies in the intensive care unit: a scoping review. BMJ Open Respir Res 2020;7:e000651.

48. Hernandez G, Pedrosa A, Ortiz R, et al. The effects of increasing effective airway diameter on weaning from mechanical ventilation in tracheostomized patients: a randomized controlled trial. Intensive Care Med 2013;39:1063–70.

49. Pryor L, Ward E, Cornwell P, et al. Clinical indicators associated with successful tracheostomy cuff deflation. Aust Crit Care 2016;29:132–7.

50. McGowan S, Potter L, Carmichael A, et al. A decision making tool and protocol for early cuff deflation and one way valve inline for patients who are ventilated with a tracheostomy: a case series report. J Intensive Care Soc 2022;23:169–71.

51. Brodsky M, Levy M, Jedlanek E, et al. Laryngeal injury and upper airway symptoms after oral endotracheal intubation with mechanical ventilation during critical care: a systematic review. Crit Care Med 2018;46:2010–7.

52. Istanboulian L, Rose L, Gorospe F, et al. Barriers to and facilitators for the use of augmentative and alternative communication and voice restorative strategies for adults with an advanced airway in the intensive care unit: a scoping review. J Crit Care 2020;57:168–76.

53. Freeman-Sanderson A, Togher L, Elkins M, et al. Return of voice for ventilated tracheostomy patients in ICU: a randomized controlled trial of early-targeted intervention. Crit Care Med 2016;44:1075–81.

54. Wallace S, McGrath B. Laryngeal complications after tracheal intubation and tracheostomy. BJA Educ 2021;21:250–7.

55. Wallace S, McGowan S, Sutt A. Benefits and options for voice restoration in mechanically ventilated intensive care unit patients with a tracheostomy. J Intensive Care Soc 2023;24:104–11.

56. Zuercher P, Moret C, Dziewas R, et al. Dysphagia in the intensive care unit: epidemiology, mechanisms, and clinical management. Crit Care 2019;23: 103–13.

57. Romero C, Marambio A, Larrondo J, et al. Swallowing dysfunction in nonneurologic critically ill patients who require percutaneous dilatational tracheostomy. Chest 2010;137:1278–82.

58. Jafari S, Prince R, Kim D, et al. Sensory regulation of swallowing and airway protection: a role for the internal superior laryngeal nerve in humans. J Physiol 2003; 550:287–304.

59. Skoretz S, Anger N, Wellman L, et al. A systematic review of tracheostomy modifications and swallowing in adults. Dysphagia 2020;35:935–47.

60. Morgante F, Bavikatte G, Anwar F, et al. The burden of sialorrhoea in chronic neurological conditions: current treatment options and the role of incobotulinumtoxinA (Xeomin®). Ther Adv Neurol Disord 2019;12. 1756286419888601.

61. Kang Y, Chun M, Lee S. Evaluation of salivary aspiration in brain-injured patients with tracheostomy. Ann Rehabil Med 2013;37:96–102.

62. Harbottle J, Carlin H, Payne-Doris T, et al. Eveloping an intrasalivary gland botox service for patients receiving long-term non-invasive ventilation at home: a single-centre experience. BMJ Open Resp Res 2022;9:e001188.

63. Anand R, McAuley D, Blackwood B, et al. Mucoactive agents for acute respiratory failure in the critically ill: a systematic review and meta-analysis. Thorax 2020;75:623–31.

64. Albert R, Connett J, Bailey W, et al. Azithromycin for prevention of exacerbations of COPD. N Engl J Med 2011;365:689–98.

65. Li H, Liu D, Chen L, et al. Meta-analysis of the adverse effects of long-term azithromycin use in patients with chronic lung diseases. Antimicrob Agents Chemother 2014;58:511–7.

66. Karvouniaris M, Makris D, Zygoulis P, et al. Nebulised colistin for ventilator-associated pneumonia prevention. Eur Respir J 2015;46:1732–9.

67. Xu F, He L, Che L, et al. Aerosolized antibiotics for ventilator-associated pneumonia: a pairwise and Bayesian network meta-analysis. Crit Care 2018;22:301.

68. Puthucheary Z, Rawal J, McPhail M, et al. Acute skeletal muscle wasting in critical illness. JAMA 2013;319:1591–600.

69. Herridge M, Azoulay É. Outcomes after critical illness. N Engl J Med 2023;388: 913–24.

70. Tipping C, Harrold M, Holland A, et al. The effects of active mobilisation and rehabilitation in ICU on mortality and function: a systematic review. Intensive Care Med 2017;43:171–83.

71. Devlin J, Skrobik Y, Gélinas C, et al. Clinical practice guidelines for the prevention and management of pain, agitation/sedation, delirium, immobility, and sleep disruption in adult patients in the ICU. Crit Care Med 2018;46:e825–73.
72. Lang J, Paykel M, Haines K, et al. Clinical practice guidelines for early mobilization in the ICU: a systematic review. Crit Care Med 2020;48:e1121–8.
73. Campos D, Bueno T, Anjos J, et al. Early neuromuscular electrical stimulation in addition to early mobilization improves functional status and decreases hospitalization days of critically ill patients. Crit Care Med 2022;50:1116–26.
74. Liu M, Luo J, Zhou J, et al. Intervention effect of neuromuscular electrical stimulation on ICU acquired weakness: a meta-analysis. Int J Nurs Sci 2020;7: 228–37.
75. Kho M, Molloy A, Clarke F, et al. Multicentre pilot randomised clinical trial of early in-bed cycle ergometry with ventilated patients. BMJ Open Respir Res 2019;6: e000383.
76. Chen Y, Lin H, Hsiao H, et al. Effects of exercise training on pulmonary mechanics and functional status in patients with prolonged mechanical ventilation. Respir Care 2012;57:727–34.
77. Chen S, Su C, Wu Y, et al. Physical training is beneficial to functional status and survival in patients with prolonged mechanical ventilation. J Formos Med Assoc 2011;110:572–9.
78. Schreiber A, Ceriana P, Ambrosino N, et al. Physiotherapy and weaning from prolonged mechanical ventilation. Respir Care 2019;64:17–25.
79. Costi S, Brogneri A, Bagni C, et al. Rehabilitation of difficult-to-wean, tracheostomized patients admitted to specialized unit: retrospective analyses over 10-years. Int J Environ Res Public Health 2022;19:2982.
80. Thomas S, Mehrholz J, Bodechtel U, et al. Effect of physiotherapy on regaining independent walking in patients with intensive-care-unit-acquired muscle weakness: a cohort study. J Rehabil Med 2019;51:797–804.
81. Verceles A, Wells C, Sorkin J, et al. A multimodal rehabilitation program for patients with ICU acquired weakness improves ventilator weaning and discharge home. J Crit Care 2018;204–10.
82. Dong Z, Liu Y, Gai Y, et al. Early rehabilitation relieves diaphragm dysfunction induced by prolonged mechanical ventilation: a randomised control study. BMC Pulm Med 2021;21:106.
83. Gonçalves M, Honrado T, Winck J, et al. Effects of mechanical insufflation-exsufflation in preventing respiratory failure after extubation: a randomized controlled trial. Crit Care Med 2012;16:R48.
84. Gomez-Merino E, Sancho J, Marin J, et al. Mechanical insufflation-exsufflation: pressure, volume, and flow relationships and the adequacy of the manufacturer's guidelines. Am J Phys Med Rehab 2002;81:579–83.
85. Chatwin M, Toussaint M, Goncalves MR, et al. Airway clearance techniques in neuromuscular disorders: a state of the art review. Respir Med 2018;136:98–110.
86. Rose L, Adhikari N, Leasa D, et al. Cough augmentation techniques for extubation or weaning critically ill patients from mechanical ventilation. Cochrane Database Syst Rev 2017;1:CD011833.
87. Swingwood E, Stilma W, Tume L, et al. The use of mechanical insufflation-exsufflation in invasively ventilated critically ill adults. Respir Care 2022;67: 1043–57.
88. Bissett B, Gosselink R, van Haren F. Respiratory muscle rehabilitation in patients with prolonged mechanical ventilation: a targeted approach. Crit Care 2020; 24:103.

89. Bureau C, Van Hollebeke M, Dres M. Managing respiratory muscle weakness during weaning from invasive ventilation. Eur Respir Rev 2023;32:220205.

90. Bissett B, Leditschke I, Green M, et al. Inspiratory muscle training for intensive care patients: a multidisciplinary practical guide for clinicians. Aust Crit Care 2019;32:249–55.

91. Vorona S, Sabatini U, Al-Maqbali S, et al. Inspiratory muscle rehabilitation in critically ill adults. a systematic review and meta-analysis. Ann Am Thorac Soc 2018;15:735–44.

92. Chapple L, Parry S, Schaller S. Attenuating muscle mass loss in critical illness: the role of nutrition and exercise. Curr Osteoporos Rep 2022;20:290–308.

93. Tatucu-Babet O, Ridley E. How much underfeeding can the critically ill adult patient tolerate? J Intens Med 2022;2:69–77.

94. Singer P, Blaser A, Berger M, et al. ESPEN guideline on clinical nutrition in the intensive care unit. Clin Nutr 2019;38:48–79.

95. Compher C, Bingham A, McCall M, et al. Guidelines for the provision of nutrition support therapy in the adult critically ill patient: the American Society for Parenteral and Enteral Nutrition. JPEN - J Parenter Enter Nutr 2022;46:12–41.

96. Reintam Blaser A, Rooyackers O, Bear D. How to avoid harm with feeding critically ill patients: a synthesis of viewpoints of a basic scientist, dietitian and intensivist. Crit Care 2023;27:258.

97. Ridley E, Lambell K. Nutrition before, during and after critical illness. Curr Opin Crit Care 2022;28:395–400.

98. Wischmeyer P, Bear D, Berger M, et al. Personalized nutrition therapy in critical care: 10 expert recommendations. Crit Care 2023;27:261.

99. Costigan F, Duffett M, Harris J, et al. Occupational therapy in the ICU: a scoping review of 221 documents. Crit Care Med 2019;e1014–21.

100. Rapolthy-Beck A, Fleming J, Turpin M. Occupational therapy service provision in adult intensive care units in Australia: a survey of workload practices, interventions and barriers. Aust Occup Ther J 2022;69:316–30.

101. Deemer K, Myhre B, Oviatt S, et al. Occupational therapist-guided cognitive interventions in critically ill patients: a feasibility randomized controlled trial. Can J Anaesth 2023;70:139–50.

102. Prohaska C, Sottile P, Nordon-Craft A, et al. Patterns of utilization and effects of hospital-specific factors on physical, occupational, and speech therapy for critically ill patients with acute respiratory failure in the USA: results of a 5-year sample. Crit Care 2019;23:175.

103. Twose P, Terblanche E, Jones U, et al. Therapy professionals in critical care: a UK wide workforce survey. J Intensive Care Soc 2023;24:24–31.

104. Chen Y, Jacobs W, Quan S, et al. Psychophysiological determinants of repeated ventilator weaning failure: an explanatory model. Am J Crit Care 2011;20:292–302.

105. Cohen J, Gopal A, Roberts K, et al. Ventilator-dependent patients successfully weaned with cognitive-behavioral therapy: a case series. Psychosomatics 2019;60:612–9.

106. Almeida T, Azevedo L, Nosé P, et al. Risk factors for agitation in critically ill patients. Rev Bras Ter Intensiva 2016;28:413–9.

107. Dupuis S, Brindamour D, Karzon S, et al. A systematic review of interventions to facilitate extubation in patients difficult-to-wean due to delirium, agitation, or anxiety and a meta-analysis of the effect of dexmedetomidine. Can J Anaesth 2019;66:318–27.

108. Buckley M, Smithburger P, Wong A, et al. Dexmedetomidine for facilitating mechanical ventilation extubation in difficult-to-wean ICU patients: systematic review and meta-analysis of clinical trials. J Intensive Care Med 2021;925–36.
109. Wade D, Als N, Bell V, et al. Providing psychological support to people in intensive care: development and feasibility study of a nurse-led intervention to prevent acute stress and long-term morbidity. BMJ Open 2018;8:e021083.
110. Moledina S, Shoaib A, Sun L, et al. Impact of the admitting ward on care quality and outcomes in non-ST-segment elevation myocardial infarction: insights from a national registry. Eur Heart J Qual Care Clin Outcomes 2022;8:681–91.
111. Langhorne P, Ramachandra S, Stroke Unit Trialists' Collaboration. Stroke Unit Trialists' Collaboration. Organised inpatient (stroke unit) care for stroke: network meta-analysis. Cochrane Database Syst Rev 2020;4:CD000197.
112. Lane N, Brewin K, Hartley T, et al. Specialist emergency care and COPD outcomes. BMJ Open Respir Res 2018;5:e000334.
113. Moran C, Lecky F, Bouamra O, et al. Changing the system: major trauma patients and their outcomes in the NHS (England) 2008-17. EClinicalMedicine 2018;2-3:13–21.
114. Nguyen Y, Wallace D, Yordanov Y, et al. The volume-outcome relationship in critical care: a systematic review and meta-analysis. Chest 2015;148:79–92.
115. Morche J, Mathes T, Pieper D. Relationship between surgeon volume and outcomes: a systematic review of systematic reviews. Syst Rev 2016;5:204.
116. Davies M, Quinnell T, Oscroft N, et al. Hospital outcomes and long-term survival after referral to a specialized weaning unit. Br J Anaesth 2017;118:563–9.
117. Messer B, Allen M, Antoine-Pitterson P, et al. BTS/ICS model of care for specialised weaning units. Brit Thorac Soc Rep 2023;14:1–27. https://www.brit-thoracic.org.uk/media/456179/bts-ics-model-of-care-for-specialised-weaning-units.

Physical and Cognitive Impairment in Acute Respiratory Failure

Jonathan Taylor, MD[a], Mary Elizabeth Wilcox, MD, PhD[b],*

KEYWORDS

- Physical impairment • Cognition • ARDS • Outcomes

KEY POINTS

- Recent research has brought renewed attention to the multifaceted physical and cognitive dysfunction that accompanies acute respiratory failure.
- Rehabilitation strategies and approaches to ventilator liberation have been identified as interventions to help mitigate symptoms relating to the post–intensive care syndrome.
- Comprehensive and multidisciplinary approaches to reduce experienced morbidity and accelerate recovery continue to be explored.

INTRODUCTION

Acute respiratory failure (ARF) is a critical condition characterized by the sudden inability of the respiratory system to maintain adequate oxygenation and eliminate carbon dioxide. It is a common and challenging condition both within and outside the intensive care unit (ICU), as it represents a heterogeneous syndrome associated with substantial morbidity and mortality, complex ethical dilemmas, and high health care utilization. This potentially life-threatening condition can arise from various causes, including different primary lung diseases, cardiac dysfunction, and systemic disorders. Improved understanding of respiratory physiology, advances in diagnostic tools, and the development of innovative therapeutic strategies have reshaped the management and outcomes of this syndrome.[1,2]

Although the immediate consequences are evident in the respiratory system, it is important to recognize that ARF can have profound effects on other aspects of health. New or worsening impairments in physical, psychological, or cognitive health after critical illness have collectively been termed post–intensive care syndrome (PICS), a

[a] Division of Pulmonary, Critical Care and Sleep Medicine, Mount Sinai Hospital, Icahn School of Medicine at Mount Sinai, One Gustave L. Levy Place, Box 1232, New York, NY 10029, USA;
[b] Department of Critical Care Medicine, Faculty of Medicine and Dentistry, University of Alberta, Edmonton, Canada
* Corresponding author.
E-mail address: mwilcox@ualberta.ca

Crit Care Clin 40 (2024) 429–450
https://doi.org/10.1016/j.ccc.2024.01.009
0749-0704/24/© 2024 Elsevier Inc. All rights reserved.
criticalcare.theclinics.com

constellation of symptoms that is increasingly recognized as a core component of critical care.[3] Neuromuscular and cognitive abnormalities are of particular interest given their high prevalence and substantial morbidity. This review highlights the mechanisms, risk factors, and characteristics of physical and cognitive dysfunction in ARF and comprehensively addresses notable diagnostic and therapeutic aspects pertinent to patient care.

NEUROMUSCULAR DYSFUNCTION IN ACUTE RESPIRATORY FAILURE
Overview and Epidemiology

Neuromuscular weakness during and following critical illness is common. The American Thoracic Society[4] (ATS) proposed that the term intensive care unit–acquired weakness (ICUAW) be used to describe the syndrome of generalized limb weakness that develops while the patient is critically ill for which there is no alternative explanation other than the critical illness itself.[4] In patients admitted for ARF requiring mechanical ventilation, cohorts have reported high rates of neuromuscular dysfunction.[5] An analysis of 31 studies of ICUAW used to formulate the guidelines (n = 3905) reported a prevalence of 33% in a general ICU patient population; more than a third of patients included in this analysis had respiratory failure, which was the single most common reason for ICU admission.[4] Pooled epidemiologic assessments focusing on those requiring invasive mechanical ventilation (IMV) of 1-week duration or longer suggest that independent of underlying diagnosis and illness severity, longer duration of mechanical ventilation is associated with greater risk of ICUAW.[4] In the United States, greater than 750,000 people receive mechanical ventilation annually, and approximately 300,000 individuals will require prolonged ventilatory support.[4] More than 100,000 patients survive an admission for acute respiratory distress syndrome (ARDS) each year.[6] Using these figures, more than 75,000 patients in the United States and up to 1 million worldwide are at risk of experiencing ICUAW each year.[4,7] Interventions to mitigate ICUAW are a public health priority.

Clinical consequences of this syndrome are well defined. It is associated in generalized populations of the critically ill with short- and long-term mortality,[8,9] duration of IMV, and increased ICU and hospital length of stay.[10–13] These findings have specifically been identified and replicated in survivors of ARF.[14–16] Long-term consequences of ARF in survivors are well described, including a decrease in the distance walked in 6 minutes, functional disability (ie, limitations in instrumental activities of daily living), increased health care utilization, and impaired health-related quality of life.[17–21]

Mechanisms and Risk Factors

ICUAW is an umbrella term encompassing a variety of conditions, among them critical illness myopathy (CIM), critical illness polyneuropathy (CIP), weakness, and deconditioning.[4] ARF has been independently associated with both muscle wasting and weakness. Exacerbations of asthma and chronic obstructive pulmonary disease have been specifically associated with myopathies for decades.[22,23] CIM is a result of sarcopenia and impaired muscle contractility that develops through distinct pathways, and detailed biological mechanisms and hypotheses have been summarized in previously published reviews.[24,25] Muscle atrophy begins within hours of mechanical ventilation.[26] Puthucheary and colleagues[27] demonstrated in a multimodal fashion using serial ultrasound measurement of the rectus femoris cross-sectional area and histopathologic analysis of muscle biopsies that rapid muscle wasting occurs early in critical illness and is more pronounced in those with multiorgan failure. A direct correlation was also demonstrated between the ultrasound measurements/histopathology and ICU length of stay and the severity of acute lung injury as measured by a ratio of Pao_2/Fio_2.[27]

No standard laboratory or imaging tests exist in making the diagnosis of CIM. Weakness has been measured in different ways, with most studies using some assessment of the physical examination.[4] The predominant clinical sign is flaccid, symmetric weakness. The Medical Research Council (MRC) scale is a standardized assessment of muscle strength in awake and attentive patients, grading strength in 12 different muscle groups, with variable thresholds and composite scores used in different trials. Ali and colleagues[8] demonstrated in a prospective multicenter cohort that in patients receiving IMV, handgrip strength was independently associated with hospital mortality and may serve as a simple test to identify ICU-acquired paresis. Electromyography can also be used to localize the neuromuscular lesion, although this technique may not be readily available. Pathology from muscle biopsy remains the reference standard, with classic histopathologic features of selective myosin loss, myofiber atrophy, and myofibrillar disorganization. Muscle biopsies of patients with ARDS variably showed type 2 myofiber atrophy, myosin thick filament loss, or immune cell infiltrates.[27]

The muscle atrophy of CIM demonstrates a breakdown of the contractile structure, and electrical hypoexcitability.[28–30] Models have demonstrated increasing activation of proteolysis pathways in response to common circumstances found in ARF, including muscular inactivity, inflammation, and food deprivation.[31] Decreased muscle protein synthesis has been well described in response to stressors like immobility, inflammation, and age, inhibiting muscular regenerative potential.[31] Inflammation and hyperglycemia induce loss of mitochondrial function, insulin resistance, and alterations in calcium metabolism. Microcirculatory disturbances and cytokine release result in muscle denervation.[31,32]

CIP refers to weakness related to dysfunction in multiple peripheral nerves. It portends worse outcomes as compared with CIM,[13,33] and its pathophysiology is more poorly understood. In CIP, the clinical deficits are mediated by loss of individual nerve fibers. Electrodiagnostic findings typically show an axonal sensorimotor polyneuropathy that can be seen early in critical illness. Involvement of sensory nerves can result in distal loss of pain, temperature, and vibration sensitivity.[34,35] Characteristic nerve conduction studies have been summarized elsewhere[36] and involve the loss of amplitudes of both sensory nerve action potentials and compound muscle action potentials without significant slowing.

Several mechanisms for CIP have been proposed; hypotheses include distal nerve ischemia stemming from microcirculatory inflammatory changes, and neural edema because of increased vascular permeability.[26,20] Some evidence implicates the role of channelopathies and sodium channel inactivation resulting in nerve hypoexcitability.[37,38] Nerve biopsies may sometimes be normal.[29] It can be difficult to fully distinguish CIP from CIM, and these conditions often overlap.[39] Many of these peripheral neuropathies persist at long-term follow-up in ARDS survivors.[40] There is significant overlap in the identified risk factors for the development of CIM and CIP. Multiorgan failure,[9] immobilization,[41] bed rest, and systemic inflammation[42] are well-established associated risk factors. Multiple randomized controlled trials focusing on blood glucose control have demonstrated more intense glycemic control to be associated with lower rates of CIM and CIP.[43–45] A Cochrane review concluded that intensive insulin therapy significantly reduced rates of CIP and CIM, duration of mechanical ventilation, and ICU length of stay, although the concurrent side effects and tradeoffs that come with strict glucose control are recognized.[46] Overall duration of mechanical ventilation has been associated with ICUAW,[47] and a pooled analysis of 14 studies suggested that increasing duration of mechanical ventilation is associated with a higher incidence of ICUAW.[4]

The contribution of medications to the development of ICUAW, namely corticosteroids and neuromuscular blocking agents, remains unclear. In a prospective cohort of ARDS survivors at 3 months after hospital discharge, systemic corticosteroids administration was a major determinant of measured muscular weakness.[18] This finding was supported in a meta-analysis of 12 observational studies using IMV as part of the inclusion criteria (n = 1384); the overall event rate of ICUAW in the corticosteroid group was 50% as compared with 40% in the control population.[48] Significant practice change is anticipated, as the beneficial therapeutic effects of steroids in the treatment of COVID-19 pneumonia,[49] the potential role for steroids in ARDS,[50] and the strengthening evidence for the use of hydrocortisone in severe community-acquired pneumonia[51] are likely to contribute to an increase in steroid-prescribing practices.

The association between neuromuscular blocking agents and ICUAW remains controversial. A recent large, randomized control trial of patients with moderate to severe ARDS reported that the addition of early continuous neuromuscular blockade resulted in no difference in muscle strength at day 7 or day 28 as assessed by the MRC scale.[52] Although no current evidence supports that sedatives or analgesics directly impact ICUAW, immobility as a consequence of deep sedation does increase the risk of ICUAW,[41] and hypoactive delirium as a side effect of continuous infusions can interfere with physical rehabilitation.

DIAPHRAGMATIC DYSFUNCTION

Myopathy and weakness specifically of respiratory muscles are recognized as important causes of failure to wean from the ventilator,[53,54] and recent years have brought a renewed focus on the role of the diaphragm.[55] Multimodal research using physiologic, histologic, and ultrasonographic analyses has demonstrated that diaphragmatic weakness, injury, and atrophy occur rapidly during IMV, and these injuries are correlated with the duration of ventilator support[56,57] and even mortality.[58] There are suggestions that diaphragmatic dysfunction in the critically ill may be independent of ICUAW[59] and that it can be observed in the hours following the initiation of mechanical ventilation.[26] Even when peripheral muscle function is preserved, short-term exposure to mechanical ventilation and sedating medications has been shown to have negative impacts on diaphragm contractile function, a process termed ventilator-induced diaphragm dysfunction (VIDD)[60–63] that has been comprehensively reviewed elsewhere.[63] In a population of mechanically ventilated patients deemed ready for extubation, Dres and colleagues[64] demonstrated a differential prevalence of diaphragm dysfunction as compared with ICUAW. Furthermore, the more prevalent diaphragm dysfunction and not ICUAW negatively impacted passing a spontaneous breathing trial.[64]

Assessment of transdiaphragmatic pressure in combination with phrenic nerve stimulation is considered the gold standard for measuring diaphragmatic function, although given the need for esophageal and gastric balloons, this is rarely used in clinical practice owing to its invasiveness.[65] Ultrasound measurements of diaphragmatic motion (termed dome excursion)[66] and contractile thickness (termed thickening fraction) are noninvasive, can be done at the bedside during spontaneous breathing, and have been shown to be predictive of ventilator weaning.[67] Others are investigating novel measurements of diaphragmatic electromyographic activity[68] to assess for

VIDD. Titrating ventilatory support to maintain normal levels of inspiratory effort may prevent changes in the diaphragm associated with mechanical ventilation, and programs targeting inspiratory muscle strength may offer therapeutic promise.

JOINT DYSFUNCTION

Loss of range of motion of skeletal joints occurs during prolonged immobility, when the joints are not subjected to normal movement and stress.[69] Contractures, pathologic changes that reduce joint flexibility and mobility, are a known consequence of ICU care and directly affect ambulation, increase the risk for falls, increase the likelihood of discharge to a long-term care facility, and may pose irreversible disability after critical illness.[70,71] A retrospective review of a general population of ICU patients, more than half of whom were admitted for pulmonary conditions, found at least one joint contracture in 39% of the cohort at the time of ICU transfer.[72] Follow-up of a specific population of ARDS survivors similarly noted the presence of contractures and frozen joints, although rates of these complications were less common.[18] Greater incorporation of prone positioning as a management strategy for moderate to severe ARDS may result in more unintended joint-related side effects.[73] Both shoulder and hip contractures are reported as complications of prone positioning, in addition to positional musculocutaneous nerve palsies, primarily in the brachial plexus.[74,75] Reports of heterotopic ossification following mechanical ventilation have also been published,[76] with one cohort reporting up to a 5% prevalence of large joint heterotopic ossification in ARDS survivors.[18,77] Recognition of these adverse events has led to specific interdisciplinary professional guidelines to direct pronating and supinating maneuvers to facilitate the safe and effective management of patients in the prone position.[78]

PRESSURE ULCERS, SKIN BREAKDOWN, AND SCARRING

Friction, shear forces, moisture, and malnutrition contribute to skin and tissue breakdown, and as a result, pressure injuries (PIs) are common in the ICU. Impaired tissue oxygenation and hypoxia are recognized as risk factors,[79] and the Cubbin-Jackson risk tool directly includes oxygenation in its calculation of PI risk.[80] Invasive respiratory and ventilatory support has been identified to contribute to these injuries, with IMV noted to be the most common iatrogenic risk factor in a large retrospective cohort of more than 40,000 critical care patients (27% prevalence).[81] Airway device–related PIs are common, and although rarely used, patients with nasotracheal tubes are particularly susceptible to iatrogenic harm.[82] Securing the endotracheal tube with a commercial tube holder that adheres to the cheeks has been associated with facial PIs.[83] In more severe forms of ARF, such as severe ARDS requiring proning, skin and tissue damage are recognized complications of placing patients in the prone position; similarly, specific international guidelines exist to guide standard of care.[84]

Noninvasive positive pressure ventilation (NIPPV) is a valuable treatment in the management of ARF, used most commonly in treating hypercapnic respiratory failure, in which there has been a demonstrated mortality benefit.[85] NIPPV is generally delivered through an oronasal interface or a full-face mask, although helmet modalities also exist. The facial pressure exerted by the device is known to lead to pressure lesions and nasal bridge pressure ulcers, with some studies describing incidence rates of 5% to 30%, particularly in long-term use greater than 48 hours.[86–88] These lesions can directly result in device intolerance and treatment failure, and strategies to decrease the incidence of nasal skin lesions should be considered at the start of NIPPV therapy.

In prolonged illness, tracheostomies are frequently required for patients with ARF. These patients are also at risk of PIs, specifically involving skin in the peristomal area and under tracheostomy ties and flanges.[89] Finally, stria from anasarca and iatrogenic scarring from common procedures, such as central venous catheters and pleural chest drains, are other recognized skin lesions following ARF that persist years following critical illness.[90,91]

PHYSICAL REHABILITATION THERAPY IN THE INTENSIVE CARE UNIT

Clinical practice guidelines recommend implementation of rehabilitation and mobilization therapies in the critically ill to prevent the physical complications of critical illness.[92] The Society of Critical Care Medicine Clinical Practice Guidelines for the Prevention and Management of Pain, Agitation/Sedation, Delirium, Immobility, and Sleep Disruption in Adult Patients in the ICU (PADIS)[92] are recommended to serve as a foundation for clinical practice, recommendations operationalized as part of the ICU Liberation Campaign, which furthers knowledge and implementation of the ABCDEF bundle[93] (**Fig. 1**). The PADIS guidelines defined rehabilitation as a "set of interventions designed to optimize functioning and reduce disability in individuals with a health condition,"[93] while also establishing the concept of mobilization as a "type of intervention within rehabilitation that facilitates the movement of patients and expends energy with a goal of improving patient outcomes."[93] Emphasized in these guidelines was a conditional recommendation for performing rehabilitation or mobilization in critically ill adults, over usual care or over similar interventions with a reduced duration, reduced

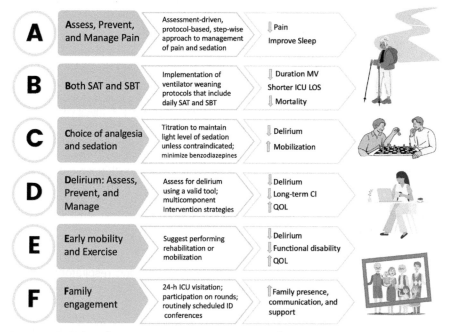

Fig. 1. ABCDEF bundle components, recommendations for incorporation into care of patients with ARF, and some of the associated benefits with regards to patient outcomes. CI, cognitive impairment; ID, interdisciplinary; LOS, length of stay; MV, mechanical ventilation; QOL, quality of life; SAT, spontaneous awakening trial; SBT, spontaneous breathing trial.

frequency, or later onset.[93] Explicitly in an ungraded statement, mechanical ventilation was determined to not be a barrier in and of itself to initiating rehabilitation/mobilization interventions.[93]

Although timely (ie, early) rehabilitation is encouraged for all patients with ARF, the optimal delivery of rehabilitation and mobilization in ARF is unknown,[93] as is a comprehensive understanding of factors limiting the consistent translation of guidelines into bedside practice.[94] Despite its demonstrated safety in landmark studies,[95] and an ungraded guideline statement concluding that serious safety events or harms do not occur commonly during physical rehabilitation or mobilization,[93] care must be taken to prevent and avoid rare respiratory-related adverse events. The PADIS guidelines, assessing 13 different studies (n = 12,200 sessions), found 15 total adverse events: four desaturation events that required an increase in FiO_2 and 3 unplanned extubations.[93] In a recent meta-analysis by Paton and colleagues[96] focusing exclusively on randomized trials involving adults requiring IMV, the use of early active mobilization did not significantly affect days alive and out of hospital at day 180 but was associated with improved physical function in survivors at 6 months. The TEAM trial recently conducted a large international, multicenter randomized controlled trial involving 192 adults who were undergoing mechanical ventilation, most of whom had sepsis.[97] The number of days that patients were alive and out of the hospital at 180 days were similar in the early-mobilization group (sessions were individually tailored to achieve highest possible level of mobilization deemed safe following randomization on day 0) and the usual-care group, with serious adverse events reported more commonly in the early-mobilization group.[97] Discordantly, a smaller single-center randomized control trial with 99 patients in both protocol arms found that early physical and occupational therapy within the first 96 hours of mechanical ventilation was associated with substantial improvements in cognitive impairment, neuromuscular weakness, and physical-related quality of life, including substantially lower rates of long-term cognitive impairment at 1 year (24% with early mobilization compared with 43% with usual care).[98] These findings suggest that early mobilization may have the potential to mitigate long-term cognitive dysfunction after critical illness. Despite large trials completed in this arena, appropriate timing of rehabilitation and mobilization in ARF remains a domain that requires further study.

LIBERATION FROM MECHANICAL VENTILATION

As a patient's ARF improves, respiratory support modalities can be weaned. Traditionally, this was considered a "weaning" process, although an alternative concept focused on the idea of "liberation" from the burden of mechanical ventilation has since been adopted.[99] Many ICUs use guideline-based protocols to assist in this liberation. The landmark "Wake Up and Breathe" study demonstrated in a multicenter, randomized controlled trial how a protocol centered on spontaneous awakening trials involving daily interruption of sedatives and protocolized spontaneous breathing trials resulted in patients spending more time off mechanical ventilation, less time in coma, less time in the ICU, decreased hospital length of stay, and improved 1-year survival.[100] Systematic reviews of protocol-driven ventilator weaning have previously been published,[101] and summative collaborative guidelines endorsed by multiple professional societies exist to help guide clinical practice.[102]

The need for sufficient respiratory muscle strength to maintain spontaneous breathing after ARF gave rise to the concept of inspiratory muscle training, whereby an extra load is applied to the diaphragm and accessory inspiratory muscles to increase their strength and endurance. This generally consists of a threshold pressure device or adjustment of the ventilator pressure trigger sensitivity. A previous systematic review including 10 studies (n = 394) concluded that such training significantly improved maximal inspiratory pressure and weaning success.[103] In smaller studies, significant benefits have also included decreased ICU and hospital length of stay.[103,104]

Focus has similarly shifted in recent years to the diaphragm, with a movement to encourage safe diaphragmatic activation during IMV to attempt to mitigate against VIDD and diaphragm disuse atrophy. A comprehensive diaphragm-protective approach to mechanical ventilation was recently proposed by Goligher and colleagues[105] on behalf of the Acute Respiratory Failure Section of the European Society of Intensive Care Medicine (ESICM), detailing strategies to optimize respiratory effort and synchrony to prevent diaphragmatic injury and improve patient outcomes. Close monitoring of respiratory drive in this setting is critical, as respiratory effort is often excessive in patients with ARF, with the potential for subsequent high lung-distending pressures to further worsen lung injury (termed patient self-inflicted lung injury, or P-SILI) and cause diaphragm myotrauma.[106] These complex interventions have for the most part not yet been tested in the clinical setting.

NEUROCOGNITIVE DYSFUNCTION IN ACUTE RESPIRATORY FAILURE
Overview and Epidemiology

Delirium is a neuropsychiatric syndrome characterized by acute, fluctuating disturbances of consciousness and cognition and is the most common manifestation of critical illness–related brain dysfunction.[107] It is the most common organ dysfunction in the medical and surgical ICU.[107] The prevalence in an ICU patient population ranges from 32% to 87%.[108–112] Prevalence appears to vary significantly depending on whether the population studied received mechanical ventilation.[108] In a large multicenter, prospective cohort of 1040 ICU patients with ARF, shock, or both, subjects developed multiple clinical phenotypes of delirium, including sedative-associated, hypoxic, septic, metabolic, and unclassified (ie, delirium in the absence of all other clinical risk factor phenotypes).[112] Longer durations of sedative-associated delirium, the most experienced phenotype, predicted worse long-term cognitive performance at both 3 and 12 months.[112] Recently, in a prospective cohort of 564 adult ICU patients, patients with ARDS (n = 48; 9%) were found to have a higher risk of ICU delirium than critically ill patients requiring mechanical ventilation alone or admission without intubation (73% vs 52% vs 21%, respectively; $P<.001$).[113] In a separate prospective cohort (n = 140) of critically ill patients from 2 ICUs in France, delirium was diagnosed in 80% of patients at least once during their ICU stay; hyperactive delirium was more common (87%) than hypoactive (13%) delirium.[114] Of patients, 69% experienced agitation requiring prolonged use of neuroleptic and sedative agents, which was associated with a statistically significant increase in the duration of mechanical ventilation (mean ratio, 1.49; 95% CI, 1.01–2.20; $P = .045$).[115]

Mechanisms and Risk Factors

Several of the physiologic derangements experienced by patients with ARDS (eg, hypoxemia, metabolic abnormalities), concomitant sepsis, and the treatments that they receive (eg, IMV, sedation-induced coma) have been identified as risk factors for ICU delirium. A systematic review of 33 studies identified 11 risk factors for delirium in the ICU, supported by medium to strong evidence.[116] Delirium risk factors can be broadly categorized into the following 3 categories: (a) features of the acute illness, (b) patient or host factors, and (c) environmental or iatrogenic factors.[117,118] Acute illness or precipitating variables would include coma, severity of illness (eg, measured by the Acute Physiology and Chronic Health Evaluation II or the Sequential Organ Failure Assessment), emergency surgery, polytrauma and mechanical ventilation; patient characteristics that are related to a higher risk of developing delirium include higher age, chronic pathologic condition (eg, dementia, hypertension); most environmental or iatrogenic variables, such as medication administration, were inconclusive based on the available evidence at the time.[119,120] Of the 11 more definitive risk factors identified in the systematic review,[18] the potentially modifiable ones include minimizing the duration of sedative-associated coma,[110,121–126] reducing days of mechanical ventilation,[122,124,127–130] and promoting the use of dexmedetomidine.[131–134] More recently, a systematic review investigated the association between risk factors among delirium subtypes; 20 studies were included.[135] Neither age nor sex were associated with a delirium subtype, although heterogeneity in study design and inconsistent reporting of subtype-specific risk factors limited data synthesis.[135]

Treatment

Numerous studies have reported improved patient-centered outcomes with implementation of evidence-based bundles aimed at reducing ICU-acquired delirium. The 2018 PADIS guidelines consist of 37 recommendations, 2 good clinical practice statements, and 32 ungraded, nonactionable statements having expanded to provide insight on the rehabilitation, mobilization, and sleep disruption in critical illness.[93] Briefly, multimodal analgesia was recognized as an impetus to reduce opioid consumption and improve long-term outcomes, including cognition.[93] Analgosedation was again reemphasized in the 2018 guideline update supporting the concept that not all mechanically ventilated patients require a sedative agent throughout the duration of intubation.[93] Furthermore, light sedation versus deep sedation, if needed, should be provided either by daily sedative interruption or by nurse-protocolized sedation.[93] Such clinical practices are components of multicomponent methods that include pharmacologic and nonpharmacologic modalities (eg, improved sleep, enhanced mobility) in reducing incident delirium or mitigating its severity and duration.[93] The ICU Liberation Bundle (ABCDEF) affords the opportunity to integrate the PADIS guidelines into clinical practice (see **Fig. 1**).[93] Numerous multifaceted implementation programs have involved the implementation of processes of care and clinical outcomes focusing on delirium screening, limited use of benzodiazepines, light sedation targets, and early mobilization.[136–139]

Unfortunately, several publications have reported poor adherence to guideline implementation, with routine delirium assessment being the most consistently reported shortfall. For example, over 1101 patient-days, Maximous and colleagues found that 39% of delirium assessments were performed as compared with 78% agitation assessments.[140] Similarly, Aparanji and colleagues found assessments were performed approximately 30% of the time, with a greater number of assessments being performed during day shifts.[141] Balas and colleagues reported on the challenge of incorporating the ABCDEF bundle into everyday practice as part of a 20-month nationwide multicenter quality improvement intervention.[142] Storytelling was recommended as a powerful tool to help successfully implement the A2F bundle, as was recognizing that each member of the ICU team including patients and their families offer unique contributions essential to implementation. Routine collection of detailed implementation data is essential for program evaluation and generalizability.[143] In a systematic review and meta-analysis, 12 multilevel causal factors impacting the implementation outcomes were categorized and subdivided into patient, provider, and organizational factors. Organizational factors were rarely reported (eg, hospital type, daily screening frequency, and assessment method used).[143]

Organizational factors, such as educational strategies, staff knowledge, motivation, and screening compliance, may influence reported delirium incidence. Moving forward, a standardized framework for reporting such factors would facilitate further insights into different processes of care and their subsequent impact.

POST–INTENSIVE CARE SYNDROME, RECOVERY TRAJECTORIES, AND PROGNOSIS AFTER ACUTE RESPIRATORY FAILURE

PICS has been recognized as a core component of critical care and has been covered comprehensively in a recent narrative review.[3] Survivors of ARF frequently experience persistent impairments in physical, psychological, and/or cognitive domains, coupled with reduced quality of life. In a cohort of 222 survivors of acute lung injury across 13 different ICUs, Fan and colleagues[15] demonstrated that muscle weakness is common in survivors and is associated with substantial impairments in physical function and quality of life that continue beyond 24 months, independent of corticosteroids or neuromuscular blockade. A multicenter population of relatively young survivors of ARDS in the Toronto ARDS Outcomes study (median age, 44) showed that survivors at 1 year could achieve just two-thirds of their predicted exercise capacity, despite nearly normal lung volume and spirometric measures, albeit with persistently mild reduction in diffusion capacity.[18,20] Despite improvements in muscle strength, these deficits persisted for years; at 5-years follow-up, the median distance walked in 6 minutes remained 76% of that walked in an age- and sex-matched control population,[19] independent of lung function. In an analysis of the ARDS Net Long-Term Outcomes Study (ALTOS), during the first year following ARDS, more than two-thirds of survivors reported clinically significant fatigue symptoms with little association with critical illness variables.[144] Increased prevalence of pain has been found in this population in a similar pattern, as one analysis of more than 800 ARDS survivors found the prevalence of pain to be 45% and 42% at 6 and 12 months, respectively, which was further associated with in-ICU opioid use during the initial episode of ARF.[145]

In a multicenter cohort of 821 critically ill patients with respiratory failure or shock, one of 4 ICU survivors, across all adult age groups, had cognitive impairment 1 year after discharge equating in severity to that of suffering mild Alzheimer disease or moderate traumatic brain injury. In a recent systematic review of 46 studies, aggregated frequency of cognitive impairment after critical illness was 35% and 45% at 3- and 6-months follow-up, respectively.[146] Interestingly, ARDS survivors had a higher prevalence of cognitive impairment as compared with a mixed ICU survivor population (approximately 80% as compared with 50% prevalence at 3-months follow-up).[146] Cognitive impairment seems to improve on average, however, from 3- to 6-months follow-up,[146,147] and any existing differences between survivor populations do not persist beyond 3 months.[146] Regardless of improvements that might be seen in early recovery, a substantial percentage of patients experience persistent long-term cognitive impairment, as high as 42% and 46% at 1 and 2 years after ICU discharge.[147–151] A limited number of studies to date have examined interventions designed to hasten recovery and/or prevent decrements in cognitive function after critical illness.[152] Most research has focused on intervening during ICU admission to reduce cognitive impairment. Treatments have included strategies for optimizing enteral nutrition, fluids, sedation, weaning, mobilization, cognitive activities, statins, and sleep quality.[132,148,153–157]

The ALTOS study prospectively collected posthospitalization outcomes for ARDS survivors from 3 ARDS Network multicenter trials, enrolling participants from 41 hospitals throughout the United States. With long-term follow-up, 4 distinct subtypes were identified, independent of degree of critical illness and baseline functional status.[158] Survivors were categorized as mildly impaired physical and mental health status (22%), moderately impaired in both domains (39%), severely impaired physical and moderately impaired mental health status (15%), and finally, severely impaired in both physical and mental health status (24%).[158] These persistent physical and cognitive deficits contribute to ongoing disability and poor quality of life. One systematic review and meta-analysis of 52 studies including more than 10,000 previously employed survivors of critical illness demonstrated that delayed return to work is common after critical illness, with up to two-thirds of patients still not working at 3 months.[159] Even at 1 year from hospitalization, one-third of previously employed survivors remain jobless.[159] No significant difference was noted when stratified by diagnosis of ARDS (vs non-ARDS) or by geographic region.[159]

Post-ICU clinics have become a vital service at many centers offering focused interdisciplinary care to survivors of critical illness. Shaped by care models in the ICU, physicians, nurses, psychologists, pharmacists, case managers, physical therapists, occupational therapists, and dieticians work together to provide comprehensive, goal-directed critical care to address the lingering effects of organ failure and may prove in the future to help mitigate symptoms of PICS and PICS-Family[160]. Further studies evaluating the impact of follow-up care of ICU survivors on patient-reported outcomes are needed.

Box 1.

Box 1

Physical and cognitive recovery after extracorporeal membrane oxygenation

The use of venovenous (VV) extracorporeal membrane oxygenation (ECMO) as therapy for ARF and severe ARDS has increased exponentially because of simultaneous advances in technology, the influenza H1N1 and SARS-CoV-2 pandemics, and emerging high-quality evidence.[160] The recently released 2023 ESICM ARDS Clinical Practice Guidelines strongly recommend in favor of ECMO for the treatment of severe ARDS.[161] Conceptually, the management of pain, sedation, and delirium for patients receiving VV-ECMO should be similar in approach to other critically ill patients of similar illness severity.[162] International cross-sectional surveys have revealed that deep sedation is more often prioritized at the initiation of VV-ECMO, and lipophilic and highly protein bound drugs may sequester within circuits, necessitating higher dosages to achieve adequate pain control and sedation.[162,163] A retrospective cohort study of one high-volume center found the incidence of delirium to be 58% while on VV-ECMO, with a concurrent high usage of antipsychotic medications and physical restraints.[164] Severe hypoxemia and fear of inadvertent cannula removal may encourage deep sedation and immobility, and changes in patient position can compromise ECMO blood flow and worsen oxygenation.[164] However, others have called for a change in approach, arguing that physical activity is significantly underdelivered to patients on ECMO.[165] Single-center cohort studies suggest that early rehabilitation can contribute to the functional recovery of patients on ECMO, with more patients likely to achieve higher levels of function and more patients able to be discharged home after ECMO support.[166] These suggestions have given rise to the "Awake ECMO" strategy, with minimized sedation time as able, to allow an awake patient to participate in functional recovery safely and actively. Much of this has been driven by the lung transplantation literature, where physical deconditioning is a relative contraindication to transplantation and thoracic surgery.[167] Immobilized patients receiving VV-ECMO as a bridge to lung transplantation are at greater risk for developing ICUAW,[168] and a strong signal for an association between pretransplantation ambulation during the ECMO bridge and improved survival posttransplant has been repeatedly demonstrated in a convincing fashion.[169-175] Benefits of physiotherapy during ECMO have similarly been shown to be feasible and beneficial in those undergoing ECMO as a bridge to recovery.[176] One recent systematic review focusing on "awake" extracorporeal life support (ECLS) of all different modalities (ie, not limited to respiratory failure) concluded that an awake ECLS strategy was safe with different cannula approaches to promote physical therapy.[177] Ambulation during mechanical ventilation and

ECMO are both feasible strategies and are evolving to become standard of care if achievable.[178,179] An integral part of any awake, mobilization strategy during ECMO support in respiratory failure is an interprofessional team approach, following the guidelines laid out by Hodgson and colleagues[180] regarding safety criteria for mobilization. Much less is known about the long-term neuromuscular and cognitive morbidity associated with ECMO therapy. Observational studies have associated the receipt of ECLS with a modestly increased risk of new mental health diagnosis or social problem diagnosis after discharge, as compared with ICU hospitalization without ECMO.[181] A multicenter collaboration across academic medical centers looked at posthospitalization recovery in survivors of respiratory failure from COVID-19 treated with VV-ECMO versus IMV alone.[182] Of those with documented follow-up at 4 months, ICUAW was present in 35% of ECMO survivors, and all survivors who were assessed (100%) had an abnormal 6-minute walk distance.[182] Alarmingly, 88% of the ECMO cohort tested positive for cognitive dysfunction, although this was not statistically significant when compared with the cohort of survivors of ARDS that required IMV alone ($P = .26$).[182] Other small studies have demonstrated no significant differences in sleep or cognitive outcomes between ECLS and non-ECLS survivors up to 1 year following discharge.[183,184] Increasing focus on PICS and long-term cognitive outcomes, and the rise of post-ICU survivorship clinics for survivors of critical illness is sure to bring renewed focus to the postdischarge outcomes of survivors of extracorporeal support.[185,186]

FUTURE DIRECTIONS

ARF has undeniable profound effects on patients' physical and cognitive function beyond pulmonary illness. Synthesizing a wide array of contemporary research, this review underscores the immediate and long-term impacts of respiratory compromise on physical, motor, and cognitive faculties and emphasizes the critical need for interdisciplinary intervention. There is an imperative for a multidisciplinary approach that integrates medical, rehabilitative, and psychosocial interventions to effectively address mitigate long-term morbidity. A dual focus is required, with interventions targeted in the ICU during critical respiratory failure and continuing following hospital discharge in outpatient survivorship clinics. Future investigations aimed at the prevention, assessment, and management of physical and neurocognitive dysfunction will allow for improved patient outcomes and quality of life in this challenging clinical context.

CLINICS CARE POINTS

- Acute respiratory failure can lead to new or worsening impairments in physical, psychological, or cognitive health after critical illness, a constellation of symptoms termed post–intensive care syndrome, which is increasingly recognized as a core component of critical care.

- Intensive care unit–acquired weakness is an umbrella term encompassing a variety of conditions, among them critical illness myopathy, critical illness polyneuropathy, weakness, and deconditioning, and is associated with morbidity and mortality.

- The Pain, Agitation/Sedation, Delirium, Immobility, and Sleep Disruption guidelines serve as the foundation for intensive care unit liberation strategies and emphasize recommendations for delirium prevention, rehabilitation, and mobilization in critically ill patients, including those with respiratory failure requiring invasive mechanical ventilation.

DISCLOSURE

The authors have nothing to disclose.

REFERENCES

1. Bos LD, Martin-Loeches I, Schultz MJ. ARDS: challenges in patient care and frontiers in research. Eur Respir Rev 2018;27(147). https://doi.org/10.1183/16000617.0107-2017.
2. Scala R, Heunks L. Highlights in acute respiratory failure. Eur Respir Rev Off J Eur Respir Soc 2018;27(147):180008.
3. Schwitzer E, Jensen KS, Brinkman L, et al. Survival ≠ recovery. CHEST Crit Care 2023;1(1):100003.
4. Fan E, Cheek F, Chlan L, et al. An official American Thoracic Society clinical practice guideline: the diagnosis of intensive care unit–acquired weakness in adults. Am J Respir Crit Care Med 2014;190(12):1437–46.
5. Qin ES, Hough CL, Andrews J, et al. Intensive care unit-acquired weakness and the COVID-19 pandemic: a clinical review. PM&R. 2022;14(2):227–38.
6. Rubenfeld GD, Caldwell E, Peabody E, et al. Incidence and outcomes of acute lung injury. N Engl J Med 2005;353(16):1685–93.
7. Ambrosino N, Vitacca M. The patient needing prolonged mechanical ventilation: a narrative review. Multidiscip Respir Med 2018;13:6.
8. Ali NA, O'Brien JM, Hoffmann SP, et al. Acquired weakness, handgrip strength, and mortality in critically ill patients. Am J Respir Crit Care Med 2008;178(3):261–8.
9. De Jonghe B, Sharshar T, Lefaucheur JP, et al. Paresis acquired in the intensive care unit: a prospective multicenter study. JAMA 2002;288(22):2859–67.
10. Tortuyaux R, Davion JB, Jourdain M. Intensive care unit-acquired weakness: Questions the clinician should ask. Rev Neurol (Paris) 2022;178(1):84–92.
11. Visser LH. Critical illness polyneuropathy and myopathy: clinical features, risk factors and prognosis. Eur J Neurol 2006;13(11):1203–12.
12. Barlas I, Oropello JM, Benjamin E. Neurologic complications in intensive care. Curr Opin Crit Care 2001;7(2):68.
13. Garnacho-Montero J, Madrazo-Osuna J, García-Garmendia J, et al. Critical illness polyneuropathy: risk factors and clinical consequences. A cohort study in septic patients. Intensive Care Med 2001;27(8):1288–96.
14. Hermans G, Van Mechelen H, Clerckx B, et al. Acute outcomes and 1-year mortality of intensive care unit–acquired weakness. a cohort study and propensity-matched analysis. Am J Respir Crit Care Med 2014;190(4):410–20.
15. Fan E, Dowdy DW, Colantuoni E, et al. Physical complications in acute lung injury survivors: a 2-year longitudinal prospective study. Crit Care Med 2014;42(4):849–59.
16. Dowdy DW, Eid MP, Dennison CR, et al. Quality of life after acute respiratory distress syndrome: a meta-analysis. Intensive Care Med 2006;32(8):1115–24.
17. Pfoh ER, Wozniak AW, Colantuoni E, et al. Physical declines occurring after hospital discharge in ARDS survivors: a 5-year longitudinal study. Intensive Care Med 2016;42(10):1557–66.
18. Herridge MS, Cheung AM, Tansey CM, et al. One-year outcomes in survivors of the acute respiratory distress syndrome. N Engl J Med 2003;348(8):683–93.
19. Herridge MS, Tansey CM, Matté A, et al. Functional disability 5 years after acute respiratory distress syndrome. N Engl J Med 2011;364(14):1293–304.
20. Cheung AM, Tansey CM, Tomlinson G, et al. Two-year outcomes, health care use, and costs of survivors of acute respiratory distress syndrome. Am J Respir Crit Care Med 2006;174(5):538–44.

21. Needham DM, Wozniak AW, Hough CL, et al. Risk factors for physical impairment after acute lung injury in a national, multicenter study. Am J Respir Crit Care Med 2014;189(10):1214–24.

22. Amaya-Villar R, Garnacho-Montero J, García-Garmendía JL, et al. Steroid-induced myopathy in patients intubated due to exacerbation of chronic obstructive pulmonary disease. Intensive Care Med 2005;31(1):157–61.

23. Douglass JA, Tuxen DV, Horne M, et al. Myopathy in severe asthma. Am Rev Respir Dis 1992;146(2):517–9.

24. Schefold JC, Wollersheim T, Grunow JJ, et al. Muscular weakness and muscle wasting in the critically ill. J Cachexia Sarcopenia Muscle 2020;11(6):1399–412.

25. Cheung K, Rathbone A, Melanson M, et al. Pathophysiology and management of critical illness polyneuropathy and myopathy. J Appl Physiol 2021;130(5): 1479–89.

26. Levine S, Nguyen T, Taylor N, et al. Rapid disuse atrophy of diaphragm fibers in mechanically ventilated humans. N Engl J Med 2008;358(13):1327–35.

27. Puthucheary ZA, Rawal J, McPhail M, et al. Acute skeletal muscle wasting in critical illness. JAMA 2013;310(15):1591–600.

28. Lad H, Saumur TM, Herridge MS, et al. Intensive care unit-acquired weakness: not just another muscle atrophying condition. Int J Mol Sci 2020;21(21):7840.

29. Lacomis D. Neuromuscular disorders in critically ill patients: review and update. J Clin Neuromuscul Dis 2011;12(4):197.

30. Shepherd S, Batra A, Lerner DP. Review of critical illness myopathy and neuropathy. Neurohospitalist 2017;7(1):41–8.

31. Batt Jane, Herridge Margaret S, Dos Santos Claudia C. From skeletal muscle weakness to functional outcomes following critical illness: a translational biology perspective. Thorax 2019;74(11):1091–8.

32. Puthucheary ZA, Astin R, Mcphail MJW, et al. Metabolic phenotype of skeletal muscle in early critical illness. Thorax 2018;73(10):926–35.

33. Koch S, Spuler S, Deja M, et al. Critical illness myopathy is frequent: accompanying neuropathy protracts ICU discharge. J Neurol Neurosurg Psychiatry 2011; 82(3):287–93.

34. de Sèze M, Petit H, Wiart L, et al. Critical illness polyneuropathy: a 2-year follow-up study in 19 severe cases. Eur Neurol 2000;43(2):61–9.

35. Zifko UA, Zipko HT, Bolton CF. Clinical and electrophysiological findings in critical illness polyneuropathy. J Neurol Sci 1998;159(2):186–93.

36. Lacomis D. Electrophysiology of neuromuscular disorders in critical illness. Muscle Nerve 2013;47(3):452–63.

37. Z'Graggen WJ, Lin CSY, Howard RS, et al. Nerve excitability changes in critical illness polyneuropathy. Brain 2006;129(9):2461–70.

38. Friedrich O, Reid MB, Van den Berghe G, et al. The sick and the weak: neuropathies/myopathies in the critically ill. Physiol Rev 2015;95(3):1025–109.

39. Latronico N, Bertolini G, Guarneri B, et al. Simplified electrophysiological evaluation of peripheral nerves in critically ill patients: the Italian multi-centre CRIMYNE study. Crit Care 2007;11(1):R11.

40. Li NY, Murthy NK, Franz CK, et al. Upper extremity neuropathies following severe COVID-19 infection: a multicenter case series. World Neurosurg 2023; 171:e391–7.

41. Llano-Diez M, Renaud G, Andersson M, et al. Mechanisms underlying ICU muscle wasting and effects of passive mechanical loading. Crit Care 2012;16(5): R209.

42. Bednarík J, Vondracek P, Dusek L, et al. Risk factors for critical illness polyneuromyopathy. J Neurol 2005;252(3):343–51.
43. Hermans G, Vanhorebeek I, Derde S, et al. Metabolic aspects of critical illness polyneuromyopathy. Crit Care Med 2009;37(10):S391.
44. Berghe GV den, Schoonheydt K, Becx P, et al. Insulin therapy protects the central and peripheral nervous system of intensive care patients. Neurology 2005; 64(8):1348–53.
45. Hermans Greet, Wilmer A, Meersseman W, et al. Impact of intensive insulin therapy on neuromuscular complications and ventilator dependency in the medical intensive care unit. Am J Respir Crit Care Med 2007;175(5):480–9.
46. Hermans G, Jonghe BD, Bruyninckx F, et al. Interventions for preventing critical illness polyneuropathy and critical illness myopathy. Cochrane Database Syst Rev 2014;1. https://doi.org/10.1002/14651858.CD006832.pub3.
47. Garnacho-Montero J, Amaya-Villar R, García-Garmendía JL, et al. Effect of critical illness polyneuropathy on the withdrawal from mechanical ventilation and the length of stay in septic patients. Crit Care Med 2005;33(2):349.
48. Yang T, Li Z, Jiang L, et al. Corticosteroid use and intensive care unit-acquired weakness: a systematic review and meta-analysis. Crit Care 2018;22:187.
49. RECOVERY Collaborative Group. Dexamethasone in hospitalized patients with Covid-19. N Engl J Med 2021;384(8):693–704.
50. Villar Jesús, Ferrando C, Martínez D, et al. Dexamethasone treatment for the acute respiratory distress syndrome: a multicentre, randomised controlled trial. Lancet Respir Med 2020;8(3):267–76.
51. Dequin PF, Meziani F, Quenot JP, et al. Hydrocortisone in severe community-acquired pneumonia. N Engl J Med 2023;388(21):1931–41.
52. National Heart, Lung, and Blood Institute PETAL Clinical Trials Network, Moss M, Huang DT, et al. "Early neuromuscular blockade in the acute respiratory distress syndrome.". N Engl J Med 2019;380(21):1997–2008.
53. De Jonghe B, Bastuji-Garin S, Durand MC, et al. Respiratory weakness is associated with limb weakness and delayed weaning in critical illness. Crit Care Med 2007;35(9):2007.
54. De Jonghe, Bernard, Sharshar T, et al. Does ICU-acquired paresis lengthen weaning from mechanical ventilation? Intensive Care Med 2004;30:1117–21.
55. Latronico N, Bolton CF. Critical illness polyneuropathy and myopathy: a major cause of muscle weakness and paralysis. Lancet Neurol 2011;10(10):931–41.
56. Hermans G, Agten A, Testelmans D, et al. Increased duration of mechanical ventilation is associated with decreased diaphragmatic force: a prospective observational study. Crit Care 2010;14(4):R127.
57. Jaber S, Petrof BJ, Jung B, et al. Rapidly progressive diaphragmatic weakness and injury during mechanical ventilation in humans. Am J Respir Crit Care Med 2011;183(3):364–71.
58. Supinski GS, Ann Callahan L. Diaphragm weakness in mechanically ventilated critically ill patients. Crit Care 2013;17(3):R120.
59. Jung B, Moury PH, Mahul M, et al. Diaphragmatic dysfunction in patients with ICU-acquired weakness and its impact on extubation failure. Intensive Care Med 2016;42(5):853–61.
60. Vassilakopoulos T, Petrof BJ. Ventilator-induced diaphragmatic dysfunction. Am J Respir Crit Care Med 2004;169(3):336–41.
61. Demoule A, Jung B, Prodanovic H, et al. Diaphragm dysfunction on admission to the intensive care unit. prevalence, risk factors, and prognostic impact—a prospective study. Am J Respir Crit Care Med 2013;188(2):213–9.

62. Ochala J, Renaud G, Diez ML, et al. Diaphragm muscle weakness in an experimental porcine intensive care unit model. PLoS One 2011;6(6):e20558.
63. Berger David, Bloechlinger S, von Haehling S, et al. Dysfunction of respiratory muscles in critically ill patients on the intensive care unit. Journal of cachexia, sarcopenia and muscle 2016;7(4):403–12.
64. Dres M, Dubé BP, Mayaux J, et al. Coexistence and impact of limb muscle and diaphragm weakness at time of liberation from mechanical ventilation in medical intensive care unit patients. Am J Respir Crit Care Med 2017;195(1):57–66.
65. Doorduin J, van Hees HWH, van der Hoeven JG, et al. Monitoring of the respiratory muscles in the critically ill. Am J Respir Crit Care Med 2013;187(1):20–7.
66. Zambon M, Greco M, Bocchino S, et al. Assessment of diaphragmatic dysfunction in the critically ill patient with ultrasound: a systematic review. Intensive Care Med 2017;43(1):29–38.
67. Qian Z, Yang M, Li L, et al. Ultrasound assessment of diaphragmatic dysfunction as a predictor of weaning outcome from mechanical ventilation: a systematic review and meta-analysis. BMJ Open 2018;8(9):e021189.
68. Dres M, Goligher EC, Heunks LMA, et al. Critical illness-associated diaphragm weakness. Intensive Care Med 2017;43(10):1441–52.
69. Brower RG. Consequences of bed rest. Crit Care Med 2009;37(10):S422.
70. Clavet H, Hébert PC, Fergusson DA, et al. Joint contractures in the intensive care unit: association with resource utilization and ambulatory status at discharge. Disabil Rehabil 2011;33(2):105–12.
71. Clavet H, Doucette S, Trudel G. Joint contractures in the intensive care unit: quality of life and function 3.3 years after hospital discharge. Disabil Rehabil 2015;37(3):207–13.
72. Clavet Heidi, Hébert PC, Fergusson D, et al. Joint contracture following prolonged stay in the intensive care unit. CMAJ (Can Med Assoc J) 2008;178(6):691–7.
73. Johnson SW, Garcia MA, Sisson EKQ, et al. Hospital variation in management and outcomes of acute respiratory distress syndrome due to COVID-19. Crit Care Explor 2022;4(2):e0638.
74. Goettler CE, Pryor JP, Reilly PM. Brachial plexopathy after prone positioning. Crit Care 2002;6(6):540–2.
75. Mano T, Fujimura S. Brachial plexus injury and musculocutaneous nerve palsy during prone positioning in a patient with COVID-19. Cureus 2022;14(5):e24931.
76. Aziz A, Choudhari R, Alexander AJ, et al. Heterotopic ossification post COVID-19: report of two cases. Radiol Case Rep 2021;16(2):404–9.
77. Hudson SJ, Brett SJ. Heterotopic ossification – a long-term consequence of prolonged immobility. Crit Care 2006;10(6):174.
78. Rowe C. Development of clinical guidelines for prone positioning in critically ill adults. Nurs Crit Care 2004;9(2):50–7.
79. Kottner J, Cuddigan J, Carville K, et al. Prevention and treatment of pressure ulcers/injuries: the protocol for the second update of the international clinical practice guideline 2019. J Tissue Viability 2019;28(2):51–8.
80. Delawder JM, Leontie SL, Maduro RS, et al. Predictive validity of the Cubbin-Jackson and Braden skin risk tools in critical care patients: a multisite project. Am J Crit Care 2021;30(2):140–4.
81. Cox J, Edsberg LE, Koloms K, et al. Pressure injuries in critical care patients in US hospitals. J Wound Ostomy Continence Nurs 2022;49(1):21–8.

82. Moser CH, Peeler A, Long R, et al. Prevention of endotracheal tube–related pressure injury: a systematic review and meta-analysis. Am J Crit Care 2022; 31(5):416–24.
83. Rastogi V, Layon AJ. Endotracheal tube fastening device-related facial pressure ulcers. Cureus 2021;13(7):e16796.
84. Fourie A, Ahtiala M, Black J, et al. Skin damage prevention in the prone ventilated critically ill patient: a comprehensive review and gap analysis (PRONEtect study). J Tissue Viability 2021;30(4):466–77.
85. Plant P, Owen J, Elliott M. Early use of non-invasive ventilation for acute exacerbations of chronic obstructive pulmonary disease on general respiratory wards: a multicentre randomised controlled trial. Lancet 2000;355(9219):1931–5.
86. Yamaguti WP, Moderno EV, Yamashita SY, et al. Treatment-related risk factors for development of skin breakdown in subjects with acute respiratory failure undergoing noninvasive ventilation or CPAP. Respir Care 2014;59(10):1530–6.
87. Carron M, Freo U, BaHammam AS, et al. Complications of non-invasive ventilation techniques: a comprehensive qualitative review of randomized trials. BJA Br J Anaesth 2013;110(6):896–914.
88. Schallom M, Cracchiolo L, Falker A, et al. Pressure ulcer incidence in patients wearing nasal-oral versus full-face noninvasive ventilation masks. Am J Crit Care 2015;24(4):349–56.
89. Moser CH, Peeler A, Long R, et al. Prevention of tracheostomy-related pressure injury: a systematic review and meta-analysis. Am J Crit Care 2022;31(6): 499–507.
90. Badia M, Trujillano J, Serviá L, et al. Skin lesions after intensive care procedures: results of a prospective study. J Crit Care 2008;23(4):525–31.
91. Hough CL, Herridge MS. Long-term outcome after acute lung injury. Curr Opin Crit Care 2012;18(1):8.
92. Lang JK, Paykel MS, Haines KJ, et al. Clinical practice guidelines for early mobilization in the ICU: a systematic review. Crit Care Med 2020;48(11):e1121.
93. Devlin JW, Skrobik Y, Gélinas C, et al. Clinical practice guidelines for the prevention and management of pain, agitation/sedation, delirium, immobility, and sleep disruption in adult patients in the ICU. Crit Care Med 2018;46(9):e825.
94. The TEAM Study Investigators, Hodgson C, Bellomo R, et al. Early mobilization and recovery in mechanically ventilated patients in the ICU: a bi-national, multicentre, prospective cohort study. Crit Care 2015;19(1):81.
95. Schweickert WD, Pohlman MC, Pohlman AS, et al. Early physical and occupational therapy in mechanically ventilated, critically ill patients: a randomised controlled trial. Lancet 2009;373(9678):1874–82.
96. Paton M, Chan S, Tipping CJ, et al. The effect of mobilization at 6 months after critical illness — meta-analysis. NEJM Evid 2023;2(2). https://doi.org/10.1056/EVIDoa2200234. EVIDoa2200234.
97. TEAM Study Investigators and the ANZICS Clinical Trials Group, Hodgson CL, Bailey M, Bellomo R, et al. Early active mobilization during mechanical ventilation in the ICU. N Engl J Med 2022;387(19):1747–58. PMID: 36286256.
98. Patel BK, Wolfe KS, Patel SB, et al. Effect of early mobilisation on long-term cognitive impairment in critical illness in the USA: a randomised controlled trial. Lancet Respir Med 2023;11(6):563–72.
99. McConville JF, Kress JP. Weaning patients from the ventilator. N Engl J Med 2012;367(23):2233–9.
100. Girard TD, Kress JP, Fuchs BD, et al. Efficacy and safety of a paired sedation and ventilator weaning protocol for mechanically ventilated patients in intensive

care (Awakening and Breathing Controlled trial): a randomised controlled trial. Lancet 2008;371(9607):126–34.

101. Girard TD, Ely EW. Protocol-driven ventilator weaning: reviewing the evidence. Clin Chest Med 2008;29(2):241–52.

102. Fan E, Zakhary B, Amaral A, et al. Liberation from mechanical ventilation in critically ill adults. An official ATS/ACCP clinical practice guideline. Ann Am Thorac Soc 2017;14(3):441–3.

103. Elkins M, Dentice R. Inspiratory muscle training facilitates weaning from mechanical ventilation among patients in the intensive care unit: a systematic review. J Physiother 2015;61(3):125–34.

104. Elbouhy MS, AbdelHalim HA, Hashem AMA. Effect of respiratory muscles training in weaning of mechanically ventilated COPD patients. Egypt J Chest Dis Tuberc 2014;63(3):679–87.

105. Goligher EC, Dres M, Patel BK, et al. Lung- and diaphragm-protective ventilation. Am J Respir Crit Care Med 2020;202(7):950–61.

106. Dianti J, Goligher EC. Monitoring respiratory effort and lung-distending pressure noninvasively during mechanical ventilation: ready for prime time. Anesthesiology 2023;138(3):235–7.

107. Ely EW, Margolin R, Francis J, et al. Evaluation of delirium in critically ill patients: validation of the confusion assessment method for the intensive care unit (CAM-ICU). Crit Care Med 2001;29(7):1370.

108. Van Rompaey B, Schuurmans MJ, Shortridge-Baggett LM, et al. Risk factors for intensive care delirium: a systematic review. Intensive Crit Care Nurs 2008; 24(2):98–107.

109. Agarwal V, O'Neill PJ, Cotton BA, et al. Prevalence and risk factors for development of delirium in burn intensive care unit patients. J Burn Care Res 2010; 31(5):706–15.

110. Roberts B, Rickard CM, Rajbhandari D, et al. Multicentre study of delirium in ICU patients using a simple screening tool. Aust Crit Care 2005;18(1):6–16.

111. Salluh JI, Soares M, Teles JM, et al. Delirium epidemiology in critical care (DECCA): an international study. Crit Care 2010;14(6):R210.

112. Girard TD, Thompson JL, Pandharipande PP, et al. Clinical phenotypes of delirium during critical illness and severity of subsequent long-term cognitive impairment: a prospective cohort study. Lancet Respir Med 2018;6(3):213–22.

113. Hsieh SJ, Soto GJ, Hope AA, et al. The association between acute respiratory distress syndrome, delirium, and in-hospital mortality in intensive care unit patients. Am J Respir Crit Care Med 2015;191(1):71–8.

114. Helms J, Kremer S, Merdji H, et al. Delirium and encephalopathy in severe COVID-19: a cohort analysis of ICU patients. Crit Care 2020;24:491.

115. Helms J, Kremer S, Merdji H, et al. Neurologic features in severe SARS-CoV-2 infection. N Engl J Med 2020;382(23):2268–70.

116. Zaal IJ, Devlin JW, Peelen LM, et al. A systematic review of risk factors for delirium in the ICU. Crit Care Med 2015;43(1):40.

117. Pandharipande P, Cotton BA, Shintani A, et al. Prevalence and risk factors for development of delirium in surgical and trauma ICU patients. J Trauma 2008; 65(1):34–41.

118. Hipp DM, Ely EW. Pharmacological and nonpharmacological management of delirium in critically ill patients. Neurotherapeutics 2012;9(1):158–75.

119. Burry LD, Williamson DR, Mehta S, et al. Delirium and exposure to psychoactive medications in critically ill adults: a multi-centre observational study. J Crit Care 2017;42:268–74.

120. van den Boogaard M, Pickkers P, Slooter AJC, et al. Development and validation of PRE-DELIRIC (PREdiction of DELIRium in ICu patients) delirium prediction model for intensive care patients: observational multicentre study. BMJ 2012; 344:e420.
121. Angles EM, Robinson TN, Biffl WL, et al. Risk factors for delirium after major trauma. Am J Surg 2008;196(6):864–70.
122. Colombo R, Corona A, Praga F, et al. A reorientation strategy for reducing delirium in the critically ill. Results of an interventional study. Minerva Anestesiol 2012;78(9):1026.
123. Dubois Marc-Jacques, Bergeron N, Dumont M, et al. Delirium in an intensive care unit: a study of risk factors. Intensive Care Med 2001;27:1297–304.
124. Ouimet S, Kavanagh BP, Gottfried SB, et al. Incidence, risk factors and consequences of ICU delirium. Intensive Care Med 2007;33(1):66–73.
125. Serafim RB, Dutra MF, Saddy F, et al. Delirium in postoperative nonventilated intensive care patients: risk factors and outcomes. Ann Intensive Care 2012; 2:51.
126. Yoshitaka S, Egi M, Morimatsu H, et al. Perioperative plasma melatonin concentration in postoperative critically ill patients: its association with delirium. J Crit Care 2013;28(3):236–42.
127. Guillamondegui OD, Richards JE, Ely EW, et al. Does hypoxia affect intensive care unit delirium or long-term cognitive impairment after multiple trauma without intracranial hemorrhage? J Trauma Acute Care Surg 2011;70(4):910.
128. mei Shi C, Wang D, sheng Chen K, et al. Incidence and risk factors of delirium in critically ill patients after non-cardiac surgery. Chin Med J (Engl). 2010;123(8):993.
129. Van Rompaey B, Elseviers MM, Schuurmans MJ, et al. Risk factors for delirium in intensive care patients: a prospective cohort study. Crit Care 2009;13(3):R77.
130. Shehabi Y, Chan L, Kadiman S, et al. Sedation depth and long-term mortality in mechanically ventilated critically ill adults: a prospective longitudinal multicentre cohort study. Intensive Care Med 2013;39(5):910–8.
131. Pandharipande PP, Pun BT, Herr DL, et al. Effect of sedation with dexmedetomidine vs lorazepam on acute brain dysfunction in mechanically ventilated patients: the MENDS randomized controlled trial. JAMA 2007;298(22):2644–53.
132. Riker RR, Shehabi Y, Bokesch PM, et al. Dexmedetomidine vs midazolam for sedation of critically ill patients: a randomized trial. JAMA 2009;301(5):489–99.
133. Ruokonen E, Parviainen I, Jakob SM, et al. Dexmedetomidine versus propofol/ midazolam for long-term sedation during mechanical ventilation. Intensive Care Med 2009;35(2):282–90.
134. Krewulak KD, Stelfox HT, Ely EW, et al. Risk factors and outcomes among delirium subtypes in adult ICUs: a systematic review. J Crit Care 2020;56: 257–64.
135. Trogrlić Z, van der Jagt M, Lingsma H, et al. Improved guideline adherence and reduced brain dysfunction after a multicenter multifaceted implementation of ICU delirium guidelines in 3,930 patients. Crit Care Med 2019;47(3):419.
136. Balas MC, Burke WJ, Gannon D, et al. Implementing the ABCDE bundle into everyday care: opportunities, challenges and lessons learned for implementing the ICU pain, agitation and delirium (PAD) guidelines. Crit Care Med 2013;41(9 0 1):S116–27.
137. Barnes-Daly MA, Phillips G, Ely EW. Improving hospital survival and reducing brain dysfunction at seven California community hospitals: implementing PAD guidelines via the ABCDEF bundle in 6,064 patients. Crit Care Med 2017; 45(2):171.

138. Pun BT, Balas MC, Barnes-Daly MA, et al. Caring for critically ill patients with the ABCDEF bundle: results of the ICU liberation collaborative in over 15,000 adults. Crit Care Med 2019;47(1):3–14.

139. Maximous R, Miller F, Tan C, et al. Pain, agitation and delirium assessment and management in a community medical-surgical ICU: results from a prospective observational study and nurse survey. BMJ Open Qual 2018;7(4):e000413.

140. Aparanji K, Kulkarni S, Metzke M, et al. Quality improvement of delirium status communication and documentation for intensive care unit patients during daily multidisciplinary rounds. BMJ Open Qual 2018;7(2):e000239.

141. Balas MC, Pun BT, Pasero C, et al. Common challenges to effective ABCDEF bundle implementation: the ICU liberation campaign experience. Crit Care Nurse 2019;39(1):46–60.

142. Rood P, Waal GH de, Vermeulen H, et al. Effect of organisational factors on the variation in incidence of delirium in intensive care unit patients: a systematic review and meta-regression analysis. Aust Crit Care 2018;31(3):180–7.

143. Neufeld KJ, Leoutsakos JMS, Yan H, et al. Fatigue symptoms during the first year following ARDS. Chest 2020;158(3):999–1007.

144. Probert JM, Lin S, Yan H, et al. Bodily pain in survivors of acute respiratory distress syndrome: a 1-year longitudinal follow-up study. J Psychosom Res 2021;144:110418.

145. Honarmand K, Lalli RS, Priestap F, et al. Natural history of cognitive impairment in critical illness survivors. a systematic review. Am J Respir Crit Care Med 2020; 202(2):193–201.

146. Wilcox ME, Brummel NE, Archer K, et al. Cognitive dysfunction in ICU patients: risk factors, predictors, and rehabilitation interventions. Crit Care Med 2013; 41(9):S81.

147. Jackson JC, Girard TD, Gordon SM, et al. Long-term cognitive and psychological outcomes in the awakening and breathing controlled trial. Am J Respir Crit Care Med 2010;182(2):183–91.

148. Hopkins RO, Weaver LK, Collingridge D, et al. Two-year cognitive, emotional, and quality-of-life outcomes in acute respiratory distress syndrome. Am J Respir Crit Care Med 2005;171(4):340–7.

149. Jackson JC, Archer KR, Bauer R, et al. A prospective investigation of long-term cognitive impairment and psychological distress in moderately versus severely injured trauma intensive care unit survivors without intracranial hemorrhage. J Trauma Acute Care Surg 2011;71(4):860.

150. Pandharipande PP, Girard TD, Jackson JC, et al. Long-term cognitive impairment after critical illness. N Engl J Med 2013;369(14):1306–16.

151. Nedergaard HK, Jensen HI, Toft P. Interventions to reduce cognitive impairments following critical illness: a topical systematic review. Acta Anaesthesiol Scand 2017;61(2):135–48.

152. Brummel NE, Girard TD, Ely EW, et al. Feasibility and safety of early combined cognitive and physical therapy for critically ill medical and surgical patients: the Activity and Cognitive Therapy in ICU (ACT-ICU) trial. Intensive Care Med 2014; 40(3):370–9.

153. Kamdar BB, King LM, Collop NA, et al. The effect of a quality improvement intervention on perceived sleep quality and cognition in a medical ICU. Crit Care Med 2013;41(3):800–9.

154. Mikkelsen ME, Christie JD, Lanken PN, et al. The adult respiratory distress syndrome cognitive outcomes study. Am J Respir Crit Care Med 2012;185(12): 1307–15.

155. Needham DM, Colantuoni E, Dinglas VD, et al. Rosuvastatin versus placebo for delirium in intensive care and subsequent cognitive impairment in patients with sepsis-associated acute respiratory distress syndrome: an ancillary study to a randomised controlled trial. Lancet Respir Med 2016;4(3):203–12.
156. Needham DM, Dinglas VD, Morris PE, et al. Physical and cognitive performance of patients with acute lung injury 1 year after initial trophic versus full enteral feeding. EDEn trial follow-up. Am J Respir Crit Care Med 2013;188(5):567–76.
157. Brown SM, Wilson EL, Presson AP, et al. Understanding patient outcomes after acute respiratory distress syndrome: identifying subtypes of physical, cognitive, and mental health outcomes. Thorax 2017;72(12):1094–103.
158. Kamdar BB, Suri R, Suchyta MR, et al. Return to work after critical illness: a systematic review and meta-analysis. Thorax 2020;75(1):17–27.
159. Sevin CM, Bloom SL, Jackson JC, et al. Comprehensive care of ICU survivors: Development and implementation of an ICU recovery center. J Crit Care 2018; 46:141148.
160. Tonna JE, Abrams D, Brodie D, et al. Management of adult patients supported with venovenous extracorporeal membrane oxygenation (VV ECMO): guideline from the extracorporeal life support organization (ELSO). ASAIO J 2021;67(6): 601–10.
161. Grasselli Giacomo, Calfee CS, Camporota L, et al. ESICM guidelines on acute respiratory distress syndrome: definition, phenotyping and respiratory support strategies. Intensive Care Med 2023;49(7):727–59.
162. Dzierba AL, Abrams D, Madahar P, et al. Current practice and perceptions regarding pain, agitation and delirium management in patients receiving venovenous extracorporeal membrane oxygenation. J Crit Care 2019;53:98–106.
163. Dzierba AL, Abrams D, Brodie D. Medicating patients during extracorporeal membrane oxygenation: the evidence is building. Crit Care 2017;21:66.
164. deBacker J, Tamberg E, Munshi L, et al. Sedation practice in extracorporeal membrane oxygenation–treated patients with acute respiratory distress syndrome: a retrospective study. ASAIO J 2018;64(4):544.
165. Tonna JE. Is active mobility the most underdelivered care component for patients on extracorporeal membrane oxygenation? Ann Am Thorac Soc 2022; 19(1):9–11.
166. Wells CL, Forrester J, Vogel J, et al. Safety and feasibility of early physical therapy for patients on extracorporeal membrane oxygenator: University of Maryland Medical Center experience. Crit Care Med 2018;46(1):53.
167. Weill D, Benden C, Corris PA, et al. A consensus document for the selection of lung transplant candidates: 2014—an update from the pulmonary transplantation Council of the International Society for Heart and Lung Transplantation. J Heart Lung Transplant 2015;34(1):1–15.
168. Hayes K, Hodgson CL, Pellegrino VA, et al. Physical function in subjects requiring extracorporeal membrane oxygenation before or after lung transplantation. Respir Care 2018;63(2):194–202.
169. Chicotka S, Pedroso FE, Agerstrand CL, et al. Increasing opportunity for lung transplant in interstitial lung disease with pulmonary hypertension. Ann Thorac Surg 2018;106(6):1812–9.
170. Abrams D, Brodie D, Arcasoy SM. Extracorporeal life support in lung transplantation. Clin Chest Med 2017;38(4):655–66.
171. Biscotti M, Gannon WD, Agerstrand C, et al. Awake extracorporeal membrane oxygenation as bridge to lung transplantation: a 9-year experience. Ann Thorac Surg 2017;104(2):412–9.

172. Fuehner T, Kuehn C, Hadem J, et al. Extracorporeal membrane oxygenation in awake patients as bridge to lung transplantation. Am J Respir Crit Care Med 2012;185(7):763–8.

173. Hoopes CW, Kukreja J, Golden J, et al. Extracorporeal membrane oxygenation as a bridge to pulmonary transplantation. J Thorac Cardiovasc Surg 2013; 145(3):862–8.

174. Tipograf Y, Salna M, Minko E, et al. Outcomes of extracorporeal membrane oxygenation as a bridge to lung transplantation. Ann Thorac Surg 2019; 107(5):1456–63.

175. Benazzo A, Schwarz S, Frommlet F, et al. Twenty-year experience with extracorporeal life support as bridge to lung transplantation. J Thorac Cardiovasc Surg 2019;157(6):2515–25.e10.

176. Munshi L, Kobayashi T, DeBacker J, et al. Intensive care physiotherapy during extracorporeal membrane oxygenation for acute respiratory distress syndrome. Ann Am Thorac Soc 2017;14(2):246–53.

177. Cucchi M, Mariani S, De Piero ME, et al. Awake extracorporeal life support and physiotherapy in adult patients: a systematic review of the literature. Perfusion 2023;38(5):939–58.

178. Turner David A, Cheifetz IM, Rehder KJ, et al. Active rehabilitation and physical therapy during extracorporeal membrane oxygenation while awaiting lung transplantation: a practical approach. Crit Care Med 2011;39(12):2593–8.

179. Bailey Polly, Thomsen GE, Spuhler VJ, et al. Early activity is feasible and safe in respiratory failure patients. Crit Care Med 2007;35(1):139–45.

180. Hodgson CL, Stiller K, Needham DM, et al. Expert consensus and recommendations on safety criteria for active mobilization of mechanically ventilated critically ill adults. Crit Care 2014;18(6):658.

181. Fernando SM, Scott M, Talarico R, et al. Association of extracorporeal membrane oxygenation with new mental health diagnoses in adult survivors of critical illness. JAMA 2022;328(18):1827–36.

182. Taylor LJ, Jolley SE, Ramani C, et al. Early posthospitalization recovery after extracorporeal membrane oxygenation in survivors of COVID-19. J Thorac Cardiovasc Surg 2023;166(3):842–51.e1.

183. Sylvestre A, Adda M, Maltese F, et al. Long-term neurocognitive outcome is not worsened by of the use of venovenous ECMO in severe ARDS patients. Ann Intensive Care 2019;9:82.

184. Daou M, Lauzon C, Bullen EC, et al. Long-term cognitive outcomes and sleep in adults after extracorporeal life support. Crit Care Explor 2021;3(4):e0390.

185. Mayer KP, Jolley SE, Etchill EW, et al. Long-term recovery of survivors of coronavirus disease (COVID-19) treated with extracorporeal membrane oxygenation: the next imperative. JTCVS Open 2021;5:163–8.

186. Higa KC, Mayer K, Quinn C, et al. Sounding the alarm: what clinicians need to know about physical, emotional, and cognitive recovery after venoarterial extracorporeal membrane oxygenation. Crit Care Med 2023;51(9):1234.

Moving?

Make sure your subscription moves with you!

To notify us of your new address, find your **Clinics Account Number** (located on your mailing label above your name), and contact customer service at:

Email: journalscustomerservice-usa@elsevier.com

800-654-2452 (subscribers in the U.S. & Canada)
314-447-8871 (subscribers outside of the U.S. & Canada)

Fax number: 314-447-8029

Elsevier Health Sciences Division
Subscription Customer Service
3251 Riverport Lane
Maryland Heights, MO 63043

*To ensure uninterrupted delivery of your subscription, please notify us at least 4 weeks in advance of move.

9780443129179